# Advanced Materials for Energy Applications: From Fuels to Batteries and Beyond

# Advanced Materials for Energy Applications: From Fuels to Batteries and Beyond

Guest Editors

**Zhao Ding**
**Liangjuan Gao**
**Shicong Yang**

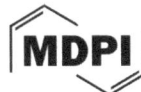

Basel • Beijing • Wuhan • Barcelona • Belgrade • Novi Sad • Cluj • Manchester

*Guest Editors*

Zhao Ding
College of Materials Science
and Engineering
Chongqing University
Chongqing
China

Liangjuan Gao
College of Materials Science
and Engineering
Sichuan University
Chengdu
China

Shicong Yang
Metallurgical and Energy
Engineering
Kunming University of
Science and Technology
Kunming
China

*Editorial Office*
MDPI AG
Grosspeteranlage 5
4052 Basel, Switzerland

This is a reprint of the Special Issue, published open access by the journal *Molecules* (ISSN 1420-3049), freely accessible at: www.mdpi.com/journal/molecules/special_issues/nanomaterials_fuel.

For citation purposes, cite each article independently as indicated on the article page online and as indicated below:

Lastname, A.A.; Lastname, B.B. Article Title. *Journal Name* **Year**, *Volume Number*, Page Range.

ISBN 978-3-7258-3810-3 (Hbk)
ISBN 978-3-7258-3809-7 (PDF)
https://doi.org/10.3390/books978-3-7258-3809-7

© 2025 by the authors. Articles in this book are Open Access and distributed under the Creative Commons Attribution (CC BY) license. The book as a whole is distributed by MDPI under the terms and conditions of the Creative Commons Attribution-NonCommercial-NoDerivs (CC BY-NC-ND) license (https://creativecommons.org/licenses/by-nc-nd/4.0/).

# Contents

About the Editors .................................................................... vii

Preface ............................................................................. ix

**Zhao Ding, Liangjuan Gao and Shicong Yang**
Advanced Materials for Energy Applications: From Fuels to Batteries and Beyond
Reprinted from: *Molecules* **2025**, *30*, 1405, https://doi.org/10.3390/molecules30071405 ...... 1

**Yaohui Xu, Yuting Li and Zhao Ding**
Network–Polymer–Modified Superparamagnetic Magnetic Silica Nanoparticles for the Adsorption and Regeneration of Heavy Metal Ions
Reprinted from: *Molecules* **2023**, *28*, 7385, https://doi.org/10.3390/molecules28217385 ...... 4

**Yunxuan Zhou, Hao Lv, Tao Chen, Shijun Tong, Yulin Zhang, Bin Wang, et al.**
Probing the Effect of Alloying Elements on the Interfacial Segregation Behavior and Electronic Properties of Mg/Ti Interface via First-Principles Calculations
Reprinted from: *Molecules* **2024**, *29*, 4138, https://doi.org/10.3390/molecules29174138 ...... 26

**Zhongting Wang, Rongrui Deng, Yumei Wang and Fusheng Pan**
Comparison of Construction Strategies of Solid Electrolyte Interface (SEI) in Li Battery and Mg Battery—A Review
Reprinted from: *Molecules* **2024**, *29*, 4761, https://doi.org/10.3390/molecules29194761 ...... 43

**Lin Zhu, Dandan Wu, Shicong Yang, Keqiang Xie, Kuixian Wei and Wenhui Ma**
Silicon Extraction from a Diamond Wire Saw Silicon Slurry with Flotation and the Flotation Interface Behavior
Reprinted from: *Molecules* **2024**, *29*, 5916, https://doi.org/10.3390/molecules29245916 ...... 67

**Zaiqiong Liu, Yiren Xu, Xurundong Kan, Mei Chen, Jingyang Dai, Yanli Zhang, et al.**
An Electrochemical Sensor for Detection of Lead (II) Ions Using Biochar of Spent Coffee Grounds Modified by $TiO_2$ Nanoparticles
Reprinted from: *Molecules* **2024**, *29*, 5704, https://doi.org/10.3390/molecules29235704 ...... 83

**Zhaoyang Wang, Zihan Zhou, Xing Gao, Qian Liu, Jianzong Man, Fanghui Du, et al.**
Natural Silkworm Cocoon-Derived Separator with Na-Ion De-Solvated Function for Sodium Metal Batteries
Reprinted from: *Molecules* **2024**, *29*, 4813, https://doi.org/10.3390/molecules29204813 ...... 96

**Alisher Abdisattar, Meir Yerdauletov, Mukhtar Yeleuov, Filipp Napolskiy, Aleksey Merkulov, Anna Rudnykh, et al.**
The Impact of Biowaste Composition and Activated Carbon Structure on the Electrochemical Performance of Supercapacitors
Reprinted from: *Molecules* **2024**, *29*, 5029, https://doi.org/10.3390/molecules29215029 ...... 109

**Yaohui Xu, Yang Zhou, Yuting Li and Yang Zheng**
Bridging Materials and Analytics: A Comprehensive Review of Characterization Approaches in Metal-Based Solid-State Hydrogen Storage
Reprinted from: *Molecules* **2024**, *29*, 5014, https://doi.org/10.3390/molecules29215014 ...... 120

**Jiangang Liu, Lu Wang and Guohuan Wu**
Sintering Behavior of Molybdenite Concentrate During Oxidation Roasting Process in Air Atmosphere: Influences of Roasting Temperature and K Content
Reprinted from: *Molecules* **2024**, *29*, 5183, https://doi.org/10.3390/molecules29215183 ...... 149

**Li Wang, Hongli Chen, Yuxi Zhang, Jinyu Liu and Lin Peng**
Research Progress in Strategies for Enhancing the Conductivity and Conductive Mechanism of LiFePO$_4$ Cathode Materials
Reprinted from: *Molecules* **2024**, *29*, 5250, https://doi.org/10.3390/molecules29225250 . . . . . . **169**

# About the Editors

**Zhao Ding**

Zhao Ding, PhD, Chongqing University, China. Zhao Ding earned his Ph.D. in Materials Science and Engineering from Illinois Institute of Technology, USA. He currently serves as an Associate Professor at the College of Materials Science and Engineering at Chongqing University. His research focuses primarily on the development of solid-state hydrogen storage materials. His academic contributions encompass over 60 peer-reviewed publications in prestigious energy and materials science journals. His work has garnered more than 2,500 independent citations, yielding an h-index of 28.

**Liangjuan Gao**

Dr. Liangjuan Gao has been working as Associate Researcher at the College of Materials Science and Engineering at Sichuan University since 2021. Dr. Gao obtained her B.S. degree in Applied Chemistry from Capital Normal University in 2010. Dr. Gao obtained her M.S. degree in Physical Chemistry from the University of the Chinese Academy of Science in 2013. Dr. Gao obtained her Ph.D degree in Materials Science and Engineering from Illinois Institute of Technology in 2018. Dr. Gao worked at the School of Materials Engineering at Purdue University from 2018 to 2021. Dr. Gao's research fields include interfacial wetting and corrosion, key materials for concentrated solar power plants and fuel cells, high-entropy ceramics, and catalysts for water splitting. Dr. Gao is serving as the Guest Editor for *Molecules*, *Nanomaterials*, and the *Chinese Journal of Rare Metals*. Dr. Gao is the independent reviewer for the *Journal of the European Ceramic Society*, *Ceramic International*, *Journal of Materials Science*, *Molecules*, etc.

**Shicong Yang**

Shicong Yang, PhD, Kunming University of Science and Technology, China. Shicong Yang earned his Ph.D. in Metallurgical Physical Chemistry from Kunming University of Science and Technology, China. He currently holds the position of University-appointed Professor at the Faculty of Metallurgical and Energy Engineering, Kunming University of Science and Technology. His research primarily focuses on the comprehensive utilization of silicon resources. His academic contributions include the publication of over 26 papers in renowned materials science and environmental journals. His research has garnered more than 500 independent citations, yielding an h-index of 10.

# Preface

The Special Issue "Advanced Materials for Energy Applications: From Fuels to Batteries and Beyond" brings together a curated compendium of original research and critical reviews that underscore the pivotal role of material innovation in confronting the great energy and environmental challenges of our time. As the global community navigates an era of escalating energy demands, finite resources, and stringent sustainability imperatives, the development and deployment of advanced materials across the energy value chain have emerged as both urgent and indispensable.

This Special Issue addresses a broad spectrum of topics, reflecting the multidisciplinary and integrative nature of modern materials science. The collected works are thematically organized into four synergistic domains: environmental monitoring and remediation, next-generation energy storage systems, materials processing and industrial optimization, and the integration of theoretical modeling with advanced characterization techniques. Together, these studies reveal how fundamental insights and technological innovations in materials synthesis, structural design, and functional performance can catalyze sustainable energy transitions.

The motivation for this Special Issue stems from the pressing need to accelerate the translation of materials research into real-world energy solutions. The contributors—renowned scholars and early-career researchers from diverse institutions—bring deep expertise and fresh perspectives to the forefront of this field. Their collective efforts illustrate the power of interdisciplinary collaboration in advancing science for societal benefit.

This volume is intended for a broad academic audience, including researchers in materials science, chemistry, energy engineering, nanotechnology, and environmental science, as well as stakeholders in industry and policy making. It is our sincere hope that the knowledge disseminated here will inspire continued innovation and foster meaningful dialogue across disciplinary and sectoral boundaries.

We extend our deepest appreciation to all authors for their high-quality contributions, and to the reviewers for their rigorous and constructive assessments. Special thanks are due to the editorial and publishing teams for their invaluable support throughout the process.

**Zhao Ding, Liangjuan Gao, and Shicong Yang**
*Guest Editors*

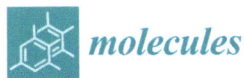 

*Editorial*

# Advanced Materials for Energy Applications: From Fuels to Batteries and Beyond

Zhao Ding [1,*], Liangjuan Gao [2] and Shicong Yang [3]

1. College of Materials Science and Engineering, National Engineering Research Center for Magnesium Alloys, Chongqing University, Chongqing 400044, China
2. College of Materials Science and Engineering, Sichuan University, Chengdu 610065, China; lgao87@scu.edu.cn
3. Faculty of Metallurgical and Energy Engineering, Kunming University of Science and Technology, Kunming 650093, China; shicongyang@kust.edu.cn
* Correspondence: zhaoding@cqu.edu.cn

The unprecedented challenges of the 21st century energy landscape necessitate a paradigm shift in materials science and engineering [1–4]. The intricate interplay between rising global energy demands and environmental sustainability has catalyzed intensive research efforts across the entire energy value chain [5–8]. This Special Issue, "Advanced Materials for Energy Applications: From Fuels to Batteries and Beyond", presents a carefully curated collection of cutting-edge research that exemplifies the transformative role of advanced materials in addressing these multifaceted challenges.

The ten papers featured in this issue collectively demonstrate the remarkable versatility and innovation in materials design, synthesis, and characterization. These contributions span multiple technological domains and can be systematically categorized into four complementary research directions: (1) advanced functional materials for environmental monitoring and remediation, (2) next-generation energy storage systems, (3) materials processing and industrial optimization, and (4) theoretical modeling coupled with advanced characterization techniques.

In the domain of environmental monitoring and remediation, two notable studies showcase innovative approaches to addressing heavy metal contamination. Liu et al. (contribution 1) developed a highly sensitive electrochemical sensing platform utilizing $TiO_2$-modified biochar derived from spent coffee grounds. The hierarchical composite structure demonstrated remarkable sensitivity toward Pb(II) detection, achieving a detection limit of 0.6268 pM under optimized conditions. This work exemplifies the synergistic integration of waste valorization and advanced materials design. Complementing this research, Xu et al. (contribution 2) engineered sophisticated network polymer-modified superparamagnetic silica nanoparticles (MSNPs-CAAQ) for heavy metal remediation. Their systematic investigation revealed impressive maximum adsorption capacities of 324.7, 306.8, and 293.3 mg/g for $Fe^{3+}$, $Cu^{2+}$, and $Cr^{3+}$ ions, respectively, with excellent recyclability maintained over multiple adsorption–desorption cycles.

Significant advances in energy storage technologies are highlighted through innovative materials development and systematic performance enhancement studies. Wang et al. (contribution 3) pioneered the development of a bio-derived separator for sodium metal batteries, utilizing natural silkworm cocoon membrane. The innovative separator design, featuring intrinsic cationic functional groups, demonstrated superior Na-ion transport kinetics and enhanced electrochemical performance, achieving an initial capacity of 79.3 mAh g$^{-1}$ at 10C with 93.6% retention after 1000 cycles. Abdisattar et al. (contribution 4) conducted a comprehensive investigation into biomass-derived activated carbons for supercapacitor applications, establishing critical structure–property relationships between lignocellulosic precursor composition and electrochemical performance. Their findings revealed that wheat bran-derived electrodes exhibited optimal performance characteristics, attributed to their unique hierarchical pore structure and surface chemistry. Wang et al. (contribution 5) further contributed to this domain through a comprehensive review of strategies for enhancing LiFePO$_4$ cathode conductivity, while Wang et al. (contribution 6) provided an in-depth comparative analysis of solid electrolyte interface formation mechanisms in Li and Mg batteries.

In the realm of materials processing and industrial optimization, several significant contributions advance our understanding of crucial manufacturing processes. Liu et al. (contribution 7) conducted a detailed investigation of the sintering behavior in molybdenite concentrate oxidation, elucidating the complex relationships between processing parameters and product characteristics. Their systematic study revealed the critical influence of temperature and potassium content on sintering mechanisms, providing valuable insights for process optimization. Additionally, Zhu et al. (contribution 8) developed an innovative flotation technique for high-purity silicon recovery from diamond wire saw silicon slurry, achieving remarkable recovery rates of 98.2% under optimized conditions, thereby addressing both resource recovery and environmental sustainability challenges.

The theoretical understanding and characterization of advanced materials have been significantly enhanced through sophisticated studies employing cutting-edge analytical techniques and computational methods. Zhou et al. (contribution 9) employed density functional theory calculations to elucidate the complex interfacial phenomena in Mg/Ti systems, providing fundamental insight into the role of various alloying elements. Their computational analysis revealed that Gd exhibits the most favorable segregation behavior with a segregation energy of $-5.83$ eV, offering valuable guidance for the rational design of magnesium-based composites. Xu et al. (contribution 10) presented an authoritative review of characterization methodologies in metal-based solid-state hydrogen storage, comprehensively analyzing both conventional and emerging analytical techniques, particularly emphasizing the crucial role of in situ and operando characterization in understanding hydrogen–material interactions at atomic and molecular levels.

Looking ahead, several emerging trends and research directions are evident from these contributions. The integration of artificial intelligence with materials design, the development of multifunctional materials for energy applications, and the optimization of sustainable production methods represent particularly promising avenues for future research. The continued evolution of in situ characterization techniques and theoretical modeling capabilities will be crucial in accelerating materials discovery and optimization. As we progress toward a more sustainable and resilient energy future, the strategic development of advanced materials remains paramount. The papers in this Special Issue demonstrate the remarkable potential of innovative materials solutions in addressing global energy challenges, while simultaneously highlighting the importance of interdisciplinary approaches and sustainable methodologies in materials research and development.

**Conflicts of Interest:** The author declares no conflicts of interest.

**List of Contributions:**

1. Liu, Z.; Xu, Y.; Kan, X.; Chen, M.; Dai, J.; Zhang, Y.; Pang, P.; Ma, W.; Zhang, J. An Electrochemical Sensor for Detection of Lead (II) Ions Using Biochar of Spent Coffee Grounds Modified by TiO$_2$ Nanoparticles. *Molecules* **2024**, *29*, 5704.
2. Xu, Y.; Li, Y.; Ding, Z. Network–Polymer–Modified Superparamagnetic Magnetic Silica Nanoparticles for the Adsorption and Regeneration of Heavy Metal Ions. *Molecules* **2023**, *28*, 7385.

3. Wang, Z.; Zhou, Z.; Gao, X.; Liu, Q.; Man, J.; Du, F.; Xiong, F. Natural Silkworm Cocoon-Derived Separator with Na-Ion De-Solvated Function for Sodium Metal Batteries. *Molecules* **2024**, *29*, 4813.
4. Abdisattar, A.; Yerdauletov, M.; Yeleuov, M.; Napolskiy, F.; Merkulov, A.; Rudnykh, A.; Nazarov, K.; Kenessarin, M.; Zhomartova, A.; Krivchenko, V. The Impact of Biowaste Composition and Activated Carbon Structure on the Electrochemical Performance of Supercapacitors. *Molecules* **2024**, *29*, 5029.
5. Wang, L.; Chen, H.; Zhang, Y.; Liu, J.; Peng, L. Research Progress in Strategies for Enhancing the Conductivity and Conductive Mechanism of LiFePO$_4$ Cathode Materials. *Molecules* **2024**, *29*, 5250.
6. Wang, Z.; Deng, R.; Wang, Y.; Pan, F. Comparison of Construction Strategies of Solid Electrolyte Interface (SEI) in Li Battery and Mg Battery—A Review. *Molecules* **2024**, *29*, 4761.
7. Liu, J.; Wang, L.; Wu, G. Sintering Behavior of Molybdenite Concentrate During Oxidation Roasting Process in Air Atmosphere: Influences of Roasting Temperature and K Content. *Molecules* **2024**, *29*, 5183.
8. Zhu, L.; Wu, D.; Yang, S.; Xie, K.; Wei, K.; Ma, W. Silicon extraction from diamond wire saw silicon slurry with flotation and the flotation interface behavior. *Molecules* **2024**, *29*, 5916.
9. Xu, Y.; Zhou, Y.; Li, Y.; Zheng, Y. Bridging Materials and Analytics: A Comprehensive Review of Characterization Approaches in Metal-Based Solid-State Hydrogen Storage. *Molecules* **2024**, *29*, 5014.
10. Zhou, Y.; Lv, H.; Chen, T.; Tong, S.; Zhang, Y.; Wang, B.; Tan, J.; Chen, X.; Pan, F. Probing the Effect of Alloying Elements on the Interfacial Segregation Behavior and Electronic Properties of Mg/Ti Interface via First-Principles Calculations. *Molecules* **2024**, *29*, 4138.

# References

1. Chu, S.; Majumdar, A. Opportunities and challenges for a sustainable energy future. *Nature* **2012**, *488*, 294–303. [PubMed]
2. Hassan, Q.; Viktor, P.; Al-Musawi, T.J.; Ali, B.M.; Algburi, S.; Alzoubi, H.M.; Al-Jiboory, A.K.; Sameen, A.Z.; Salman, H.M.; Jaszczur, M. The renewable energy role in the global energy Transformations. *Renew. Energy Focus* **2024**, *48*, 100545. [CrossRef]
3. Abdin, Z. Shaping the stationary energy storage landscape with reversible fuel cells. *J. Energy Storage* **2024**, *86*, 111354. [CrossRef]
4. Ding, Z.; Li, Y.; Yang, H.; Lu, Y.; Tan, J.; Li, J.; Li, Q.; Chen, Y.; Shaw, L.L.; Pan, F. Tailoring MgH$_2$ for hydrogen storage through nanoengineering and catalysis. *J. Magnes. Alloys* **2022**, *10*, 2946–2967. [CrossRef]
5. Centi, G.; Quadrelli, E.A.; Perathoner, S. Catalysis for CO$_2$ conversion: A key technology for rapid introduction of renewable energy in the value chain of chemical industries. *Energy Environ. Sci.* **2013**, *6*, 1711–1731.
6. Dubey, R.; Gunasekaran, A.; Ali, S.S. Exploring the relationship between leadership, operational practices, institutional pressures and environmental performance: A framework for green supply chain. *Int. J. Prod. Econ.* **2015**, *160*, 120–132. [CrossRef]
7. Garcia-Navarro, J.; Isaacs, M.A.; Favaro, M.; Ren, D.; Ong, W.; Grätzel, M.; Jiménez-Calvo, P. Updates on hydrogen value chain: A strategic roadmap. *Glob. Chall.* **2024**, *8*, 2300073. [CrossRef] [PubMed]
8. Le, T.T.; Sharma, P.; Bora, B.J.; Tran, V.D.; Truong, T.H.; Le, H.C.; Nguyen, P.Q.P. Fueling the future: A comprehensive review of hydrogen energy systems and their challenges. *Int. J. Hydrogen Energy* **2024**, *54*, 791–816. [CrossRef]

**Disclaimer/Publisher's Note:** The statements, opinions and data contained in all publications are solely those of the individual author(s) and contributor(s) and not of MDPI and/or the editor(s). MDPI and/or the editor(s) disclaim responsibility for any injury to people or property resulting from any ideas, methods, instructions or products referred to in the content.

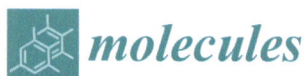 

*Article*

# Network–Polymer–Modified Superparamagnetic Magnetic Silica Nanoparticles for the Adsorption and Regeneration of Heavy Metal Ions

Yaohui Xu [1,2], Yuting Li [3] and Zhao Ding [4,*]

[1] Laboratory for Functional Materials, School of New Energy Materials and Chemistry, Leshan Normal University, Leshan 614000, China; xuyaohui1986@163.com
[2] Leshan West Silicon Materials Photovoltaic New Energy Industry Technology Research Institute, Leshan 614000, China
[3] The State Key Laboratory of Refractories and Metallurgy, Institute of Advanced Materials and Nanotechnology, Wuhan University of Science and Technology, Wuhan 430081, China; lyt@wust.edu.cn
[4] College of Materials Science and Engineering, National Engineering Research Center for Magnesium Alloys, Chongqing University, Chongqing 400044, China
* Correspondence: zhaoding@cqu.edu.cn; Tel.: +86-023-65127881

**Abstract:** Superparamagnetic magnetic nanoparticles (MNPs, $Fe_3O_4$) were first synthesized based on a chemical co–precipitation method, and the core–shell magnetic silica nanoparticles (MSNPs, $Fe_3O_4@SiO_2$) were obtained via hydrolysis and the condensation of tetraethyl orthosilicate onto $Fe_3O_4$ seed using a sol–gel process. Following that, MSNPs were immobilized using a three–step grafting strategy, where 8-hloroacetyl–aminoquinoline (CAAQ) was employed as a metal ion affinity ligand for trapping specific heavy metal ions, and a macromolecular polymer (polyethylenimine (PEI)) was selected as a bridge between the surface hydroxyl group and CAAQ to fabricate a network of organic networks onto the MSNPs' surface. The as–synthesized MSNPs–CAAQ nanocomposites possessed abundant active functional groups and thus contained excellent removal features for heavy metal ions. Specifically, the maximum adsorption capacities at room temperature and without adjusting pH were 324.7, 306.8, and 293.3 mg/g for $Fe^{3+}$, $Cu^{2+}$, and $Cr^{3+}$ ions, respectively, according to Langmuir linear fitting. The adsorption–desorption experiment results indicated that $Na_2EDTA$ proved to be more suitable as a desorbing agent for $Cr^{3+}$ desorption on the MSNPs–CAAQ surface than HCl and $HNO_3$. MSNPs–CAAQ exhibited a satisfactory adsorption capacity toward $Cr^{3+}$ ions even after six consecutive adsorption–desorption cycles; the adsorption efficiency for $Cr^{3+}$ ions was still 88.8% with 0.1 mol/L $Na_2EDTA$ as the desorbing agent. Furthermore, the MSNPs–CAAQ nanosorbent displayed a strong magnetic response with a saturated magnetization of 24.0 emu/g, and they could be easily separated from the aqueous medium under the attraction of a magnet, which could facilitate the sustainable removal of $Cr^{3+}$ ions in practical applications.

**Keywords:** nanoparticles; magnetic; surface modification; adsorption; regeneration; heavy metal ion

**Citation:** Xu, Y.; Li, Y.; Ding, Z. Network–Polymer–Modified Superparamagnetic Magnetic Silica Nanoparticles for the Adsorption and Regeneration of Heavy Metal Ions. *Molecules* **2023**, *28*, 7385. https://doi.org/10.3390/molecules28217385

Academic Editor: Maria Luisa Saladino

Received: 23 September 2023
Revised: 29 October 2023
Accepted: 30 October 2023
Published: 1 November 2023

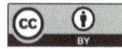

**Copyright:** © 2023 by the authors. Licensee MDPI, Basel, Switzerland. This article is an open access article distributed under the terms and conditions of the Creative Commons Attribution (CC BY) license (https://creativecommons.org/licenses/by/4.0/).

## 1. Introduction

Heavy metal ions (HMIs) can easily spread through the food chain and seriously threaten human health [1–3], as well as negatively influencing the ecological environment of sustainable development [4–6]. Chromium ($Cr^{3+}$), arsenic ($As^{3+}$), cadmium ($Cd^{2+}$), mercury ($Hg^{2+}$), and plumbum ($Pd^{2+}$) ions were considered to be the five most toxic HMIs, with intense toxicity and the tendency to cause serious diseases even at very low concentrations [7]. Therefore, HMI pollution in water caused by modern industry is an important issue due to its toxicity, complex components, and non–biodegradability. Usually, HMI pollution in water has the characteristics of a large pollution area, so it is difficult to enrich HMIs in water using extraction methods. This has been presented as a simple and effective method to fix HMIs in situ to reduce their toxicity in water due to the obvious repair effect, simple construction technology, short construction period, reasonable repair costs, and other characteristics. Among the technologies used to cure or stabilize HMIs in water, the adsorption method is the most economical and effective method [8–10]. Reasonable and efficient adsorbents are the key to determining the feasibility of the purification and recovery of HMIs in water by adsorption. The primary adsorbents used in wastewater treatment are categorized as carbon [11], silica [12], zeolite [13], metal–based [14] nano–adsorbents, and magnetic nanoparticles [15]. In addition to the above main classes of adsorbents, several economical bio–adsorbents have been produced from agricultural waste, food waste, cellulose waste, and industrial by–products [16,17].

The non–magnetic nanosorbents are easy to lose in the process of use, which is not conducive to recovery. In any case, exhausted non–magnetic nano–adsorbents have to be removed from the liquid, and magnetic extraction appears to be the most frequently adopted solution [10]. Therefore, magnetic nanomaterials, especially superparamagnetic nanomaterials, have received extensive attention from researchers. Magnetic nanoparticles (MNPs, $Fe_3O_4$) are an excellent candidate nanosorbent because of their small size effect and apparent superparamagnetism [18]. The greatest strength of MNPs is that they are easily attracted to the target zone under the guidance of an external magnetic field [19–23]. An inconvenient disadvantage of MNPs is that they are prone to oxidative degradation when directly exposed to the environment. In order to reduce the instability of MNPs, a core–shell structure of magnetic silica nanoparticles (MSNPs) is proposed, in which the MNPs, as the core, can facilitate targeted control and recyclable separation under an applied magnetic field, while the silica ($SiO_2$), as the shell, can prevent the magnetic core from oxidation and corrosion [24].

Surface modification proved to be an effective way to improve the adsorption performance of nanosorbents. At present, many studies are focused on the surface modification of MSNPs to improve their adsorptive capacity by grafting the end–reactive functional groups. Generally, the grafted organic molecules, such as iminodiacetic acid, (3–aminopropyl)triethoxysilane, N–(trimethoxysilylpropyl)ethylenediamine triacetic acid, and 3–mercaptopropyltrimethoxysilane, had a distinct affinity for combining with $Zn^{2+}$ [25], $Cu^{2+}$ [26], $Pb^{2+}$ [27], $Cd^{2+}$ [28], and $Hg^{2+}$ [29] ions. However, the single–stranded grafting of small organic molecules still cannot meet the actual application demand. On this basis, polymer grafting has been proposed to increase the amount of end–reactive functional groups, which yields MSNPs/polymers with excellent adsorptive features [30–32]. Despite this progress in the synthesis of MSNPs–based absorbents, it is still challenging to further improve their adsorptive capacity since further increases in the amount of ligands or the introduction of large macromolecules are restrained by the steric hindrance, limiting their actual applications.

In this regard, we proposed network polymer (8–chloroacetyl–aminoquinoline, CAAQ)–modified MSNPs to remove HMIs using a three–step grafting strategy, as shown in Figure 1a. In the design of this network structure on MSNPs' surfaces, the selected macromolecular polymer was key. Polyethylenimine (PEI) possessed numerous branched chains of $-NH_2$ groups, which formed the framework of a network structure. MSNPs were like a tree, and CAAQ was the final fruit (end–active group), while PEI was like a branch with rich twigs ($-NH_2$ group), providing numerous sites for the growth of the final fruit. The network design could effectively increase the quantity of active functional groups in the limited space and thus improve their adsorption capacity. The key process of this synthesis was to achieve a controllable bridge of MTCS/CPTCS and PEI, allowing for more CAAQ to become immobilized onto MSNPs. Moreover, the removal and regeneration of HMIs by MSNPs–CAAQ from aqueous solutions was investigated, as shown in Figure 1b.

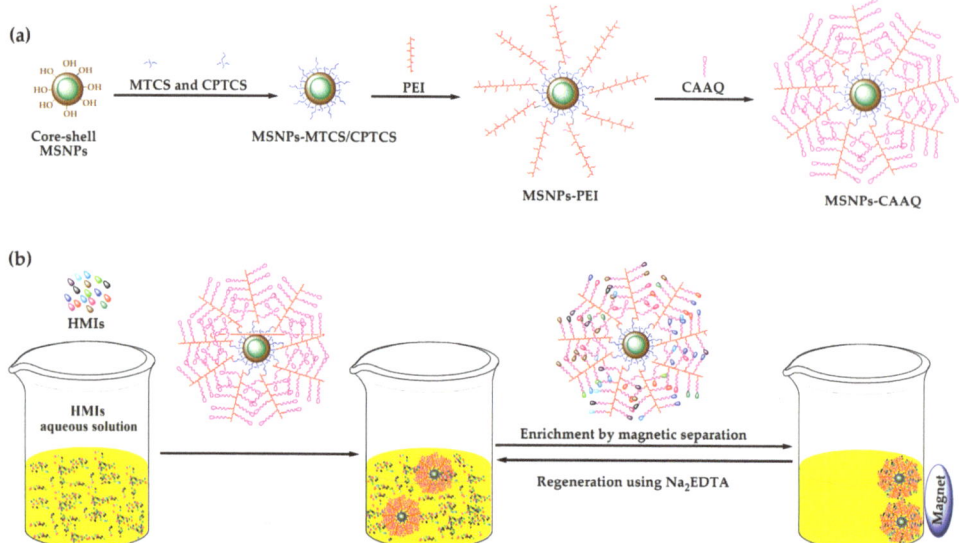

**Figure 1.** (**a**) Synthesis scheme of MSNPs–CAAQ nanocomposites; (**b**) schematic diagram of HMIs adsorption and magnetic separation.

## 2. Results and Discussion

### 2.1. Characterizations of MNPs and MSNPs

Figure 2a,b show the XRD patterns of the as–synthesized MNPs and MSNPs, respectively. The XRD pattern of MNPs in Figure 2a displays several well–resolved diffraction peaks that could match well with the (111), (220), (311), (222), (400), (422), (511), (440), (533) and (622) planes of cubic spinel $Fe_3O_4$ (JCPDS No. 65–3107). All crystal planes could be identified, indicating that the obtained $Fe_3O_4$ crystal was complete, and the average grain size of $Fe_3O_4$ was calculated with a value of about 9.0 nm according to Scherrer's formula. In addition to the diffraction peaks of the cubic spinel $Fe_3O_4$ phase, there was a weak and broad peak at $2\theta = 15\sim28°$ (yellow area in Figure 2b), which was consistent with the amorphous $SiO_2$ phase. Compared to the XRD diffraction intensity of MNPs in Figure 2a, that of MSNPs in Figure 2b was slightly reduced, further implying that the amorphous $SiO_2$ was coated onto the surface of $Fe_3O_4$ seeds. Further analysis of the core–shell structure of MSNPs was conducted by TEM analysis, as discussed later.

TEMs were employed to characterize the morphology, size, and microstructure of MNPs and MSNPs. The TEM image in Figure 3a demonstrates that the as–synthesized MNPs exhibited a uniform size of ~10 nm. Moreover, we could observe that these particles had the same direction of lattice fringes with an interplanar spacing of 0.308 nm from the high–resolution TEM (HRTEM) image in Figure 3a's inset, fitted with (220) in cubic spinel $Fe_3O_4$, which proves that the as–synthesized $Fe_3O_4$ was a single–crystalline structure. After coating with $SiO_2$, the particle size increased to ~21 nm from ~10 nm, according to the TEM image in Figure 3b. Furthermore, the obvious core–shell structure with a core size of ~10 nm and a shell thickness of ~5.5 nm could be clearly observed from the amplified TEM image in Figure 3b's inset. The XRD data in Figure 2 and TEM data in Figure 3 could prove that MNPs with a single–crystal structure can be synthesized using the chemical co–precipitation method, while MSNPs with a core–shell structure can be obtained through the hydrolysis and condensation of TEOS on a single–crystal $Fe_3O_4$ seed.

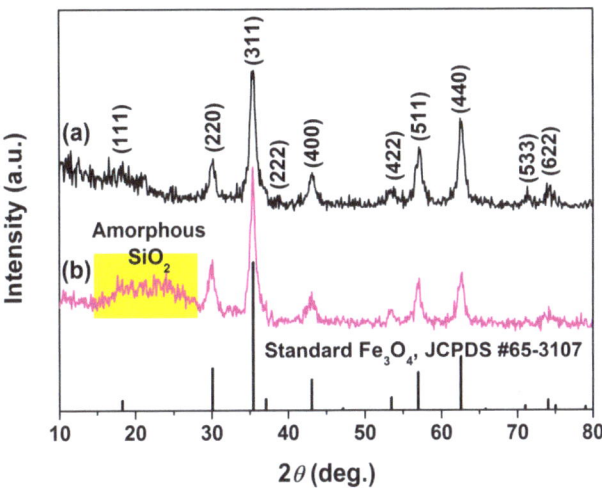

**Figure 2.** XRD spectra of (**a**) MNPs and (**b**) MSNPs contrasted with the standard Fe$_3$O$_4$ (JCPDS No. 65–3107) pattern.

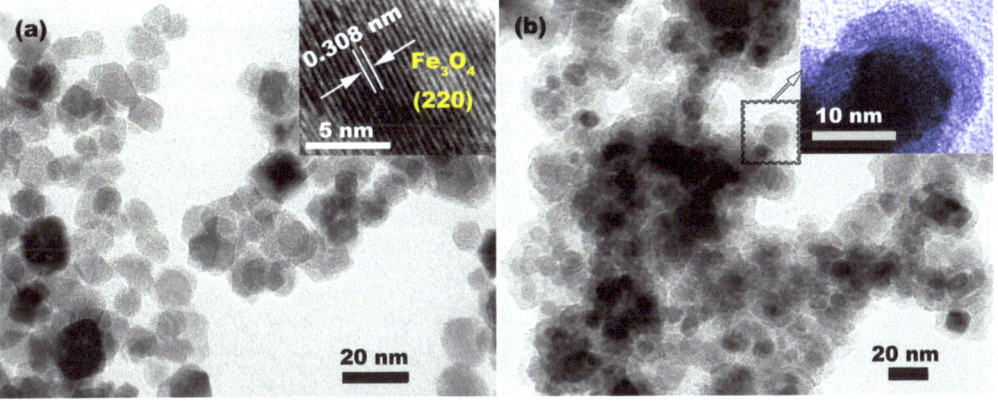

**Figure 3.** (**a**) TEM image of MNPs (inset is an HRTEM image of MNPs); (**b**) TEM image of MSNPs (inset is an amplified TEM image of MSNPs).

## 2.2. Characterizations of MSNPs–CAAQ

Figure 4a shows the XRD spectrum of as–synthesized MSNPs–CAAQ. In Figure 4a, the broad peak at $2\theta = \sim22.5°$ or other sharp little peaks at $2\theta > \sim33.0°$ imply the existence of at least two kinds of phases in the MSNPs–CAAQ samples. The broad peak at $2\theta = \sim22.5°$ could be attributed to some phases with an amorphous state, while the several sharp little peaks at $2\theta > \sim33.0°$ were indexed to the (311), (400), (511), and (440) planes of the standard Fe$_3$O$_4$ (JCPDS No. 65–3107) pattern, indicating the presence of the cubic spinel Fe$_3$O$_4$ phase. Compared with the XRD patterns of MNPs and MSNPs in Figure 2, the diffraction peak intensity of the Fe$_3$O$_4$ phase was reduced dramatically, while the broad featureless peak of SiO$_2$ was clearly increased, becoming even stronger than that of the Fe$_3$O$_4$ phase, indicating that organic molecules were coated on the MSNPs' surface after modification. Figure 4b shows the TEM image of MSNPs–CAAQ. In Figure 4b, an extra amorphous coating can be observed around the particles, further implying successful CAAQ modification.

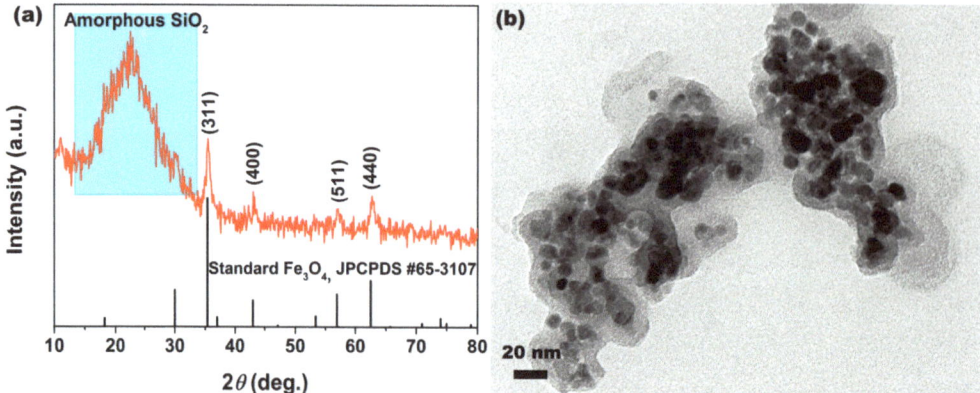

**Figure 4.** (a) XRD spectrum contrasted with standard Fe$_3$O$_4$ (JCPDS NO. 65–3107) pattern and (b) TEM image of MSNPs–CAAQ.

The thermal decomposition behaviors of MSNPs and MSNPs–CAAQ were determined using a TG instrument at a heating rate of 10 °C/min under a flow of air within the temperature range of 25 to 600 °C. For the TG curve of MSNPs in Figure 5a, a relative weight loss of 8.6% was detected over the entire temperature range, which was probably caused by the evaporation of adsorbed water and the decomposition of hydroxyl groups (–OH) on the MSNPs' surface, while a far higher weight loss of 31.7% over the entire temperature range was observed for MSNPs–CAAQ in Figure 5b, which could mainly be attributed to the evaporation of adsorbed water and the decomposition of the grafted organic molecules layer, including MTCS, CPTCS, PEI, and CAAQ. Below ~150 °C, the TG curves of MSNPs and MSNPs–CAAQ almost coincided, indicating that the water content on the surface of MSNPs and MSNPs–CAAQ was basically the same. Therefore, the weight percentage of grafted organic molecules on MSNPs' surface could be calculated by subtracting the weight loss of MSNPs from that of MSNPs–CAAQ, and the value was ~23.1%.

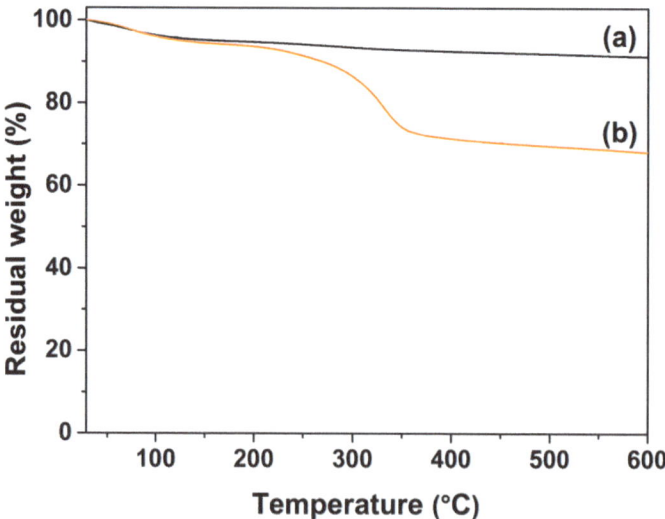

**Figure 5.** TG curves of (a) MSNPs and (b) MSNPs–CAAQ.

To determine the organic composition of MSNPs' surfaces, FTIR and XPS analyses were employed. Figure 6a–d shows the FTIR spectra of MSNPs, MSNPs–MTCS/CPTCS, MSNPs–PEI, and MSNPs–CAAQ, respectively. For all FTIR spectra in Figure 6, there were several apparent absorption peaks at 3433, 1088, and 584 cm$^{-1}$, corresponding to the stretching of –OH [33], Si–O [34], and Fe–O [35] bonds, respectively. This further demonstrated the successful synthesis of Fe$_3$O$_4$/SiO$_2$ composites with numerous –OH groups, which was consistent with the XRD analysis results in Figure 2. Compared with the FTIR spectrum of MSNPs in Figure 6a, two new absorption peaks at 2970 cm$^{-1}$ (C–H bond) and 1274 cm$^{-1}$ (Si–C bond) [36] were observed. For the FTIR spectrum of MSNPs–MTCS/CPTCS in Figure 6b. In addition to the absorption peaks of C–H and Si–C bonds, the FTIR spectrum of MSNPs–PEI presented in Figure 6c showed a new peak at 1392 cm$^{-1}$ [37], ascribed to the stretching of the C–N bond. In addition to the above–mentioned absorption peaks in Figure 6a–c, there were also three new absorption peaks at 1695, 1551, and 1437 cm$^{-1}$ for the FTIR spectrum of MSNPs–CAAQ in Figure 6b, ascribed to the stretching of HN–C=O, C=N, and –NH bonds [38], respectively. This indicates that MTCS/CPTCS, PEI, and CAAQ were successfully grafted onto the MSNPs' surface.

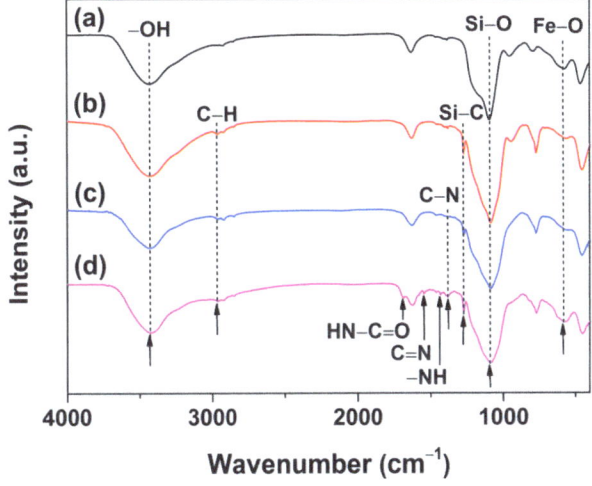

**Figure 6.** FTIR spectra of (a) MSNPs, (b) MSNPs–MTCS/CPTCS, (c) MSNPs–PEI, and (d) MSNPs–CAAQ.

Figure 7a shows the XPS spectra of MSNPs, MSNPs–MTCS/CPTCS, MSNPs–PEI, and MSNPs–CAAQ. By comparing the XPS spectrum of MSNPs, that of MSNPs–MTCS/CPTCS showed a clear new peak in the Cl signal at ~200.0 eV, which probably derived from the MTCS and CPTCS grafted onto the MSNPs' surface. The XPS spectra of MSNPs–PEI and MSNPs–CAAQ both showed a clear new peak in N element at ~400.0 eV, which probably derived from the nitrogenous organic matter grafted onto MSNPs' surfaces, including PEI and CAAQ. In addition, the absence of a Cl signal for the XPS spectrum of MSNPs–PEI suggested a successful dechlorination coupling reaction between MSNPs–MTCS/CPTCS and the PEI molecule. Moreover, the detailed N 1s core–level spectrum of MSNPs–CAAQ could be curve–fitted into four peak components, as shown in Figure 7b. The binding energies at 401.8, 400.8, 399.7, and 398.9 eV could be attributed to pyridinic N species, N–C species, HN–C=O species, and aromatic N species, respectively [39–41]. Figure 7c also shows the XPS spectrum of C 1s core levels for MSNPs–CAAQ. From Figure 7c, the C 1s core–level spectrum is shown to present four peaks with binding energies of 286.7, 285.8, 284.8, and 284.1 eV, attributable to the NH–C=O, C–N, –(CH$_2$)$_n$–, and –C$_6$H$_5$– species, respectively [42–45]. This further confirms that the CAAQ–modified MSNPs were successfully yielded using the three–step grafting method (see Figure 1a), involving MTCS/CPTCS co–modification, PEI grafting, and CAAQ grafting.

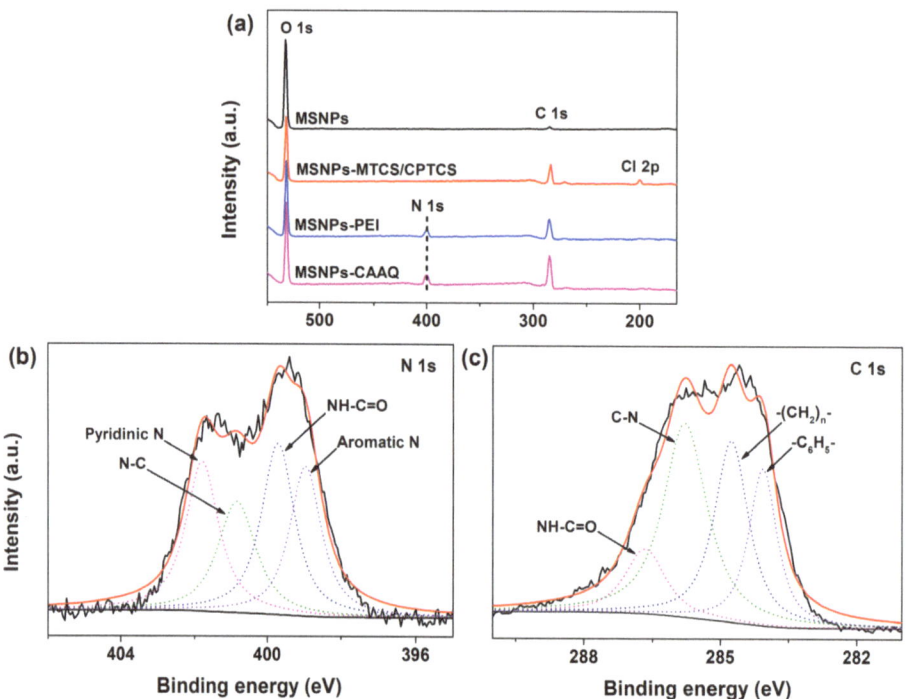

**Figure 7.** XPS wide scan of (**a**) MSNPs, MSNPs–MTCS/CPTCS, MSNPs–PEI, and MSNPs–CAAQ; (**b**) C 1s and (**c**) N 1s core levels of MSNPs–CAAQ.

### 2.3. Magnetic Analysis of MNPs, MSNPs and MSNPs–CAAQ

The magnetic properties were measured using a vibrating sample magnetometer. As displayed in Figure 8a, the saturated magnetizations ($M$) of MNPs, MSNPs, and MSNPs–CAAQ were 61.0, 38.1, and 24.0 emu/g, respectively. Compared with MNPs, the reduced $M$ values for MSNPs and MSNPs–CAAQ were mainly attributed to the increased weight of non–magnetic layers, including amorphous $SiO_2$ and grafted organic molecules [46]. Figure 8b shows the magnified curve of the surrounding origin in Figure 8a (the area inside the pink box of Figure 8a). All three samples of MNPs, MSNPs, and MSNPs–CAAQ could be regarded as superparamagnetic with negligible hysteresis. This suggests that MNPs encapsulated in the $SiO_2$ shell could preserve their superparamagnetism. In practical applications, it is extremely important that the magnetic carriers or supports exhibit rapid responsiveness under an applied magnetic field without retaining any magnetism after withdrawing the applied magnetic field. Moreover, Figure 8c shows the time–dependence of the magnetic response behavior of MSNPs–CAAQ suspension by adding an external magnet to the right side of the bottle. In Figure 8c, these particles are shown to be well dispersed in an aqueous medium without a magnet (Blank in Figure 8c), and they were easily separated from the solution under the attraction of the magnet. The solution appeared clear and transparent within 28 s. However, the Tyndall effect can be observed by the naked eye in Figure 8d, indicating that some MSNPs–CAAQ nanoparticles were still floating in the aqueous solution. As the magnetic separation continued, the Tyndall effect disappeared at 111 s, indicating that the solid–liquid separation was complete. This is a potential drawback of the MSNPs–CAAQ nano–adsorbent due to its low saturation magnetization, which risks leaving behind some nanoparticles that were uncaught by the applied magnetic field. In order to minimize this shortcoming, it was necessary to extend the operation time of the applied magnetic field.

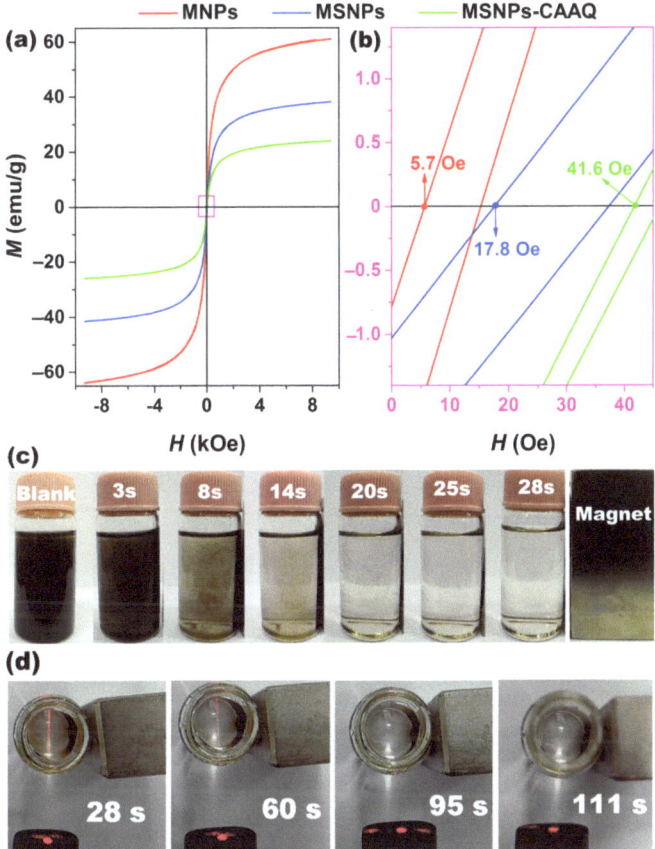

**Figure 8.** (**a**) Room–temperature magnetic hysteresis loops of MNPs, MSNPs, and MSNPs–CAAQ; (**b**) the amplified curves around the coercive value (the area inside the pink box in Figure 8a); (**c**) time–dependence of the magnetic response behavior of MSNPs–CAAQ suspension after adding an external magnet to the right side of the bottle; (**d**) the clear liquid of the Tyndall effect over time.

### 2.4. Adsorption Characteristics

The adsorption capacity of MSNPs–CAAQ for the selected HMIs, including $Ag^+$, $Zn^{2+}$, $Cu^{2+}$, $Co^{2+}$, $Cd^{2+}$, $Mn^{2+}$, $Pb^{2+}$, $Hg^{2+}$, $Cr^{3+}$ and $Fe^{3+}$ ions, was evaluated at room temperature without pH pre–adjustments. Figure 9 shows the time–dependence of the adsorption profiles of the selected HMIs onto MSNPs–CAAQ composites. Figure 9 shows that the as–synthesized MSNPs–CAAQ exhibited strong and rapid adsorption features for HMIs within the first 1.0 h, and the adsorption process was mostly completed within 1.5 h of the reaction. For $Fe^{3+}$, $Cu^{2+}$ and $Cr^{3+}$ ions, the adsorption efficiencies within 1.5 h could reach 98.9%, 96.4%, and 95.9%, respectively. Moreover, MSNPs–CAAQ exhibited universal adsorption capacities for $Zn^{2+}$, $Mn^{2+}$ and $Pb^{2+}$ ions, with adsorption efficiencies of over 70% within 1.5 h. The sequence and values of the adsorption efficiency within 2.5 h were as follows: $Fe^{3+}$ (98.5%) > $Cu^{2+}$ (96.1%) > $Cr^{3+}$ (95.3%) > $Mn^{2+}$ (75.3%) > $Zn^{2+}$ (72.9%) > $Pb^{2+}$ (71.8%) > $Cd^{2+}$ (65.6%) > $Hg^{2+}$ (55.7%) > $Co^{2+}$ (52.2%) > $Ag^+$ (47.1%). As a comparison, the adsorption efficiency of MSNPs without CAAQ modifications was also tested and is shown in the inset of Figure 9. As observed, the adsorption efficiencies of MSNPs within 2.5 h were below 6.0% for all HMIs under the same conditions, indicating that the absorption of HMIs was mainly attributed to the grafted CAAQ rather than MSNPs. The high adsorption efficiencies of MSNPs–CAAQ could be due to the abundant adsorption sites from the CAAQ network that were transferred onto the MSNPs' surface, which also demonstrates the superiority of our design.

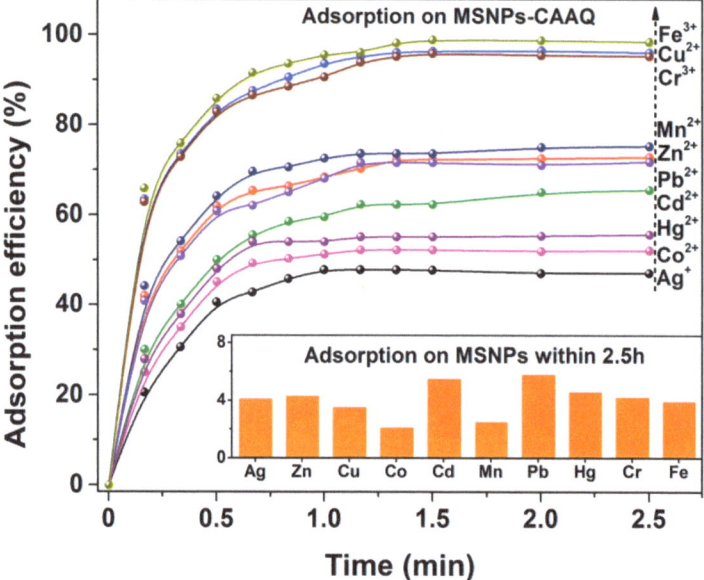

**Figure 9.** Adsorption profiles onto MSNPs–CAAQ for HMIs (inset shows the adsorption efficiencies within 2.5 h of MSNPs without CAAQ modifications for HMIs). (Adsorbent dose was 1.0 g/L; adsorbate dose was 200 mg/L; $V$ = 50 mL; reaction temperature was 298.15 K; no pH pre-adjustments).

The experimental data of the adsorption of $Fe^{3+}$, $Cu^{2+}$, and $Cr^{3+}$ ions onto MSNPs–CAAQ were analyzed by the Langmuir isotherm model and Freundlich isotherm model; their Langmuir linear fittings and Freundlich plots are shown in Figure 10a,b, and the corresponding Langmuir and Freundlich parameters that were calculated are listed in Table 1. From Figure 10a, it is shown that the Langmuir isotherm model was a good fit for modeling the adsorption of $Fe^{3+}$, $Cu^{2+}$, and $Cr^{3+}$ ions onto the MSNPs–CAAQ surface. However, the experimental data considerably deviated from the Freundlich model in Figure 10b, suggesting that it was not appropriate to use the Freundlich model to predict the adsorption isotherms of $Fe^{3+}$, $Cu^{2+}$, and $Cr^{3+}$ ions onto MSNPs–CAAQ. As observed in Table 1, the Langmuir isotherm model had high correlation coefficients ($R^2$ > 0.9980), implying that the adsorption of $Fe^{3+}$, $Cu^{2+}$, and $Cr^{3+}$ ions could be better described by the Langmuir model. The saturated adsorption amounts ($q_m$) of $Fe^{3+}$, $Cu^{2+}$, and $Cr^{3+}$ ions were 324.7, 306.8, and 293.3 mg/g, respectively, according to the Langmuir linear fitting. Moreover, a comparison of the maximum adsorption capacities of $Fe^{3+}$, $Cu^{2+}$, and $Cr^{3+}$ ions onto other adsorbents is shown in Table 2 [47–51]. Except for the adsorption of $Cu^{2+}$ and $Cr^{3+}$ ions onto EDTA–inspired polydentate hydrogels, the adsorption capacities were significantly higher for the MSNPs–CAAQ sorbents used in this study.

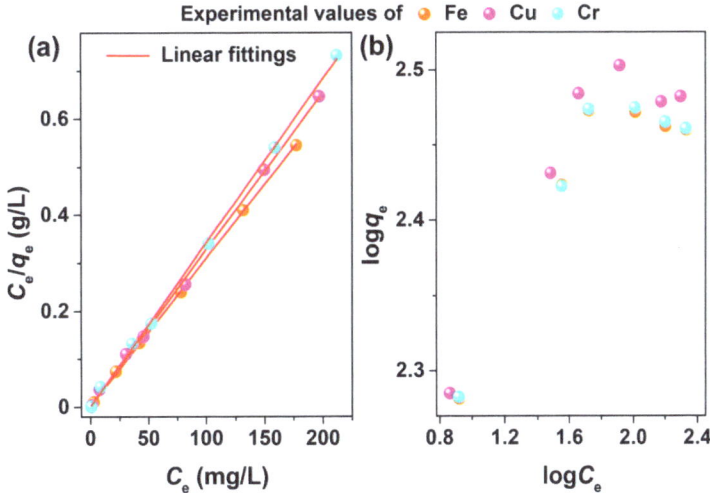

**Figure 10.** (**a**) Langmuir linear fittings and (**b**) Freundlich plots of $Fe^{3+}$, $Cu^{2+}$, and $Cr^{3+}$ ions onto MSNPs–CAAQ.

**Table 1.** Relevant parameters of Langmuir isotherms for the adsorption of $Fe^{3+}$, $Cu^{2+}$, and $Cr^{3+}$ ions.

| Langmuir Isotherm Model | $\frac{C_e}{q_e} = \frac{1}{q_m}C_e + \frac{1}{K_L q_m}$ | | |
|---|---|---|---|
| Parameters | $q_m$ (mg/g) | $K_L$ | $R^2$ |
| $Fe^{3+}$ | 324.7 | 0.7016 | 0.9997 |
| $Cu^{2+}$ | 306.8 | 0.6981 | 0.9988 |
| $Cr^{3+}$ | 293.3 | 0.7894 | 0.9990 |

**Table 2.** Comparison of maximum adsorption capacities of various adsorbents for $Fe^{3+}$, $Cu^{2+}$, and $Cr^{3+}$ ions.

| Adsorbent | HMIs | Adsorption Capacity ($q_m$, mg/g) | Reference |
|---|---|---|---|
| Manganese dioxide–modified biochar | $Fe^{3+}$ | 52.39 | [47] |
| Activated biochars prepared by leucaena leucocephala | $Fe^{3+}$ | 32.89 | [48] |
| Phosphorylated nanocellulose (Phos–CNCSL) | $Fe^{3+}$ $Cu^{2+}$ | 115 117 | [49] |
| $Fe_3O_4$/$FeMoS_4$/MgAl–LDH nanocomposite | $Cu^{2+}$ | 108.28 | [50] |
| Core–shell magnetic $Fe_3O_4$@zeolite NaA | $Cu^{2+}$ | 86.54 | [51] |
| EDTA–inspired polydentate hydrogels | $Cu^{2+}$ $Cr^{3+}$ | 436.5 340.6 | [52] |
| Organosulphur–modified biochar | $Cr^{3+}$ | 35.2 | [53] |
| Porous carbon materials derived from rice wastes | $Cr^{3+}$ | 9.23 | [54] |
| MSNPs–CAAQ nanocomposite | $Fe^{3+}$ $Cu^{2+}$ $Cr^{3+}$ | 324.7 306.8 293.3 | This work |

In actual industrial wastewater, the coexistence of multiple HMIs is common, so it was necessary to investigate the influence of competing ions on adsorption. An adsorption experiment in a mixed–HMIs solution was also carried out, in which the mass of each HMI was 20 mg, the mass of the MSNPs–CAAQ adsorbent was 0.5 g, and the total volume of solution was 500 mL. The adsorption efficiency of the matrixed HMIs is shown in Figure 11. As observed, MSNPs–CAAQ exhibited universal and excellent adsorption capacities for all HMIs; the adsorption efficiencies could reach over 92.0% within 1.5 h, mainly due to the large adsorption capacity of the MSNPs–CAAQ adsorbent and the low initial concentration of each HMI in the mixed solution. It could be concluded from the above adsorption experiments that MSNPs–CAAQ is suitable as an adsorbent for the removal of HMIs, especially when the concentration of HMIs is low. In view of the strong toxicity of the $Cr^{3+}$ ion, the adsorption characteristics of $Cr^{3+}$ ions on MSNPs–CAAQ will be explored in the following research.

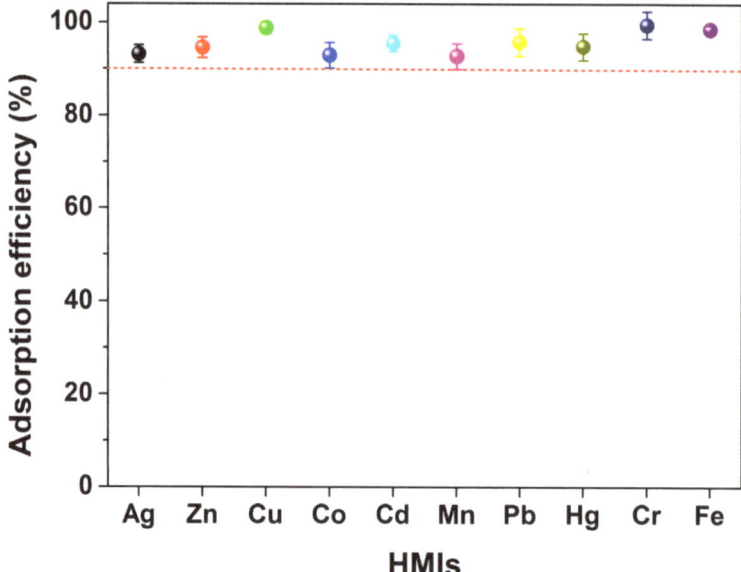

**Figure 11.** Adsorption efficiency of MSNPs–CAAQ for mixed–HMIs solution. (Mixed HMIs contained $Ag^+$, $Zn^{2+}$, $Cu^{2+}$, $Co^{2+}$, $Cd^{2+}$, $Mn^{2+}$, $Pb^{2+}$, $Hg^{2+}$, $Cr^{3+}$, and $Fe^{3+}$ ions; the mass of each HMI was 20 mg; MSNPs–CAAQ was 0.5 g; $V$ = 500 mL; $t$ = 1.5 h; reaction temperature was 298.15 K; no pH pre-adjustments). (Note: the different color ball represent was the adsorption efficiency of MSNPs–CAAQ for different HMIs in the mixed solution).

*2.5. Effect of pH on Adsorption*

Figure 12 shows the adsorption efficiencies of MSNPs–CAAQ at various pH values by plotting the normalized adsorption efficiency at different pH values. The initial concentration and volume of $Cr^{3+}$ ions were 250 mg/L and 50 mL; the mass of MSNPs–CAAQ was 1.0 g/L; and the pH value (1~8) of the aqueous solution was adjusted using HCl and NaOH aqueous solutions. Figure 12 shows that the pH value of the aqueous solution has a great influence on the adsorption efficiency of MSNPs–CAAQ. Below pH = 2.0, the adsorption efficiency of $Cr^{3+}$ ions was very low, which could be attributed to the electrostatic repulsion between the positively charged $Cr^{3+}$ ions and the protonated surface of MSNPs–CAAQ under strong acidic conditions. However, the adsorption efficiency increased steeply starting from pH = 3.0 and reached its maximum at around pH = 6.0, which could be attributed to the formation of a metal complex on the MSNPs–CAAQ surface. The decrease at around pH = 7.0 and 8.0 could be attributed to the dissociation of the loaded $Cr^{3+}$ ions on the MSNPs–CAAQ surface under strong basic conditions.

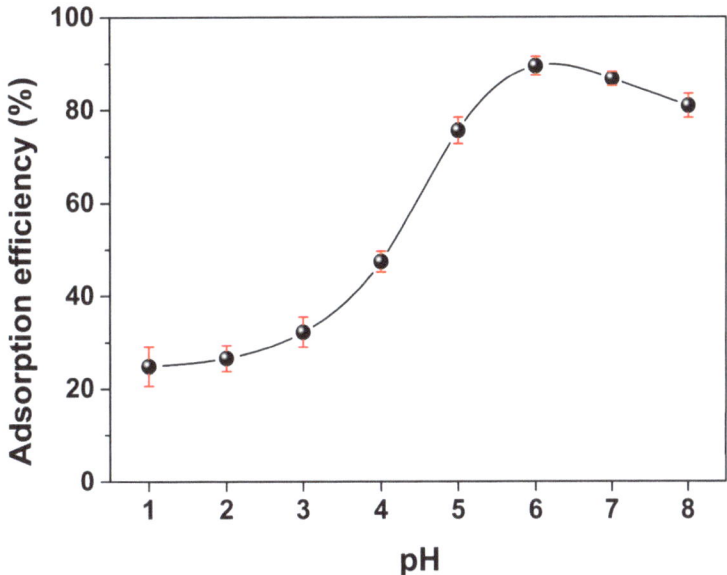

**Figure 12.** Effect of pH on the adsorption of $Cr^{3+}$ ions by MSNPs–CAAQ. (The adsorbent dose was 0.05 g; the initial concentration and volume of $Cr^{3+}$ ions were 250 mg/L and 50 mL; $t$ = 1.5 h; the reaction temperature was 298.15 K).

*2.6. Effect of Temperature on Adsorption*

For chemical adsorption, the degree of adsorption for the adsorbent would increase with the increase in adsorption reaction temperature, and the opposite rule would hold for physical absorption. Therefore, the effects of temperature on the adsorption of $Cr^{3+}$ ions were investigated in the range of 298.15~338.15 K in this work. In Figure 13a, the adsorption efficiency of the $Cr^{3+}$ ion on MSNPs–CAAQ is shown to slowly increase with an increase in temperature, which implies the possibility of a chemical–reaction–led adsorption process. Moreover, these experimental data on adsorption were fitted using the Van't Hoff equation, as shown in Figure 13b. Moreover, thermodynamic parameters such as $\Delta H^0$ and $\Delta S^0$ were calculated and are summarized in Table 3. In Table 3, a highly associated correlation coefficient ($R^2$) of 0.9993 was obtained, suggesting the reliability of the thermodynamic fitting result in this work. The positive value of $\Delta H^0$ (2.31 KJ/mol) indicates that the adsorption reaction was endothermic, while the positive value of $\Delta S^0$ (45.00 J/mol·K) implies that the disorder and randomness at the solid solution interface of the $Cr^{3+}$ ion with MSNPs–CAAQ increase during the adsorption process.

*2.7. Adsorption Kinetics*

The sorption kinetics of the $Cr^{3+}$ ion onto MSNPs–CAAQ were tested with the pseudo–first–order and pseudo–second–order kinetic models by plotting $\log(q_e-q_t)$ versus $t$ (Figure 14a) and plotting $t/q_t$ versus $t$ (Figure 14b), and the kinetic parameters calculated by fitting with these two models are listed in Table 4. In Table 4, the pseudo–second–order equation showed a higher correlation coefficient ($R^2$ = 0.9989) than that of the pseudo–second–order equation ($R^2$ = 0.9841). Moreover, the adsorption values calculated at equilibrium ($q_{e,cal}$, 206.61 mg/g) from the pseudo–second–order kinetic model were much closer to those of the experimental model ($q_{e,exp}$, 191.8 mg/g). Therefore, the pseudo–second–order model was more suitable for describing the adsorption kinetics of the $Cr^{3+}$ ion onto MSNPs–CAAQ, indicating that the chemisorption was the rate–controlling step during the attachment process. Furthermore, the three plausible interaction modes of MSNPs–CAAQ with the $Cr^{3+}$ ion that were proposed are shown in Figure 15, in which the $Cr^{3+}$ ions were selectively coordinated with carbonyl "O" and three "N" atoms. Similar coordination modes have been reported previously [55–57].

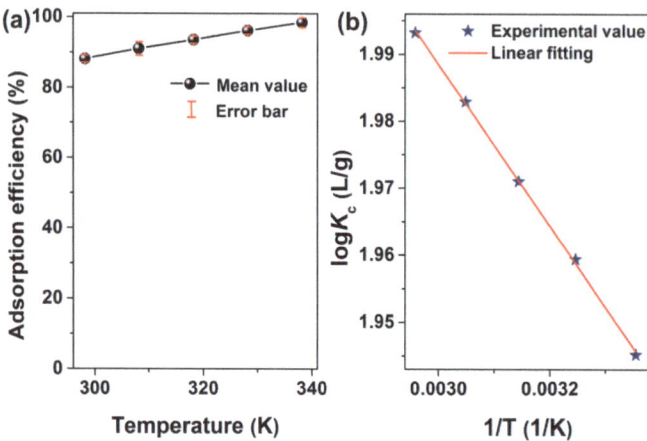

**Figure 13.** (a) Effects of temperature on the adsorption efficiency of the $Cr^{3+}$ ion on MSNPs–CAAQ; (b) experimental data of adsorption of the $Cr^{3+}$ ion at a set temperature of 298.15, 308.15, 318.15, 328.15, and 338.15 K on MSNPs–CAAQ fitted using the Van't Hoff equation. (Adsorbent dose was 1.0 g/L; adsorbate dose was 300 mg/L; $V$ = 50 mL; $t$ = 1.5 h; no pH pre–adjustments).

**Table 3.** Thermodynamic parameters for the adsorption of $Cr^{3+}$ ions onto MSNPs–CAAQ.

| Van't Hoff Thermodynamic Equation | $\log \frac{q_e}{c_e} = -\frac{\Delta H^0}{2.303R} \times \frac{1}{T} + \frac{\Delta S^0}{2.303R}$ | | |
|---|---|---|---|
| **Parameters** | $\Delta H^0$ (KJ/mol) | $\Delta S^0$ (J/mol·K) | $R^2$ |
| | 2.31 | 45.00 | 0.9993 |

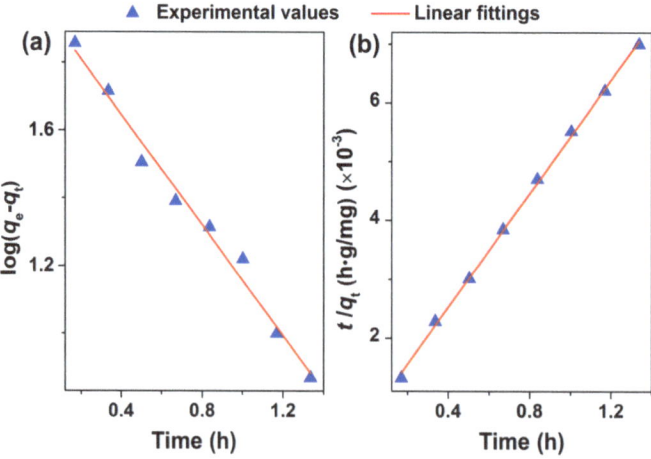

**Figure 14.** Linear fittings by (a) pseudo–first–order and (b) pseudo–second–order kinetic models for the adsorption of $Cr^{3+}$ ions onto MSNPs–CAAQ.

Table 4. Kinetic parameters for the adsorption of $Cr^{3+}$ ions onto MSNPs–CAAQ surfaces.

| Kinetic Model | Pseudo–First–Order $\log(q_{e1,cal}-q_t)=-\frac{k_1}{2.303}t+\log q_{e1,cal}$ | | | Pseudo–Second–Order $\frac{t}{q_t}=\frac{1}{q_{e2,cal}}t+\frac{1}{k_2 q_{e2,cal}^2}$ | | |
|---|---|---|---|---|---|---|
| Parameters | $q_{e1,cal}$ (mg/g) | $K_1$ (1/h) | $R^2$ | $q_{e2,cal}$ (mg/g) | $K_1$ (g/mg·h) | $R^2$ |
| | 93.61 | 1.8801 | 0.9841 | 206.61 | 0.03839 | 0.9989 |

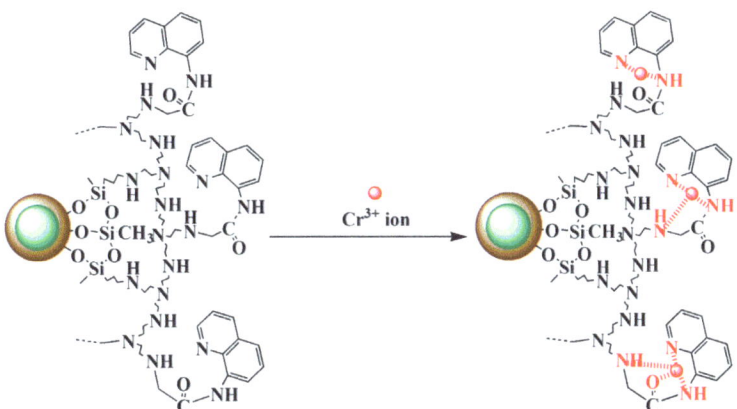

**Figure 15.** The proposed coordination modes between MSNPs–CAAQ and $Cr^{3+}$ ions.

## 2.8. Desorption and Reusability

A suitable desorbing agent was needed for the quantitative recovery of the adsorbed $Cr^{3+}$ ions onto MSNPs–CAAQ. For this purpose, several desorbing agents with different concentrations, including HCl, $HNO_3$, and $Na_2EDTA$, were examined and are shown in Figure 16a–c, respectively. As observed in Figure 16a,b, the use of HCl and $HNO_3$ with concentrations of less than 0.10 mol/L did not quantitatively recover the retained $Cr^{3+}$ ion. The higher concentration of HCl and $HNO_3$ (0.20 mol/L) was effective, and HCl with a concentration of 0.20 mol/L was more effective than the same concentration, as well as $HNO_3$; the desorption for $Cr^{3+}$ ions could reach 95.6% for the first cycle. When using $Na_2EDTA$ as a desorbing agent in Figure 16c, the higher concentration above 0.10 mol/L was more effective than the low concentration of 0.05 mol/L, and the desorption for $Cr^{3+}$ ions could reach 97.5%. Therefore, based on the experimental results and economic considerations, 0.2 mol/L HCl, 0.2 mol/L $HNO_3$, and 0.1 mol/L $Na_2EDTA$ were selected as the desorbing agents to desorpt HMIs on the surface of MSNPs–CAAQ.

The adsorption–desorption experiments were conducted using HCl, $HNO_3$, and $Na_2EDTA$ as the desorbing agents for six successive cycles at room temperature, and the regenerated MSNPs–CAAQ was reused in the next cycle of adsorption experiments. Figure 17a–c shows the regeneration plot of MSNPs–CAAQ for the re-adsorption of $Cr^{3+}$ ions using HCl (0.2 mol/L), $HNO_3$ (0.2 mol/L), and $Na_2EDTA$ (0.1 mol/L) as desorbing agents, respectively. When using 0.2 mol/L HCl and 0.2 mol/L $HNO_3$ as desorbing agents, as shown in Figure 17a,b, the adsorption efficiencies of $Cr^{3+}$ ions on regenerated MSNPs–CAAQ were 91.6% and 83.3% in the first cycle and reduced to 50.3% and 38.9% after six consecutive regeneration cycles. These results indicated that neither HCl nor $HNO_3$ were suitable desorbing agents for HMIs–loaded MSNPs–CAAQ, which could be due to the deformation effects on the MSNPs–CAAQ sorbent surface during desorption and the mass loss caused by demagnetization. When 0.1 mol/L $Na_2EDTA$ was used as an adsorbing agent, as shown in Figure 17c, the adsorption efficiency of the first regenerated MSNPs–CAAQ for $Cr^{3+}$ ions reached 94.5%. Moreover, there was a certain degree of decline, but the removal efficiency for $Cr^{3+}$ ions was maintained at 88.8% after six cycles, implying that the as–synthesized MSNPs–CAAQ nano–sorbent has a great economic value.

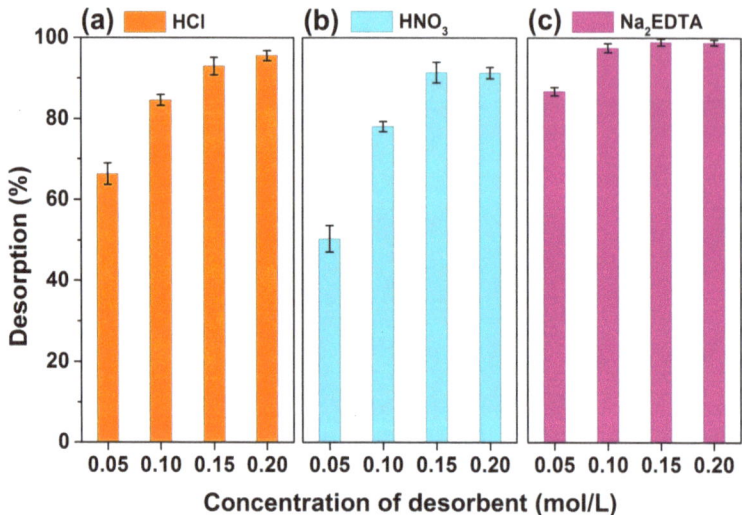

**Figure 16.** Effect of some desorbing afents (**a**) HCl, (**b**) $HNO_3$, and (**c**) $Na_2EDTA$ with different concentrations (0.05~0.20 mol/L) on the desorption of $Cr^{3+}$ ions from the MSNPs–CAAQ surface.

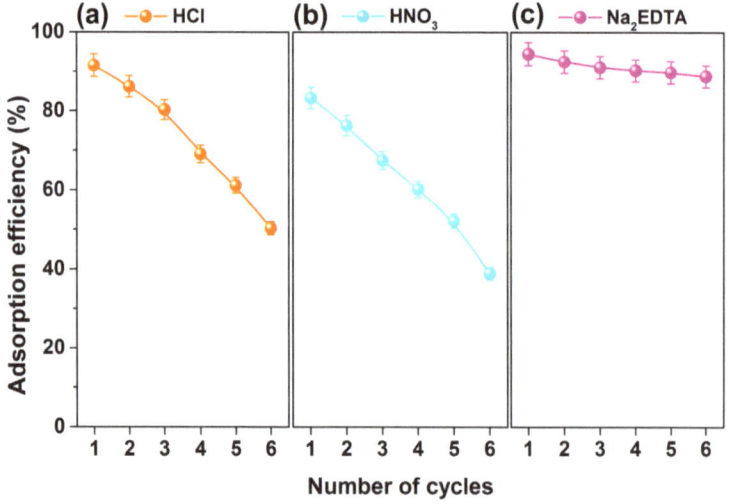

**Figure 17.** Effect of adsorbent regeneration times on the adsorption efficiencies using (**a**) 0.2 mol/L HCl, (**b**) 0.2 mol/L $HNO_3$, and (**c**) 0.1 mol/L $Na_2EDTA$ as desorbing agents. (Initial adsorbent was 1.0 g/L; $Cr^{3+}$ concentration was 200 mg/L; $V$ = 50 mL; desorption time was 12 h; re–adsorption time was 1.5 h; 298.15 K).

## 3. Experimental Procedure

### 3.1. Starting Materials

$FeCl_2·4H_2O$ (AR), $FeCl_3·6H_2O$ (AR), tetraethyl orthosilicate (TEOS, >99.0%), 3–chloro propyltrichlorosilane (CPTCS, >97.0%), triethylamine (99%), and EDTA disodium salt dihydrate ($Na_2EDTA$, 99.999%) were obtained from Shanghai Macklin Biochemical Co., Ltd.

(Shanghai, China). Methyltrichlorosilane (MTCS, >98.0%) and branched polyethylenimine (PEI, Mw ~25,000) were obtained from Tokyo (Shanghai, China) Chemical Industry Co., Ltd. (Shanghai, China) and Sigma–Aldrich (Shanghai, China) Trading Co., Ltd. (Shanghai, China), respectively. Ethanol, hexane, dichloromethane, acetonitrile, $NH_3 \cdot H_2O$ (25~28 wt.%), and 8–aminoquinoline (98%) were purchased from Chengdu Kelong Chemical Co., Ltd. (Chengdu, China) and Shanghai Civi Chemical Technology Co., Ltd. (Shanghai, China), respectively. Chloroacetyl chloride (98%) was purchased from Shanghai Xianding Biological Science and Technology Co., Ltd. (Shanghai, China).

*3.2. Synthesis*

3.2.1. Synthesis of Core–Shell MSNPs

Firstly, MNPs with hydroxyl groups (–OH) were synthesized based on a simple chemical co–precipitation method. $FeCl_2 \cdot 4H_2O$ (10 mmol) and $FeCl_3 \cdot 6H_2O$ (20 mmol) were dissolved into 120 mL of distilled water under an $N_2$ atmosphere with mechanical stirring, to which 60 mL of $NH_3 \cdot H_2O$ was added; then, the mixture was heated to 70 °C and left for 30 min. After that, the precipitate was washed with distilled water and dispersed into a solution of sodium citrate dihydrate (150 mL, 20 mmol/L) with mechanical stirring under an $N_2$ atmosphere for 12 h at room temperature. Subsequently, the citrate–modified MNPs were washed with distilled water and ethanol.

Following that, the core–shell MSNPs were synthesized via hydrolysis and the condensation of TEOS onto the MNPs' surface, as shown in Figure 18. A total of ~0.56 g citrate–modified MNPs and 5.0 mL $NH_3 \cdot H_2O$ were added to 120 mL ethanol under an $N_2$ atmosphere with mechanical stirring; then, 4.0 mL TEOS was added, and the mixture was left for 8 h at room temperature. After this reaction, the as–synthesized MSNPs were washed with ethanol.

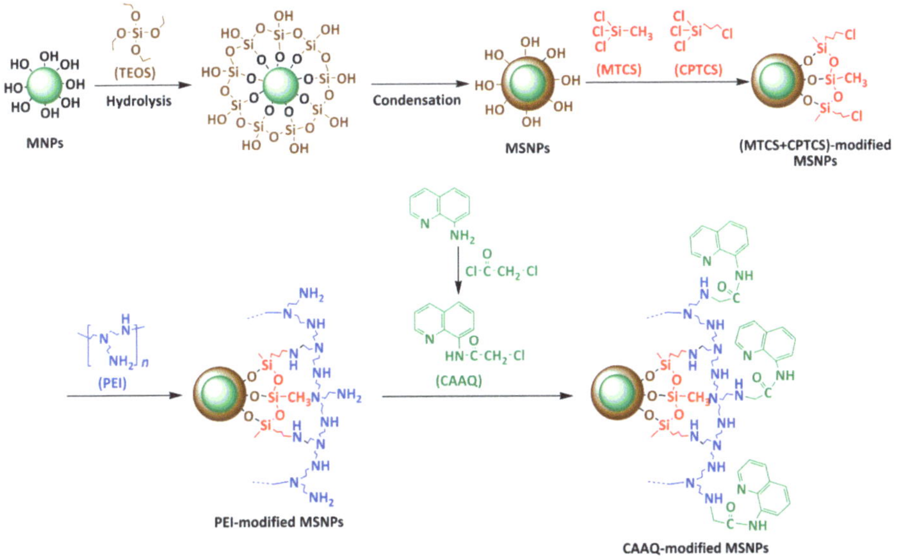

**Figure 18.** Schematic diagram illustrating the processes of the synthesis of MSNPs and surface modification with CAAQ onto MSNPs via a combined "grafting–from" and "grafting–to" approach; 3.3. synthesis of MSNPs–CAAQ using a three–step grafting strategy.

The core–shell MSNPs were modified with CAAQ to fabricate the network polymer coating through a three–step grafting strategy involving MTCS/CPTCS's co–modification, PEI–grafting, and CAAQ–grafting. As shown in Figure 18, the as–synthesized MSNPs were first modified with MTCS and CPTCS to yield chlorine groups, which provided the preconditions for subsequent surface modifications. Following that, the branched PEI was grafted onto chlorine–modified MSNPs to equip them with amino–active functional groups. Finally, the pre–synthesized CAAQ was immobilized onto MSNPs–PEI through the coupling reactions between the amines and chlorine groups.

3.2.2. Synthesis of MTCS and CPTCS co–Modified MSNPs

MSNPs (~0.5 g), MTCS (17.6 mmol), and CPTCS (1.4 mmol) were added to 150 mL of hexane, and the mixture was left for 24 h at room temperature in a hydrochloric acid atmosphere. After that, the as–synthesized MTCS and CPTCS co–modified MSNPs (labeled as MSNPs–MTCS/CPTCS) were washed with hexane, ethanol, and distilled water.

3.2.3. Synthesis of PEI–Modified MSNPs

The MSNPs–MTCS/CPTCS, PEI (1.0 mL), and methanol (5.0 mL) mentioned above were added to 120 mL of distilled water with mechanical stirring under an $N_2$ atmosphere, and the mixture was left for 48 h at 65 °C. After that, the as–synthesized PEI–modified MSNPs (labeled as MSNPs–PEI) were washed with distilled water.

3.2.4. Pre–Synthesis of CAAQ and Synthesis of CAAQ–Modified MSNPs by "Grafting–to" Approach

CAAQ can be pre–synthesized by a simple organic reaction. Briefly, 16.4 mmol 8–aminoquinoline and 2.5 mL triethylamine were mixed in 100 mL dichloromethane in an ice bath with magnetic stirring for 30 min in darkness. Then, 14.9 mmol of chloroacetyl chloride was added, and the mixture was left for 48 h at room temperature. After reaction, the crude products (8–chloroacetyl–aminoquinoline (CAAQ)) were collected by evaporating the solvent and purified by silica column chromatography ($V_{\text{Petroleum ether}}/V_{\text{Ethylacetate}} = 3/1$).

Finally, the pre–synthesized CAAQ was securely immobilized onto MSNPs–PEI through a series of coupling reactions between the amines (–$NH_2$) and chlorine (–Cl) groups. The PEI–modified MSNPs discussed above and 5.4 mmol CAAQ were added to 110 mL acetonitrile with mechanical stirring, and the mixture was refluxed at 60 °C for 24 h under $N_2$ atmosphere. After further aging for 24 h, the CAAQ–modified MSNPs (labeled as MSNPs–CAAQ) were collected and washed with acetonitrile and ethanol.

3.3. Characterization

The crystallographic phases of samples were characterized by X–ray diffraction (XRD, DX–2700, Dandong, China). The morphology and size of samples were examined by transmission electron microscopy (TEM, JEM–2100, Tokyo, Japan). Fourier transform infrared spectra (FTIR) of samples were recorded on a Nicolet iS10 spectrometer (Thermo Scientific, Waltham, MA, USA). X–ray photoelectron spectroscopy (XPS) analyses of samples were performed using an ESCALAB 250Xi spectrometer (Thermo Scientific, Waltham, MA, USA). Thermogravimetric (TG) curves of samples were collected by an SDT–2960 thermogravimetric instrument (TA Instruments, New Castle, DE, USA) at a heating rate of 10 °C/min under a flow of air. The quantitative analyses of HMIs in the adsorption and desorption experiments were performed using atomic absorption spectrometry (AAS, AA–6800, Shimadzu, Japan) and inductively coupled plasma mass spectrometry (ICP–MS, VG PQ ExCell, Thermo Electron Co., Vallejo, CA, USA). The magnetic properties of samples were obtained using a vibrating sample magnetometer (VSM, Lakeshore 7307, Novi, MI, USA) at room temperature.

3.4. Adsorption Experiments

The adsorption characteristics of MSNPs–CAAQ nanocomposites were evaluated by removing HMIs from simulated wastewaters; the selected HMIs included $Ag^+$, $Zn^{2+}$, $Cu^{2+}$, $Co^{2+}$, $Cd^{2+}$, $Mn^{2+}$, $Pb^{2+}$, $Hg^{2+}$, $Cr^{3+}$ and $Fe^{3+}$ ions. A total of 0.05 g MSNPs–CAAQ was dispersed into the set HMIs aqueous solution (50 mL, 50~500 mg/L). The mixture was stirred at a constant speed of 200 rpm at a set temperature of 298.15~338.15 K. After the adsorption reaction occurred within a given time ($t$, $t$ = 0~2.5 h), the particles were collected by magnetic separation, and the concentrations of these HMIs in the supernatant were measured using ICP–MS. The adsorption efficiency at time $t$ ($A_t$, %) and equilibrium adsorption amount ($q_m$, mg/g) of HMIs were calculated using Equation (1) and Equation (2), respectively.

$$A_t = \frac{C_0 - C_t}{C_0} \times 100\% \tag{1}$$

$$q_e = \frac{(C_0 - C_e)V}{m} \tag{2}$$

where $C_0$ (mg/L) is the initial concentration of HMIs' aqueous solution, $C_t$ (mg/L) is the concentration of HMIs at the given time $t$, $m$ (g) is the mass of MSNPs–CAAQ, and $V$ (L) is the volume of the HMIs aqueous solution.

To investigate the adsorption mechanism between MSNPs–CAAQ and HMIs, the experimental data were analyzed by the Langmuir isotherm model and the Freundlich isotherm model using Equation (3) [58] and Equation (4) [59], respectively:

$$\frac{C_e}{q_e} = \frac{1}{q_m} C_e + \frac{1}{K_L q_m} \tag{3}$$

$$\log q_e = \frac{1}{n} \log C_e + \log K_F \tag{4}$$

where $C_e$ (mg/L), $q_e$ (mg/g), and $q_m$ (mg/g) are the equilibrium concentration, equilibrium quantity, and saturated adsorption amounts, respectively. $K_L$ and $K_F$ are the Langmuir adsorption constants related to the affinity of the binding site and the Freundlich adsorption constants related to the adsorption capacity, respectively, and $n$ is the adsorption intensity. Moreover, $q_m$ and $K_L$ can be evaluated by the plot of $C_e/q_e$ against $C_e$, while $n$ and $K_F$ can be evaluated by the plot of $\log(q_e)$ against $\log(C_e)$.

To explore the thermodynamic characteristics of the adsorption process, the enthalpy change ($\Delta H^0$, KJ/mol) and entropy change ($\Delta S^0$, J/mol·K) were calculated using the Van't Hoff plot using Equation (5) [60]. To investigate the kinetic characteristics of the adsorption reaction, the experimental data of adsorption were evaluated by the pseudo–first–order and pseudo–second–order models using Equations (6) and (7) [61], respectively.

$$\log \frac{q_e}{C_e} = -\frac{\Delta H^0}{2.303R} \times \frac{1}{T} + \frac{\Delta S^0}{2.303R} \tag{5}$$

where $T$ (K) is the temperature of the adsorption reaction; $R$ (J/mol·K) is the gas constant per molecule.

$$\log(q_{e1,cal} - q_t) = -\frac{k_1}{2.303} t + \log q_{e1,cal} \tag{6}$$

where $q_{e1,\,cal}$ (mg/L), and $k_1$ (1/h) are the calculated equilibrium adsorption amount and the rate constant of the pseudo–first–order equation, respectively, which can be evaluated by the plot of $\log(q_{e1,cal} - q_t)$ against $t$:

$$\frac{t}{q_t} = \frac{1}{q_{e2,cal}} t + \frac{1}{k_2 q_{e2,cal}^2} \tag{7}$$

where $q_{e2,cal}$ (mg/L), and $k_2$ (g/mg·h) are the calculated equilibrium adsorption amount and the rate constant of the pseudo–second–order equation, respectively, which can be evaluated by the plot of $t/q_t$ against $t$.

*3.5. Desorption and Reusability Experiments*

In order to regenerate MSNPs–CAAQ nanocomposites, an elution step using a suitable desorbing agent (HCl, $HNO_3$, or $Na_2EDTA$) was carried out after each adsorption cycle. After the adsorption of the saturated HMIs, the HMIs–loaded MSNPs–CAAQ was exposed to HCl, $HNO_3$, or $Na_2EDTA$ solution with a desired concentration to allow for regeneration for 12 h under continuous mechanical stirring and was then magnetically separated from the water sample and washed several times with distilled water. The regenerated MSNPs–CAAQ were reused in the next cycle of adsorption experiments, and the adsorption–desorption experiments were conducted for six cycles at room temperature.

## 4. Conclusions

In summary, we presented a general strategy to synthesize network–polymer–modified magnetic nanomaterials. First, we designed and synthesized core–shell MSNPs with a ~10 nm core and ~5.5 nm shell through the hydrolysis and condensation of TEOS onto a single–crystal $Fe_3O_4$ seed. Following that, the core–shell MSNPs were modified with CAAQ to fabricate the network polymer coating through a three–step grafting strategy, in which polymer grafting was designed using a macromolecular polymer (PEI) to fabricate an organic network onto the MSNPs surface and to serve as a bridge between the surface hydroxyl group and CAAQ. The as–synthesized MSNPs–CAAQ nanocomposites showed a strong magnetic response under an external magnet, which made it easier to recycle quickly in practical applications. The adsorption experimental results indicated that MSNPs–CAAQ had an excellent absorption capacity for HMIs due to their abundant end–reactive functional groups: the saturated adsorption amounts of $Fe^{3+}$, $Cu^{2+}$ and $Cr^{3+}$ ions were 324.7, 306.8, and 293.3 mg/g, respectively, according to the Langmuir linear fitting. Moreover, MSNPs–CAAQ also exhibited universal adsorption capacities for $Zn^{2+}$, $Mn^{2+}$, and $Pb^{2+}$ ions, with adsorption efficiencies over 70%. The adsorption isotherm for the $Cr^{3+}$ ion fitted the experimental data well when using the Langmuir isotherm model, and its adsorption kinetics could be described by the pseudo–second–order equation. More importantly, $Na_2EDTA$ (0.10 mol/L) was more suitable as a desorbing agent for MSNPs–CAAQ regeneration than HCl (0.20 mol/L) and $HNO_3$ (0.20 mol/L). Additionally, the adsorption efficiency of the $Cr^{3+}$ ion on regenerated MSNPs–CAAQ could still be maintained at 88.8% after six adsorption–desorption cycles, showing the high economic value of the as–synthesized MSNPs–CAAQ nano–sorbent. Moreover, our design provides a general strategy for the fabrication of high–performance HMIs absorbents and can easily be extended to other absorption materials for actual applications.

**Author Contributions:** Conceptualization, Y.X. and Y.L.; validation, Y.L. and Z.D.; investigation, Y.X., Y.L. and Z.D.; resources, Y.X.; data curation, Z.D.; writing—original draft, Y.X.; writing—review and editing, Y.X. and Z.D.; supervision, Z.D.; project administration, Z.D.; funding acquisition, Y.X. and Z.D. All authors have read and agreed to the published version of the manuscript.

**Funding:** This study was financially supported by the Opening Project of Crystalline Silicon Photovoltaic New Energy Research Institute, China (2022 CHXK002), Leshan Normal University Research Program, China (KYPY2023–0001), and Fundamental Research Funds for the Central Universities, China (2023 CDJXY–019).

**Institutional Review Board Statement:** Not applicable.

**Informed Consent Statement:** Not applicable.

**Data Availability Statement:** Not applicable.

**Conflicts of Interest:** The authors declare no conflict of interest.

## References

1. Su, X.; Kushima, A.; Halliday, C.; Zhou, J.; Li, J.; Hatton, T.A. Electrochemically–mediated selective capture of heavy metal chromium and arsenic oxyanions from water. *Nat. Commun.* **2018**, *9*, 4701. [CrossRef] [PubMed]

2. Li, B.; Zhang, Y.; Ma, D.; Shi, Z.; Ma, S. Mercury nano–trap for effective, efficient removal of mercury(II) from aqueous solution. *Nat. Commun.* **2014**, *5*, 5537. [CrossRef]
3. Liu, C.; Wu, T.; Hsu, P.C.; Xie, J.; Zhao, J.; Liu, K.; Sun, J.; Xu, J.; Tang, J.; Ye, Z.; et al. Direct/alternating current electrochemical method for removing and recovering heavy metal from water using graphene oxide electrode. *ACS Nano* **2019**, *13*, 6431–6437. [CrossRef] [PubMed]
4. Wu, C.S.; Khaing Oo, M.K.; Fan, X. Highly sensitive multiplexed heavy metal detection using quantum–dot–labeled dnazymes. *ACS Nano* **2010**, *4*, 5897–5904. [CrossRef] [PubMed]
5. Ojeajiménez, I.; López, X.; Arbiol, J.; Puntes, V. Citrate–coated gold nanoparticles as smart scavengers for mercury(II) removal from polluted waters. *ACS Nano* **2012**, *6*, 2253–2260. [CrossRef]
6. Salt, D.E.; Blaylock, M.; Kumar, N.P.B.A.; Dushenkov, V.; Ensley, B.D.; Chet, I.; Raskin, I. Phytoremediation: A novel strategy for the removal of toxic metals from the environment using plants. *Nat. Biotechnol.* **1995**, *13*, 468–474. [CrossRef] [PubMed]
7. Kumar, R.; Patil, S.A. Removal of heavy metals using bioelectrochemical systems. In *Integrated Microbial Fuel Cells for Wastewater Treatment*; Butterworth–Heinemann: Oxford, UK, 2020; pp. 49–71. [CrossRef]
8. Kumar, R.; Yadav, S.; Patil, S.A. Bioanode–Assisted Removal of $Hg^{2+}$ at the Cathode of Microbial Fuel Cells. *J. Hazard. Toxic Radio.* **2020**, *24*, 04020034. [CrossRef]
9. Nazir, M.A.; Bashir, M.A.; Najam, T.; Javad, M.S.; Suleman, S.; Hussain, S.; Kumar, O.P.; Shah, S.S.A.; Rehman, A.U. Combining structurally ordered intermetallic nodes: Kinetic and isothermal studies for removal of malachite green and methyl orange with mechanistic aspects. *Microchem. J.* **2021**, *164*, 105973. [CrossRef]
10. Rauwel, P.; Rauwel, E. Towards the Extraction of Radioactive Cesium-137 from Water via Graphene/CNT and Nanostructured Prussian Blue Hybrid Nanocomposites: A Review. *Nanomaterials* **2019**, *9*, 682. [CrossRef]
11. Zhang, Y.; Niu, Q.; Gu, X.; Yang, N.; Zhao, G. Recent progress of carbon nanomaterials for electrochemical detection and removal of environmental pollutants. *Nanoscale* **2019**, *11*, 11992–12014. [CrossRef]
12. Kumar, R.; Rauwel, P.; Rauwel, E. Nanoadsorbants for the Removal of Heavy Metals from Contaminated Water: Current Scenario and Future Directions. *Processes* **2021**, *9*, 1379. [CrossRef]
13. Jha, V.K.; Nagae, M.; Matsuda, M.; Miyake, M. Zeolite formation from coal fly ash and heavy metal ion removal characteristics of thus–obtained Zeolite X in multi–metal systems. *J. Environ. Manag.* **2009**, *90*, 2507–2514. [CrossRef] [PubMed]
14. Efome, J.E.; Rana, D.; Matsuura, T.; Lan, C.Q. Metal–organic frameworks supported on nanofibers to remove heavy metals. *J. Mater. Chem. A* **2018**, *6*, 4550–4555. [CrossRef]
15. Yan, H.; Li, H.; Tao, X.; Li, K.; Yang, H.; Li, A.; Xiao, S.; Cheng, R. Rapid Removal and Separation of Iron(II) and Manganese(II) from Micropolluted Water Using Magnetic Graphene Oxide. *ACS Appl. Mater. Interfaces* **2014**, *6*, 9871–9880. [CrossRef]
16. Bolisetty, S.; Peydayesh, M.; Mezzenga, R. Sustainable technologies for water purification from heavy metals: Review and analysis. *Chem. Soc. Rev.* **2019**, *48*, 463–487. [CrossRef]
17. Zhao, W.; Chen, I.W.; Huang, F. Toward large–scale water treatment using nanomaterials. *Nano Today* **2019**, *27*, 11–27. [CrossRef]
18. Kumar, R.; Rauwel, P.; Kriipsalu, M.; Wragg, D.; Rauwel, E. Nanocobalt based ($Co@Co(OH)_2$) sand nanocomposite applied to manganese extraction from contaminated water. *J. Environ. Chem. Eng.* **2023**, *11*, 109818. [CrossRef]
19. Kulpa–Koterwa, A.; Ossowski, T.; Niedziałkowski, P. Functionalized $Fe_3O_4$ Nanoparticles as Glassy Carbon Electrode Modifiers for Heavy Metal Ions Detection—A Mini Review. *Materials* **2021**, *14*, 7725. [CrossRef]
20. Lisjak, D.; Mertelj, A. Anisotropic magnetic nanoparticles: A review of their properties, syntheses and potential applications. *Prog. Mater. Sci.* **2018**, *95*, 286–328. [CrossRef]
21. Han, X.; Deng, Z.; Yang, Z.; Wang, Y.; Zhu, H.; Chen, B.; Cui, Z.; Ewing, R.; Shi, D. Biomarkerless targeting and photothermal cancer cell killing by surface–electrically–charged superparamagnetic $Fe_3O_4$ composite nanoparticles. *Nanoscale* **2017**, *9*, 1457–1465. [CrossRef]
22. Young, K.L.; Xu, C.; Xie, J.; Sun, S. Conjugating methotrexate to magnetite ($Fe_3O_4$) nanoparticles via trichloro-s-triazine. *J. Mater. Chem.* **2009**, *19*, 6400–6406. [CrossRef]
23. Liu, S.; Guo, S.; Sun, S.; You, X.Z. Dumbbell–like Au–$Fe_3O_4$ nanoparticles: A new nanostructure for supercapacitors. *Nanoscale* **2015**, *7*, 4890–4893. [CrossRef]
24. Shi, X.; You, W.B.; Zhao, Y.; Li, X.; Shao, Z.; Che, R. Multi–scale magnetic coupling of $Fe@SiO_2@C$–Ni yolk@triple–shell microsphere for broadband microwave absorption. *Nanoscale* **2019**, *11*, 17270–17276. [CrossRef]
25. Ni, Q.; Chen, B.; Dong, S.; Tian, L.; Bai, Q. Preparation of core–shell structure $Fe_3O_4@SiO_2$ superparamagnetic microspheres immoblized with iminodiacetic acid as immobilized metal ion affinity adsorbents for His–tag protein purification. *Biomed. Chromatogr.* **2015**, *30*, 566–573. [CrossRef]
26. Jin, S.; Park, B.C.; Ham, W.S.; Pan, L.; Kim, Y.K. Effect of the magnetic core size of amino–functionalized $Fe_3O_4$ mesoporous $SiO_2$ core–shell nanoparticles on the removal of heavy metal ions. *Colloids Surf. A* **2017**, *531*, 133–140. [CrossRef]
27. Liu, Y.; Fu, R.; Sun, Y.; Zhou, X.; Baig, S.A.; Xu, X. Multifunctional nanocomposites $Fe_3O_4@SiO_2$–EDTA for Pb(II) and Cu(II) removal from aqueous solutions. *Appl. Surf. Sci.* **2016**, *369*, 267–276. [CrossRef]
28. Pogorilyi, R.; Pylypchuk, I.; Melnyk, I.; Zub, Y.; Seisenbaeva, G.; Kessler, V. Sol–gel derived adsorbents with enzymatic and complexonate functions for complex water remediation. *Nanomaterials* **2017**, *7*, 298. [CrossRef]
29. Zhang, S.; Zhang, Y.; Liu, J.; Xu, Q.; Xiao, H.; Wang, X.; Xu, H.; Zhou, J. Thiol modified $Fe_3O_4@SiO_2$ as a robust, high effective, and recycling magnetic sorbent for mercury removal. *Chem. Eng. J.* **2013**, *226*, 30–38. [CrossRef]

30. Chen, Y.; Xiong, Z.; Zhang, L.; Zhao, J.; Zhang, Q.; Peng, L.; Zhang, W.; Ye, M.; Zou, H. Facile synthesis of zwitterionic polymer–coated core–shell magnetic nanoparticles for highly specific capture of N–linked glycopeptides. *Nanoscale* **2015**, *7*, 3100–3108. [CrossRef]
31. Li, S.; Li, N.; Yang, S.; Liu, F.; Zhou, J. The synthesis of a novel magnetic demulsifier and its application for the demulsification of oil–charged industrial wastewaters. *J. Mater. Chem. A* **2014**, *2*, 94–99. [CrossRef]
32. Liu, G.; Cai, M.; Wang, X.; Zhou, F.; Liu, W. Core–shell–corona–structured polyelectrolyte brushes–grafting magnetic nanoparticles for water harvesting. *ACS Appl. Mater. Inter.* **2014**, *6*, 11625–11632. [CrossRef] [PubMed]
33. Khan, A.A.; Khan, I.A.; Siyal, M.I.; Lee, C.K.; Kim, J.O. Optimization of membrane modification using $SiO_2$ for robust anti–fouling performance with calcium–humic acid feed in membrane distillation. *Environ. Res.* **2019**, *170*, 374–382. [CrossRef] [PubMed]
34. Ruhi, G.; Bhandari, H.; Dhawan, S.K. Designing of corrosion resistant epoxy coatings embedded with polypyrrole/$SiO_2$ composite. *Prog. Org. Coat.* **2014**, *77*, 1484–1498. [CrossRef]
35. Chen, Z.; Wang, J.; Pu, Z.; Zhao, Y.; Jia, D.; Chen, H.; Wen, T.; Hu, B.; Alsaedi, A.; Hayat, T.; et al. Synthesis of magnetic $Fe_3O_4$/CFA composites for the efficient removal of U(VI) from wastewater. *Chem. Eng. J.* **2017**, *320*, 448–457. [CrossRef]
36. Duffy, E.; Mitev, D.P.; Thickett, S.C.; Townsend, A.T.; Paull, B.; Nesterenko, P.N. Assessing the extent, stability, purity and properties of silanised detonation nanodiamond. *Appl. Surf. Sci.* **2015**, *357*, 397–406. [CrossRef]
37. Zhang, S.; Kai, C.; Liu, B.; Zhang, S.; Wei, W.; Xu, X.; Zhou, Z. Facile fabrication of cellulose membrane containing polyiodides and its antibacterial properties. *Appl. Surf. Sci.* **2020**, *500*, 144046.1–144046.6. [CrossRef]
38. Karimi Shervedani, R.; Rezvaninia, Z.; Sabzyan, H. Oxinate–aluminum(III) nanostructure assemblies formed via in–situ and ex–situ oxination of gold–self–assembled monolayers characterized by electrochemical, attenuated total reflectance fourier transform infrared spectroscopy, and X–ray photoelectron spectroscopy methods. *Electrochim. Acta* **2015**, *180*, 722–736. [CrossRef]
39. Beard, B.C. Cellulose nitrate as a binding energy reference in N(1s) XPS studies of nitrogen–containing organic molecules. *Appl. Surf. Sci.* **1990**, *45*, 221–227. [CrossRef]
40. Liu, H.; Zhou, Y.; Yang, Y.; Zou, K.; Wu, R.; Xia, K.; Xie, S. Synthesis of polyethylenimine/graphene oxide for the adsorption of U(VI) from aqueous solution. *Appl. Surf. Sci.* **2019**, *471*, 88–95. [CrossRef]
41. El–Rahman, H.A.A.; Schultze, J.W. New quaternized aminoquinoline polymer films: Electropolymerization and characterization. *J. Electroanal. Chem.* **1996**, *416*, 67–74. [CrossRef]
42. Jackson, S. Determining hybridization differences for amorphous carbon from the XPS C 1s envelope. *Appl. Surf. Sci.* **1995**, *90*, 195–203. [CrossRef]
43. Choi, S.J.; Kim, S.J.; Kim, I.D. Ultrafast optical reduction of graphene oxide sheets on colorless polyimide film for wearable chemical sensors. *NPG Asia Mater.* **2016**, *8*, e315. [CrossRef]
44. Pan, N.; Li, L.; Ding, J.; Wang, R.; Jin, Y.; Xia, C. A schiff base/quaternary ammonium salt bifunctional graphene oxide as an efficient adsorbent for removal of Th(IV)/U(VI). *J. Colloid Interface Sci.* **2017**, *508*, 303–312. [CrossRef]
45. Kosa, S.A.; Al–Zhrani, G.; Abdel Salam, M. Removal of heavy metals from aqueous solutions by multi–walled carbon nanotubes modified with 8–hydroxyquinoline. *Chem. Eng. J.* **2012**, *181–182*, 159–168. [CrossRef]
46. Lv, Z.P.; Luan, Z.Z.; Cai, P.Y.; Wang, T.; Li, C.H.; Wu, D.; Zuo, J.L.; Sun, S. Enhancing magnetoresistance in tetrathiafulvalene carboxylate modified iron oxide nanoparticle assemblies. *Nanoscale* **2016**, *8*, 12128–12133. [CrossRef] [PubMed]
47. Maneechakr, P.; Karnjanakom, S. Environmental surface chemistries and adsorption behaviors of metal cations ($Fe^{3+}$, $Fe^{2+}$, $Ca^{2+}$ and $Zn^{2+}$) on manganese dioxide–modified green biochar. *RSC Adv.* **2019**, *9*, 24074–24086. [CrossRef] [PubMed]
48. Maneechakr, P.; Karnjanakom, S. The essential role of Fe(III) ion removal over efficient/low–cost activated carbon: Surface chemistry and adsorption behavior. *Res. Chem. Intermed.* **2019**, *45*, 4583–4605. [CrossRef]
49. Liu, P.; Borrell, P.F.; Božič, M.; Kokol, V.; Oksman, K.; Mathew, A.P. Nanocelluloses and their phosphorylated derivatives for selective adsorption of $Ag^+$, $Cu^{2+}$ and $Fe^{3+}$ from industrial effluents. *J. Hazard. Mater.* **2015**, *294*, 177–185. [CrossRef]
50. Behbahani, E.S.; Dashtian, K.; Ghaedi, M. $Fe_3O_4$–$FeMoS_4$: Promise magnetite LDH–based adsorbent for simultaneous removal of Pb (II), Cd (II), and Cu (II) heavy metal ions. *J. Hazard. Mater.* **2021**, *410*, 124560. [CrossRef]
51. Cao, J.; Wang, P.; Shen, J.; Sun, Q. Core–shell $Fe_3O_4$@zeolite NaA as an adsorbent for $Cu^{2+}$. *Materials* **2020**, *13*, 5047. [CrossRef]
52. Panja, S.; Hanson, S.; Wang, C. EDTA–inspired polydentate hydrogels with exceptionally high heavy metal adsorption capacity as reusable adsorbents for wastewater purification. *ACS Appl. Mater. Interfaces* **2020**, *12*, 25276–25285. [CrossRef] [PubMed]
53. Macedo, J.C.A.; Gontijo, E.S.J.; Herrera, S.G.; Rangel, E.C.; Komatsu, D.; Landers, R.; Rosa, A.H. Organosulphur–modified biochar: An effective green adsorbent for removing metal species in aquatic systems. *Surf. Interfaces* **2021**, *22*, 100822. [CrossRef]
54. Dias, D.; Bernardo, M.; Matos, I.; Fonseca, I.; Pinto, F.; Lapa, N. Activation of co–pyrolysis chars from rice wastes to improve the removal of $Cr^{3+}$ from simulated and real industrial wastewaters. *J. Clean. Prod.* **2020**, *267*, 121993. [CrossRef]
55. Deraeve, C.; Maraval, A.; Vendier, L.; Faugeroux, V.; Pitié, M.; Meunier, B. Preparation of new bis(8–aminoquinoline) ligands and comparison with bis(8–hydroxyquinoline) ligands on their ability to chelate $Cu^{II}$ and $Zn^{II}$. *Eur. J. Inorg. Chem.* **2008**, *2008*, 5622–5631. [CrossRef]
56. Huang, J.; Xu, Y.; Qian, X. Rhodamine–based fluorescent off–on sensor for $Fe^{3+}$–in aqueous solution and in living cells: 8–aminoquinoline receptor and 2:1 binding. *Dalton Trans.* **2014**, *43*, 5983–5989. [CrossRef] [PubMed]
57. Mirzaei, M.; Eshtiagh–Hosseini, H.; Bolouri, Z.; Rahmati, Z.; Esmaeilzadeh, A.; Hassanpoor, A.; Bauza, A.; Ballester, P.; Mague, J.T.; Notash, B.; et al. Rationalization of noncovalent interactions within six new MII/8–aminoquinoline supramolecular complexes (MII = Mn, Cu, and Cd): A combined experimental and theoretical DFT study. *Cryst. Growth Des.* **2015**, *15*, 1351–1361. [CrossRef]

58. Langmuir, I. The adsorption of gases on plane surfaces of glass, mica and platinum. *J. Am. Chem. Soc.* **1918**, *40*, 1361–1403. [CrossRef]
59. Freundlich, H. Uber die adsorption in lo sungen. *J. Phys. Chem.* **1907**, *57*, 385–470. [CrossRef]
60. Das, S.; Mishra, S. Insight into the isotherm modelling, kinetic and thermodynamic exploration of iron adsorption from aqueous media by activated carbon developed from *Limonia acidissima* shell. *Mater. Chem. Phys.* **2020**, *245*, 122751. [CrossRef]
61. Schiewer, S.; Patil, S.B. Pectin–rich fruit wastes as biosorbents for heavy metal removal: Equilibrium and kinetics. *Bioresour. Technol.* **2008**, *99*, 1896–1903. [CrossRef]

**Disclaimer/Publisher's Note:** The statements, opinions and data contained in all publications are solely those of the individual author(s) and contributor(s) and not of MDPI and/or the editor(s). MDPI and/or the editor(s) disclaim responsibility for any injury to people or property resulting from any ideas, methods, instructions or products referred to in the content.

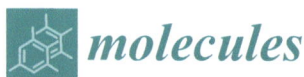
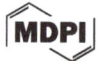

Article

# Probing the Effect of Alloying Elements on the Interfacial Segregation Behavior and Electronic Properties of Mg/Ti Interface via First-Principles Calculations

Yunxuan Zhou [1,2], Hao Lv [2], Tao Chen [1,*], Shijun Tong [1,2], Yulin Zhang [1], Bin Wang [1], Jun Tan [1,2,*], Xianhua Chen [1,2] and Fusheng Pan [1,2]

[1] Lanxi Magnesium Materials Research Institute, Lanxi 321100, China; yunxuanzhou93@gmail.com (Y.Z.); 18818276064@163.com (S.T.); zhangyulin@pku.edu.cn (Y.Z.); zjnuwangbin@163.com (B.W.); xhchen@cqu.edu.cn (X.C.); fspan@cqu.edu.cn (F.P.)
[2] National Engineering Research Center for Magnesium Alloys, College of Materials Science and Engineering, Chongqing University, Chongqing 400044, China; aicaodafu@sina.com
\* Correspondence: ct2017@cqu.edu.cn (T.C.); jun.tan@cqu.edu.cn (J.T.)

**Abstract:** The interface connects the reinforced phase and the matrix of materials, with its microstructure and interfacial configurations directly impacting the overall performance of composites. In this study, utilizing seven atomic layers of Mg(0001) and Ti(0001) surface slab models, four different Mg(0001)/Ti(0001) interfaces with varying atomic stacking configurations were constructed. The calculated interface adhesion energy and electronic bonding information of the Mg(0001)/Ti(0001) interface reveal that the HCP2 interface configuration exhibits the best stability. Moreover, Si, Ca, Sc, V, Cr, Mn, Fe, Cu, Zn, Y, Zr, Nb, Mo, Sn, La, Ce, Nd, and Gd elements are introduced into the Mg/Ti interface layer or interfacial sublayer of the HCP2 configurations, and their interfacial segregation behavior is investigated systematically. The results indicate that Gd atom doping in the Mg(0001)/Ti(0001) interface exhibits the smallest heat of segregation, with a value of −5.83 eV. However, Ca and La atom doping in the Mg(0001)/Ti(0001) interface show larger heat of segregation, with values of 0.84 and 0.63 eV, respectively. This implies that the Gd atom exhibits a higher propensity to segregate at the interface, whereas the Ca and La atoms are less inclined to segregate. Moreover, the electronic density is thoroughly analyzed to elucidate the interfacial segregation behavior. The research findings presented in this paper offer valuable guidance and insights for designing the composition of magnesium-based composites.

**Keywords:** Mg/Ti interface; elastic anisotropy; interface segregation; electronic properties; alloying elements

## 1. Introduction

Magnesium (Mg) alloys are referred to as the "green engineering materials of the 21st century" owing to their numerous outstanding properties, including superior specific strength, specific stiffness, excellent machinability, and environmental friendliness [1–5]. Consequently, they have garnered considerable attention and hold significant potential for applications in high-performance automotive, aerospace, hydrogen storage, and 3C industries [6–10]. However, in comparison to traditional materials such as aluminum alloys, Mg alloys feature a hexagonal close-packed (HCP) crystal structure with a limited number of slip systems, leading to a limited plastic deformation capability [11]; they also face challenges such as low modulus and poor formability. This limitation significantly impedes the industrial utilization of Mg alloys [12]. Developing and applying high-performance Mg alloys is crucial for bolstering and advancing the Mg alloy industry, as well as boosting manufacturing competitiveness.

Scholars in pertinent research have concentrated on enhancing the overall performance of Mg alloy materials through strategies like compositional design, alloying with

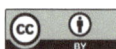

trace elements, and employing heat treatment processes [13]. The in situ formation or the incorporation of particles is also a potent method for boosting the strength and elastic modulus (stiffness) of Mg alloys [14,15]. This involves incorporating a second phase with high modulus, good toughness, high thermal stability, and excellent dynamic stability to improve the strength, modulus, and stability of Mg alloys. Whether it is externally added particles or in situ formed second phases, interfaces are formed between the enhancement phase and the Mg matrix, and the microstructure and interface bonding strength significantly affect the performance of Mg-based composite materials [16]. Ceramic particle reinforcements (like SiC, $Al_2O_3$, $B_4C$, TiC, $TiB_2$, etc.) are widely used in Mg-based composite materials [17–19]. Ding et al. [20] prepared CNTs@SiC/Mg-6Zn composites through chemical vapor deposition, semi-solid stirring combined with ultrasonic treatment, and hot extrusion deformation. Their finding revealed that while the yield strength of the composite rose from 154 MPa to 218 MPa, its room-temperature fracture elongation decreased from 15.6% to 6.1%. Although the addition of ceramic particles can enhance the corrosion resistance, strength, wear resistance, and modulus of Mg-based composite materials, it can also lead to a decrease in material fracture toughness (some composites have an elongation below 1%) due to their low plastic formability and poor thermal physical compatibility at the interface. Moreover, such an utterly incoherent interface easily generates stress concentration, leading to the initiation of microcracks. On the other hand, the ceramic reinforcement itself is a brittle phase, resulting in a low plasticity in Mg-based composites, making industrial application of such materials quite challenging. Therefore, finding reinforcements with high plastic deformation capability that closely match the Mg's crystallographic and physical characteristics is a potential method for enhancing the strength, plasticity, and modulus of Mg-based composites.

Numerous experimental results also demonstrate that titanium (Ti) can effectively enhance the strength and plasticity of Mg-based composite materials [21]. Perez et al. [22] prepared Mg-10(vol.%)Ti composite materials using powder metallurgy forming combined with hot extrusion deformation. The tensile strength at room temperature was measured to be 160 MPa, with an elongation of 8%. Furthermore, Wu et al. [23] developed Ti particle-reinforced Mg-based composite materials, where Ti particles form interfaces with the Mg alloy matrix featuring an elementally graded distribution structure. This composite material achieves a tensile strength of 327 MPa and an elongation of 20.4%. In addition, some researchers have utilized first-principles calculations to probe the interfacial properties between ceramic reinforcements (or second phases) and the Mg matrix (such as Mg/TiC, Mg/AlN, Mg/ZnO, $Mg/Al_2MgC_2$, $Mg/Mg_2Sn$, $Mg/Al_4C_3$, $Mg/TiB_2$, $Mg/ZrB_2$, $Mg/Ti_2AlC$, $Mg/Al_2MgC_2$, $Mg/Al_2CO$, etc.) [24–33]. Furthermore, the dynamic stability of some second phases was assessed through phonon spectrum analysis. The calculation results of elastic properties indicate these phases possess a high Young's modulus, suggesting their potential as reinforcing phases. Moreover, some researchers have studied the stability and elastic properties of binary (60.51 GPa for Young's modulus in $Mg_2Sn$ phase, 71–94 GPa for Young's modulus in $Mg_{17}Al_{12}$ phase) or ternary phases (72.15–98.27 GPa for Young's modulus in $Mg_{32}(Al,Zn)_{49}$ phase with different Al:Zn atomic ratio) in magnesium alloys or Mg-based composites [34–36]. There are also studies on Mg matrix composites reinforced with heterogeneous metals. For example, the adhesion strength and interfacial bonding of various Mg/X (X = Ti, Zr, Hf, V, Nd, Cr, Mo, Mn, and Fe) interface configurations were investigated by Bao et al. [37]. Relevant studies have shown that Ti, with its HCP structure matching that of Mg, can form a coherent Mg/Ti interface, thereby contributing to the enhancement of the Mg alloys' comprehensive performance. Additionally, Ti and Mg do not mix at equilibrium, indicating that there is no reaction between Ti and Mg elements, thereby inhibiting the formation of brittle intermetallic compounds at the Mg-Ti interface. This formable Ti forms a strong interface bond with Mg and exhibits fewer internal defects, thus better enhancing the material's properties. However, the segregation behavior of common alloying elements in Mg/Ti interfaces is still poorly understood. This work employs the first-principles calculations method to establish various interface configurations between the heterogeneous metal Ti and Mg matrix. Additionally, low-cost alloying elements and rare earth elements are introduced at the interface to investigate their segregation behavior. This research provides valuable insights into the development of heterogeneous metal-reinforced Mg-based composite materials.

## 2. Results and Discussion

### 2.1. Bulk and Surface Properties

The equilibrium crystal structures after geometric optimization of pure Mg and Ti are depicted in Figure 1a,b, and the green and gray spheres denote Mg and Ti atoms, respectively. The Mg has the HCP structure with a space group of P63/mmc, featuring only one standard Wyckoff site, namely 2c (0.67, 0.33, 0.75). The optimized lattice parameters of Mg are approximately a = b = 3.19 Å and c = 5.29 Å, which closely match experimental values (a = b = 3.210 Å and c = 5.211 Å; a = b = 3.209 Å, c = 5.171 Å) and other computational results (a = b = 3.159~3.228 Å and c = 5.073~5.186 Å) [31,38,39]. For titanium (Ti), generally, there are two allotropes of α-phase (with HCP structure) and the β-phase (with BCC structure), and the critical temperature of the phase transition is approximately 882.5 °C [40]. Considering the actual service of Mg alloys, the temperature is below 882.5 °C; therefore, α-Ti is chosen in this work. Moreover, α-Ti belongs to the P63/mmc space group, with theoretical lattice constants of a = b = 2.94 Å, c = 4.64 Å, α = β = 90°, and γ = 120° [41], where the Wyckoff position for Ti atoms is 2c(1/3, 2/3, 1/4). The calculated lattice parameters of this phase are a = b = 2.91 Å, c = 4.59 Å, α = β = 90°, and γ = 120°, respectively. It can be observed that the lattice constants obtained through GGA + PBE calculations exhibit a variation of approximately 1.03% compared to the theoretical values, showing the validity of the selected parameters. In addition, the calculated c/a ratio for α-Ti is approximately 1.57, while for Mg, it is 1.65, indicating that α-Ti has a better formability than Mg [42,43], which is advantageous for enhancing the formability of Mg alloys.

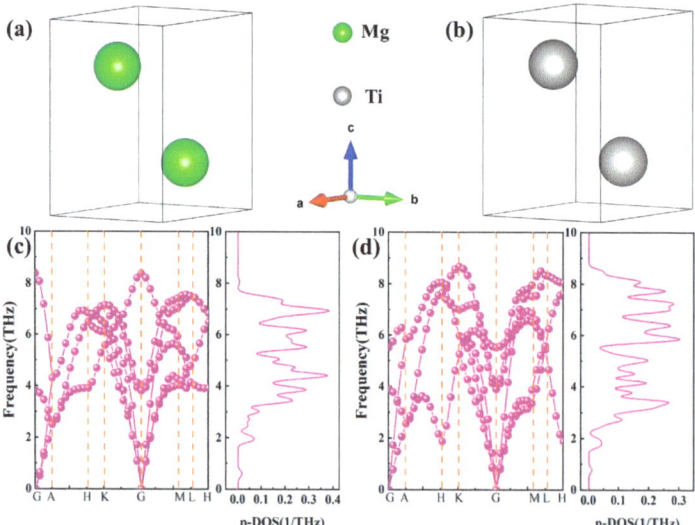

**Figure 1.** (**a,b**) The equilibrium crystal structures after geometric optimization of Mg and Ti, (**c,d**) Phonon spectra and phonon density of state of Mg and Ti, where green and gray spheres represent Mg and Ti atoms, respectively.

Phonon calculations of Mg and Ti offer a criterion for the stability of crystals. Specifically, in any high-symmetry dispersion, the absence of imaginary frequencies serves as an indicator that the crystal structure is dynamically stable. The calculated phonon spectra and phonon density of states for pure Mg and Ti with HCP structures are illustrated in

Figure 1c,d, with the phonon spectrum path being *G-A-H-K-G-M-L-H*. It can be observed from Figure 1 that the long-range coulomb interaction in the phonon spectrum results in higher frequencies for the longitudinal optical branches compared to the transverse optical branches. In other words, at the high-symmetry point *G*, the three phonon spectra with relatively lower frequencies correspond to acoustic phonon branches, while the spectra with relatively higher frequencies correspond to optical phonon branches. The phonon spectra, furthermore, do not contain imaginary frequencies at any high-symmetry point, showing that both Mg and Ti are dynamically stable. Additionally, the calculated phonon density of states, as presented in Figure 1c,d, reveals that the phonon spectra are primarily distributed within the frequency range of 2–8 THz. Moreover, the distribution of phonon spectra is similar, with only slight variations in trends around local high-symmetry points. For example, at the *K* high-symmetry point, the frequencies of Ti are notably higher than those of Mg. Noticeably, the vibrational spectrum of the phonon density of states for Mg atoms is higher than that for Ti atoms due to the lower mass of Mg atoms compared to Ti atoms, with both falling below 0.4 1/THz.

To investigate the mechanical properties of pure Mg and Ti, we employed the stress–strain method to predict the elastic stiffness matrix for each phase [44,45]. Subsequently, using the Voigt–Ruess–Hill approximation method [46], we derive the elastic constants ($C_{ij}$), elastic modulus, and hardness, as depicted in Figure 2a–c. It is important to note that the formulas for calculating elastic modulus, Poisson's ratio, and hardness can be found in Bao et al.'s work [47]. Noticeably, both the elastic constants and elastic modulus, as well as the hardness of Ti, are significantly greater than those of Mg, showing it has a strengthening effect in Mg alloys. The calculated Young's modulus of Ti is ~153.4 GPa, significantly higher than Mg's 43.9 GPa (close to the experimental value of ~45 GPa [48]), and higher than other binary or ternary phases (like $Al_2Gd$ (144.2 GPa), $Mg_2Gd_5$ (74.8 GPa), $Mg_{24}Y_5$ (66.6 GPa), MgZn (79.1 GPa), $Al_2Ca$ (94.34 GPa), $\beta'$-$Mg_7Tb$ (57.1 GPa), $Al_2Li_3$ (125.4 GPa), $Al_3CuCe$ (82.2 GPa), and $Mg_3(MnAl_9)_2$ (125.6 GPa) [49–53], indicating that Ti plays a positive role in enhancing the modulus of Mg alloys. The $C_{11}$ value for Ti is the highest, with approximately 205.9 GPa, suggesting that Ti exhibits better incompressibility than Mg (~55.4 GPa for $C_{11}$). This implies that it is more resistant to compression along the a-axis ($\varepsilon_{11}$ direction) under uniaxial stress. The smaller $C_{11}$ of Mg (approximately 19.9 GPa) indicates that Mg is more susceptible to shear deformation on the (100) crystal plane than Ti. Moreover, the predicted hardness values by Chen's and Tian's models are displayed in Figure 2c. Furthermore, the hardness of Ti predicted by both models is greater than that of Mg. According to Tian's model, the hardness values of Ti and Mg are 7.72 and 2.71 GPa, respectively, representing a difference of about three times. The Poisson's ratio, Cauchy pressure, and bulk modulus to shear modulus ($B/G$) ratio can all serve to assess the brittleness and toughness of materials. Generally, the critical values for brittleness and toughness of the Poisson ratio and $B/G$ ratio are 0.26 and 1.75, respectively. Observations from Figure 2d reveal that the $B/G$ and Poisson's ratios ($v$) of pure Ti are marginally higher than those of pure Mg, suggesting a slightly superior plasticity in Ti compared to Mg. Nonetheless, both Ti and Mg exhibit calculated values around 0.30, indicating similar metallic characteristics. Additionally, using the Cauchy pressure ($C_{12}$–$C_{44}$) to assess their ductility, it is evident that the Cauchy pressure of Ti is much greater than that of Mg, indicating that Ti has a better plastic deformation capability.

The anisotropy indices of Mg and Ti, obtained through DFT calculations, are depicted in Figure 3, and the specific elastic anisotropy calculation formulas can be described in the works of Ranganathan et al. [54]. The calculated anisotropy indices $A^U$, $A_B$, and $A_G$, and the shear anisotropy indices ($A_1$, $A_2$, and $A_3$) are depicted in Figure 3a,b. Analysis from Figure 3a,b reveal that Mg exhibits greater anisotropy than Ti, with $A^U$ values of 0.34 and 0.15 for Mg and Ti, respectively. The anisotropy of Mg is approximately twice that of Ti. The shear anisotropy factor values for Mg, $A_1$, $A_2$, and $A_3$ are 1.01, 1.01, and 1.61, respectively, which are greater than Ti's shear anisotropy indices ($A_1 = A_2 = 0.72$ and $A_3 = 0.71$), indicating Mg exhibits a more noticeable shear anisotropy. The three-dimensional (3D) surface plots of Young's modulus anisotropy for Mg and Ti, moreover, are represented in Figure 3c,d. It can be observed from the figures that the 3D plots of Young's modulus of Mg and Ti deviate from sphericity, indicating their anisotropic. Noticeably, 3D plots of Young's modulus for Mg exhibit more deviation from sphericity compared to Ti, suggesting that the anisotropy of Young's modulus for Mg is stronger than that of Ti, which aligns with the results of our calculated anisotropy index of $A^U$. In addition, Figure 3e,f illustrate the two-dimensional (2D) projections of Young's modulus anisotropy for Mg and Ti. Overall, the 2D of Ti's Young's modulus exhibits smaller differences in different directions compared to Mg's projection. This indicates that Ti has a lower anisotropy. The anisotropic Young's modulus results mentioned above play a critical role in designing the texture of Mg alloys. They have important implications for the design of laminated composite panels or Mg-based composite materials reinforced with heterogeneous metals.

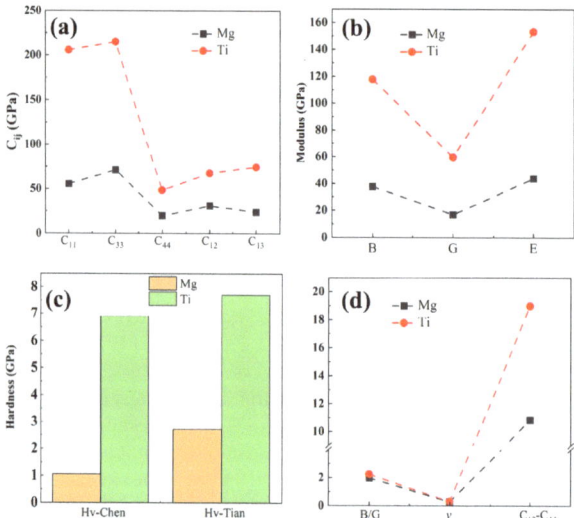

**Figure 2.** The mechanical properties of Mg and Ti calculated using first-principles calculations are (**a**) elastic constants, (**b**) elastic modulus, including bulk modulus ($B$), shear modulus ($G$), and Young's modulus ($E$), (**c**) predicted hardness by the Chen's and Tian's models, and (**d**) brittleness and toughness.

Before performing interface calculations, it is necessary to relax and compute the Mg and Ti surfaces. Generally, the greater the number of atoms in the surface model, signifying more layers of atoms, the closer the properties exhibited by the surface will be to those of the bulk material. Additionally, when constructing the model, it is essential to consider the computational capability of the server and ensure that both surfaces approximate the properties of the bulk material. Considering the space group symmetry and lattice matching of Mg and Ti, the (0001) surfaces of Mg and Ti are cleaved based on bulk phases, and a 2 × 2 supercell is created. Previous literature suggests that a slab model consisting of seven atomic layers of Mg is adequate to portray bulk-like properties. Similarly, a 2 × 2 supercell model with seven atomic layers of Ti is also deemed sufficient to capture bulk-like properties [55]. The Mg(0001) and Ti(0001) surface configurations with top and side views are displayed in Figure 4. Noticeably, the Mg(0001) and Ti(0001) surface slab models consist of 28 Mg atoms and 28 Ti atoms, with each layer containing either 4 Mg atoms or 4 Ti atoms. The relaxed lattice constants for the Mg(0001) slab model are as follows: a = b = 6.45 Å, c = 30.45 Å; α = β = 90°, γ = 120°. Similarly, for the Ti(0001) slab model, the relaxed lattice constants are: a = b = 5.92 Å, c = 28.74 Å; α = β = 90°, γ = 120°. Notably, both structures demonstrate matching in lattice parameters and angles, facilitating the establishment of interface models.

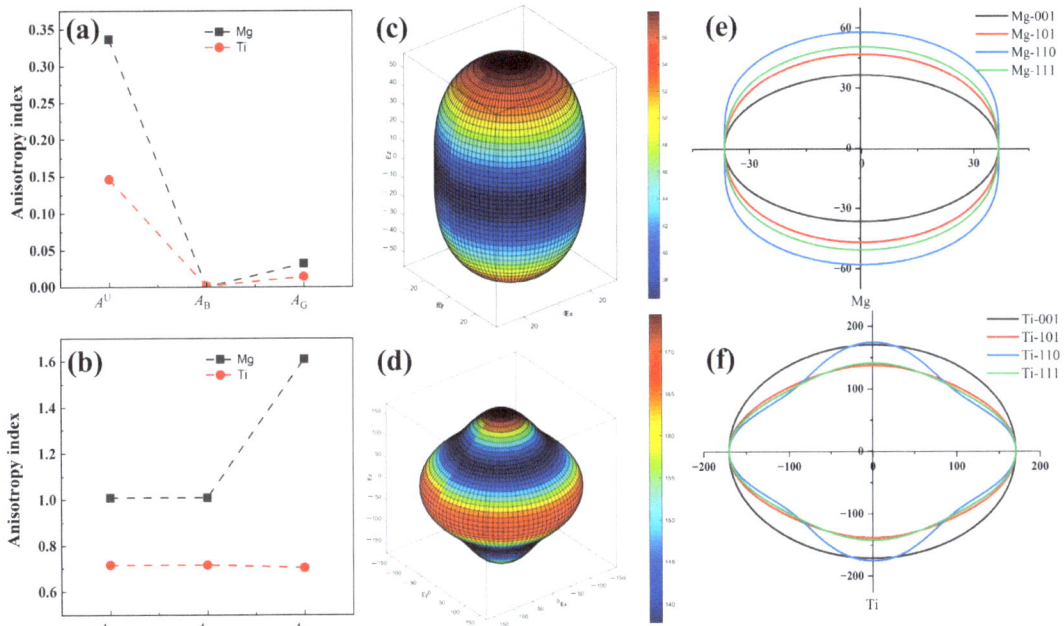

**Figure 3.** The anisotropy of Mg and Ti crystal structures is (**a**) $A^U$, $A_B$, $A_G$, (**b**) $A_1$, $A_2$, and $A_3$, three-dimensional (3D) surface plots and two-dimensional (2D) projections with different planes of Young's modulus for Mg (**c**,**e**) and Ti (**d**,**f**) crystal structures, and the unit for Young's modulus in (**c**–**f**) is GPa.

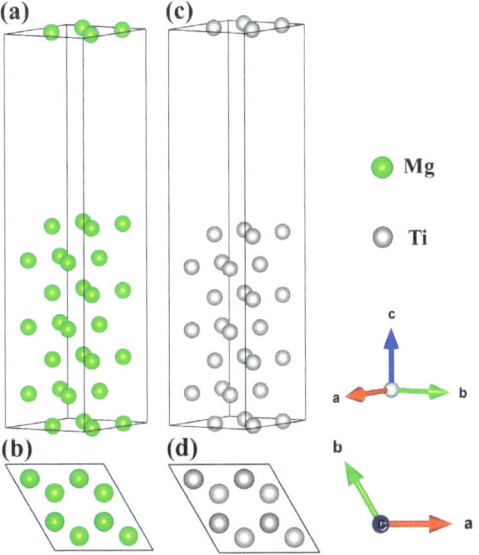

**Figure 4.** The surface configurations of Mg and Ti. Top and side views of the Mg(0001) (**a**,**b**) and Ti(0001) (**c**,**d**) surfaces.

## 2.2. Properties of the Mg/Ti Interface

### 2.2.1. Interfacial Configuration

Establishing the interface model requires consideration of the phase matching at the interface, and the mismatch of lattice parameters and angles must be calculated [56–58]. Furthermore, Ti with an HCP crystal structure possesses a higher Young's modulus of approximately 153.4 GPa and a lower anisotropy, which can serve as a reinforcement material. Based on the dynamic stability of the bulk material, we optimize the lattice constants of the bulk Mg and Ti and establish the interface structure based on the lattice constants of the bulk material. Exactly, the lower the mismatch at the interface is, the better the interface matching is [59]. Through a comparison of the lattice constants, surface, and interface areas of Mg and Ti, it was found that the interfacial mismatch was less than 5%, showing good interface matching [60,61]. There are four different configurations in the Mg/Ti interface, namely, OT, MT, HCP1, and HCP2, as shown in Figure 5. Specifically, the OT configuration indicates that Mg atoms at the interface are directly positioned on top of the first layer of Ti(0001) atoms. The MT configuration depicts Mg atoms at the interface located above the midpoint of the atomic connections in the first layer of Ti(0001) atoms. The HCP1 configuration shows Mg atoms at the interface situated in the polyhedral vacancies of the first layer of Ti(0001) atoms. Lastly, the HCP2 configuration illustrates Ti atoms at the interface occupying the polyhedral vacancies of the first layer of Mg(0001) atoms. The interface configurations of Mg(0001)/Ti(0001) with different atomic stacking sequences are illustrated in Figure 5. Here, (a, c, e, g) represent the main views of the interface stacking models. In contrast, (b, d, f, g) depict the top views of the interface stacking models. Additionally, the red dashed line represents the interface between Mg and Ti, where the area above the red line indicates the Ti(0001) surface, and the area below the red line represents the Mg(0001) surface.

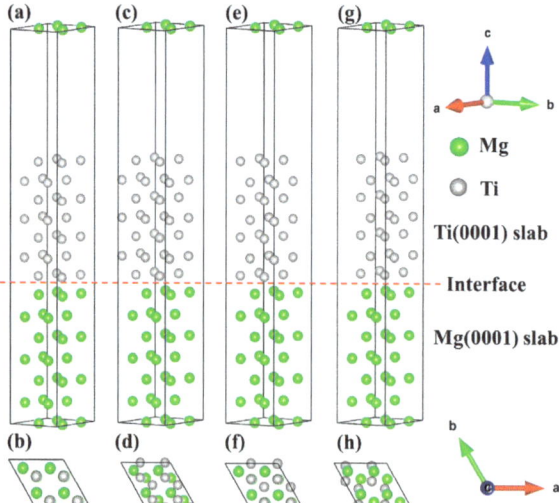

**Figure 5.** The interfacial configurations of the Mg(0001)/Ti(0001) interface with different atomic stacking sequences, (**a,b**) OT configuration, (**c,d**) MT configuration, (**e,f**) HCP1 configuration, and (**g,h**) HCP2 configuration.

The interface adhesion energy ($W_{ad}$) is the reversible work per unit area required to separate the Mg(0001)/Ti(0001) interface between condensed phases Mg(0001) and Ti(0001) to generate two free surfaces, which denotes [62,63]:

$$W_{ad} = (E_{Mg}^{slab} + E_{Ti}^{slab} - E_{Mg/Ti}^{interface})/A_i \quad (1)$$

where the $E_{Mg}^{slab}$ and $E_{Ti}^{slab}$ are total energies of a seven-layer Mg(0001) and seven-layer Ti(0001) free surface, $E_{Mg/Ti}^{interface}$ is the total energy of interface, and $A_i$ represents the interface area of Mg(0001)/Ti(0001) interface. In general, the interfacial distance significantly influences the interface performance. Hence, it is essential to conduct tests to evaluate the interfacial distance [24,64]. On the other hand, the purpose of testing the interface distance is to understand the approximate bonding length, which can be expressed by the following formula:

$$W_{ad}(d) = -W_{ad}\left[1 + \frac{(d-d_0)}{l}\right]\exp\left[-\frac{(d-d_0)}{l}\right] \quad (2)$$

where $W_{ad}$ is the ideal interface adhesion energy of the Mg(0001)/Ti(0001) interface. $d_0$ and $d$ represent the equilibrium interface separate value and the interfacial separation distance between the Mg(0001) and Ti(0001) slabs, and $l$ is a Thomas–Fermi screening length. The interface total energy and the ideal interface adhesion energy ($W_{ad}$) for various stacking models of Mg(0001)/Ti(0001) fluctuate with the separation distance of the Mg/Ti interface, as described in Figure 6. It is clear that the total interfacial energy of various atomic interface configurations of Mg(0001) and Ti(0001) decreases as the interface distance increases. Beyond a separation distance of 2.5 Å, the interfacial total energy tends to level off. Due to the energies of Mg(0001) and Ti(0001) surfaces, the area $A_i$ remains constant, with only the total energy of the Mg/Ti interface with different atomic configurations varying. As a result, Figure 6a,b exhibit similar shapes of the curves. Moreover, the OT model's interfacial total energy variation is relatively larger than the other configurations. The $W_{ad}$ exhibits an opposite trend as the interface distance increases. Initially, $W_{ad}$ increases with the interface distance and then stabilizes within the 1.5 to 4.5 Å separation distance between the two rigid free surfaces. Therefore, the interface distance can be around 2.5 Å, according to the analysis of Figure 6. Additionally, based on the predicted interface distance, the lattice parameters a, b, and the three angles of the interface were fixed while atoms were relaxed. The interfacial properties and the effect of alloying elements on the interface were then calculated.

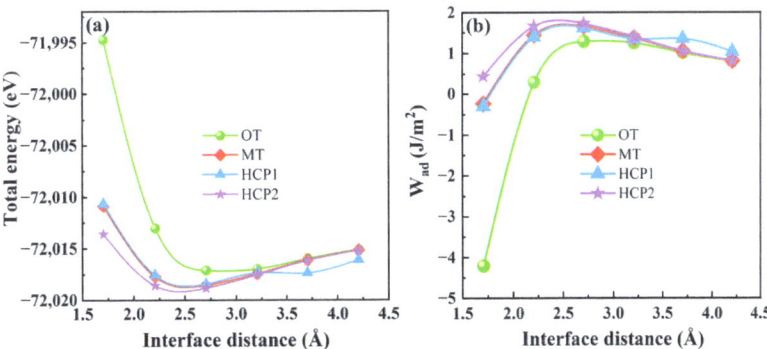

**Figure 6.** The interfacial total energy (**a**) and the ideal interface adhesion energy (**b**) of Mg(0001)/Ti(0001) interface with different atomic stacking sequences.

2.2.2. Interfacial Segregation Behavior and Interfacial Adhesion Work

To investigate the influence of different alloying elements on interface properties and consider the solubility of trace alloying elements, we further expanded the aforementioned models using a 2 × 1 supercell method, achieving an approximate alloy concentration of 1%. Here, the most stable Mg(0001)/Ti(0001) interface with HCP2 configuration is chosen to investigate the influence of different alloying elements on its interfacial segregation behavior and stability. In the doped model, the total number of atoms is 112, including 56 Mg atoms, 55 Ti atoms, and one alloying element TM commonly found in Mg alloys

(TM = Si, Ca, Sc, V, Cr, Mn, Fe, Cu, Zn, Y, Zr, Nb, Mo, Sn, La, Ce, Nd, and Gd), as shown in Figure 7, in which the green and gray spheres represent Mg and Ti atoms, respectively, and the red sphere represents the alloying atom TM. Based on the Wyckoff positions of Ti and Mg atoms in the bulk phase, it can be inferred that Ti or Mg atoms in the Mg(0001)/Ti(0001) interface models are equivalent. In the pure Mg(0001)/Ti(0001) interface model, one Ti atom is substituted by an alloying element TM, creating a doped model. Since the alloy concentration is approximately 1%, corresponding to a dilute model, its influence on lattice constants is negligible. Consequently, the interface distance is also approximately 2.5 Å.

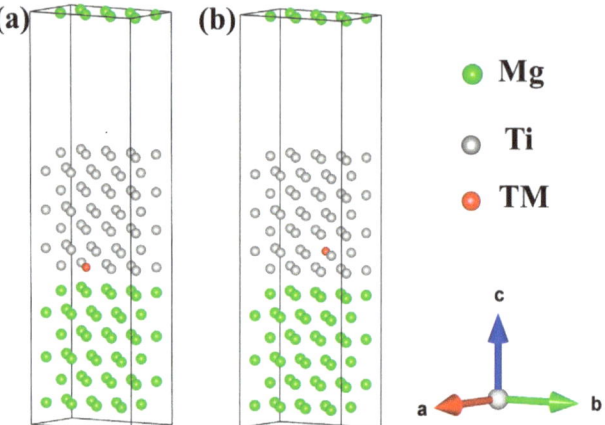

**Figure 7.** The interfacial configuration of alloy element doping at the Mg/Ti interface, (**a**) doping at the interface Ti layer, and (**b**) doping at the interface Ti sub-surface layer.

The heat of segregation is an important indicator for characterizing the preference of alloying atom positions. It can also characterize the difficulty of segregation of atoms at a specific position in the interface models. The heat of segregation ($\Delta E_{seg}$) typically reflects the difficulty of alloy element segregation at the interface, as shown in Formula (3) [65–67]:

$$\Delta E_{seg} = \frac{1}{n}\left(E^{interface}_{Mg/Ti-TM} - E^{interface}_{Mg/Ti} + n\mu_{Ti} - n\mu_{TM}\right) \quad (3)$$

In Formula (3), $E^{interface}_{Mg/Ti-TM}$ is the total energy after adding the alloying element on the interface Ti layer and Ti sub-surface layer of the Mg/Ti interface, $E^{interface}_{Mg/Ti}$ represents the total energy of the pure interface, $\mu_{Ti}$ and $\mu_{TM}$ represent the chemical potential of Ti and alloying element, which satisfy the following relationship [68,69]: $\mu_{TM} = E^{bulk}_{TM}/n_x$, and n represents the number of alloying element. Since we are considering only one alloying atom, n = 1 in this case. In general, a positive $\Delta E_{seg}$ suggests that the alloying element is less likely to segregate at the interface, while a negative $\Delta E_{seg}$ indicates a higher likelihood of segregation [70–72]. To investigate the interfacial segregation behavior of various alloying elements at the Mg(0001)/Ti(0001) interface, an alloy atom should be introduced into either the Ti layer or Ti sub-surface layer at the interface. Figure 8a depicts the calculated $\Delta E_{seg}$ values for various alloying elements at the interface. The findings reveal notable disparities in the heat of segregation, implying that these elements have the capability to segregate at the interface and impact its characteristics, even at low concentrations. Among them, after doping Gd atoms into the first layer of Ti atoms for the Mg(0001)/Ti(0001) interface, which exhibits the minimum $\Delta E_{seg}$ of approximately −5.83 eV. This suggests that, compared to other elements, Gd is most likely to segregate at this position. However, after doping Ca and La atoms into the first layer of Ti atoms, the interface exhibits larger $\Delta E_{seg}$ with values of 0.84 eV and 0.63 eV, respectively. This indicates that, compared to other alloying atoms,

Ca and La atoms are less likely to segregate at the interface. Additionally, after doping alloying elements such as V, Cr, Mn, and Nb, the $\Delta E_{\text{seg}}$ values are positive, suggesting a more incredible difficulty in segregation at the interface. The heat of segregation of interface layer Ti atoms after doping different alloying atoms at the Mg(0001)/Ti(0001) interface follows the following order: Gd > Si > Sn > Nd > Cu > Ce > Zn > Sc > Fe > Zr > Mo > Mn > Y > V > Nb > Cr > La > Ca. Similarly, we have also calculated the $\Delta E_{\text{seg}}$ of the second outermost layer Ti atoms at the Mg(0001)/Ti(0001) interface following the doping of various alloying elements. The outcomes mirror those observed for doping at the interface layer Ti atoms, demonstrating the following order: Gd > Si > Sn > Nd > Fe > Cu > Sc > Mn > Zn > Ce > Zr > Mo > Nb > V > Cr > Y > La > Ca. Comparing the $\Delta E_{\text{seg}}$ values at the positions of the first or second outermost layer Ti atoms, it is evident that Gd, Si, Sn, and Nd are prone to segregation, whereas alloying elements like Ca, La, Cr, and V are less likely to undergo segregation. The segregation behavior of the aforementioned alloying elements at the Mg/Ti interface provides valuable guidance for designing and selecting heterogeneous metal Ti-reinforced Mg-based composite materials.

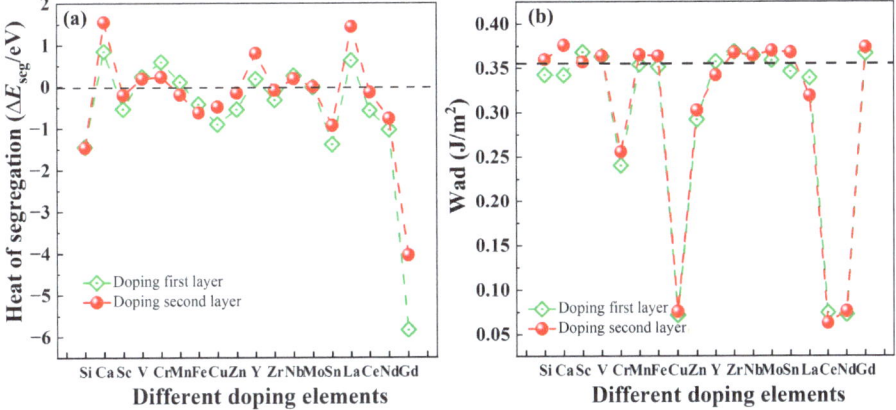

**Figure 8.** The heat of segregation ($\Delta E_{\text{seg}}$) (**a**) and work of adhesion ($W_{\text{ad}}$) (**b**) of Mg(0001)/Ti(0001) interface with different alloy elements doping the first layer and the sub-surface layer of Ti atoms, and the dashed lines in (**b**) represent the $W_{\text{ad}}$ of pure Mg/Ti interface.

After doping alloying elements to the Mg/Ti interface, the $W_{\text{ad}}$ can be used as:

$$W_{ad} = (E_{Mg}^{slab} + E_{Ti-TM}^{slab} - E_{Mg/Ti-TM}^{interface})/A_i \qquad (4)$$

where the $E_{Ti-TM}^{slab}$ is total energy of a seven-layer Ti(0001) free surface after adding an alloying element, $E_{Mg/Ti-TM}^{interface}$ is the total energy of the Mg/Ti interface after adding an alloying element. Figure 8b illustrates the $W_{\text{ad}}$ of the Mg(0001)/Ti(0001) interfaces after the introduction of alloying elements. The dashed line within the figure represents the magnitude of $W_{\text{ad}}$ for the pure Mg(0001)/Ti(0001) interface. Generally, the larger the $W_{\text{ad}}$ of the interface is, the stronger the cohesive strength of interface atoms is, whereas the opposite scenario indicates a weakening of cohesive strength. Further analysis reveals that, besides Gd, the doping of alloying elements such as Sc, V, Y, Zr, Nb, and Mo also leads to a slight increase in the $W_{\text{ad}}$ of the Mg(0001)/Ti(0001) interface. This indicates that these alloying elements also have a strengthening effect on the cohesive strength of the interface to some extent.

2.2.3. Electronic Structure

It utilizes first-principles methods to examine the electronic structure of the pure Mg/Ti interface and doping Mg/Ti interface configurations, allowing for a detailed exploration of atomic electron levels and revealing the fundamental nature of crystal structures. This capability is one of the key advantages of first-principles calculations, offering valuable insights for the advancement of materials design and engineering. The total and partial density of states for different interface configurations of the Mg(0001)/Ti(0001) are depicted in Figure 9. Evidently, based on the total density of states near the Fermi level ($E_F$), all the Mg(0001)/Ti(0001) interface configurations exhibit metallic properties. The total density of states shows little variation across different configurations. Since the primary performance differences arise from variations in the electronic configurations near the Fermi level, the partial density of states from −9 eV to 3 eV can be plotted, as shown in Figure 9b–e. The density of states near $E_F$ is predominantly influenced by Mg-$p$ and Ti-$d$ states. Notably, structural properties, such as cohesion, elastic constants, and interface energy, are primarily associated with the $d$-band within the Ti atoms. For the Mg/Ti interface with OT, MT, HCP1, and HCP2 configurations, it is evident that around the energy of −3 eV, there is a clear overlap between Mg-$s$ and Ti-$p$ orbitals, indicating the presence of $sp$ hybridization. Moreover, to clearly see the difference in the density of states near the $E_F$, we magnified the density of states in Figure 9a near the $E_F$, as shown in Figure 9(a1). Noticeably, it is apparent that the total density of states near the $E_F$ is lowest for the Mg(0001)/Ti(0001) interface with the HCP2 configuration, suggesting its highest stability. This correlates with the previously computed results for the $W_{ad}$.

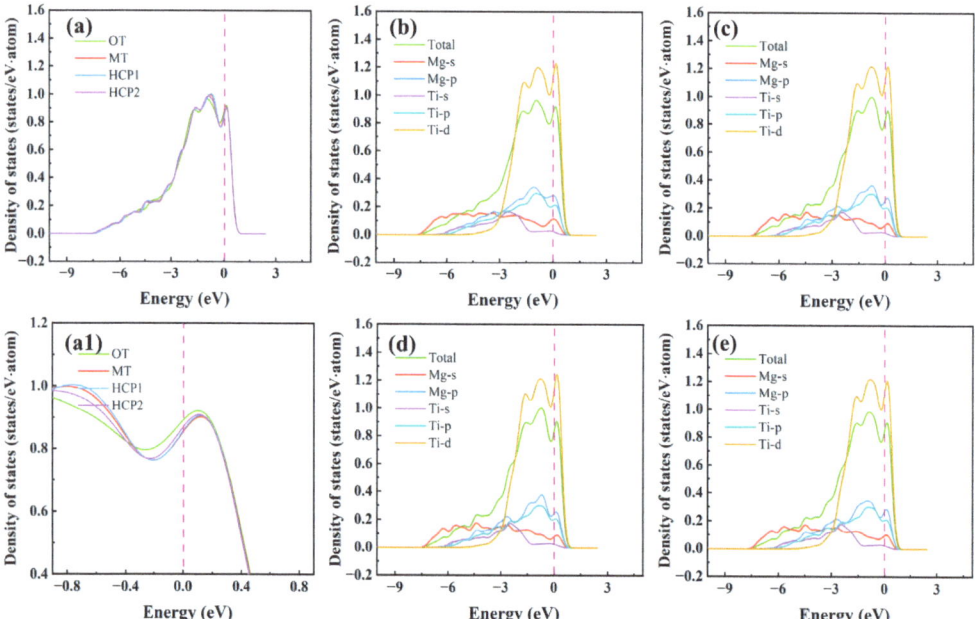

**Figure 9.** The total density of states (**a**) (where (**a1**) is a magnified view of (**a**) near the Fermi level) and partial density of states (**b**–**e**) with different interface configurations for the Mg(0001)/Ti(0001) interface. (**b**) OT configuration, (**c**) MT configuration, (**d**) HCP1 configuration, and (**e**) HCP2 configuration.

The electronic structure determines the mechanical properties of the Mg/Ti interfaces. To comprehend the microscopic mechanisms that govern the interface properties of Mg(0001)/Ti(0001), the interface's charge density difference was plotted, as depicted in Figure 10. We can observe from Figure 10 that the degree of localization near Ti atoms is higher compared to that near Mg atoms, indicating a higher degree of delocalization near Mg atoms. Furthermore, among all interface configuration structures, the HCP2 interface exhibits a higher localization at the interface, indicating stronger metallic bonding between Mg and Ti and, thus, a more stable interface structure. Furthermore, to analyze the influence of different alloying elements on the interfacial segregation behavior of the Mg(0001)/Ti(0001) interface, several typical alloying elements (including Ca, La, Cu, and Ce) are chosen, and the charge density difference in these interface models after doping is analyzed. The specific results are depicted in Figures 11 and 12. The red dashed line in Figures 11 and 12 represents the interface position, where the section on the right side corresponds to the Ti(0001) layer, and the section on the left side corresponds to the Mg(0001) layer. Indeed, it is clear that the region surrounding Ti atoms is depicted in red, whereas the area surrounding Mg atoms is shown in blue, suggesting that Ti atoms gain electrons while Mg atoms lose electrons. Compared to the interface electronic structure without doping, the distribution of electron clouds changes when introducing different alloying elements to the interface. Additionally, it can be observed that the delocalization around Ca atoms is more significant than that around Ce, Cu, and La atoms, and there is partial overlap between the electron clouds of Mg and Ca atoms, indicating the formation of strong metallic bonds between Ca atoms and Ti or Mg, thereby enhancing the interface. However, the charge density difference plots of Mg(0001)/Ti(0001) interfaces with different alloying elements doped near the sub-surface Ti atoms are notably different from those doped near the surface Ti atoms. The electronic structure around the second layer of Ti atoms has undergone significant changes, indicating the formation of TM-Ti bonds. It can be observed that the area surrounding Cu atoms is encapsulated by blue spherical shapes, while the region around Ce atoms exhibits a symmetric distribution resembling "petals", which is related to the waveforms associated with Ce atom's $d$ orbitals. Exactly during plastic deformation, the non-spherical distribution of electrons serves as a barrier, hindering the material's plastic deformation and ultimately improving its mechanical properties. In all interfaces, electrons around the bulk Mg atoms transfer to the Mg atoms at the interface, weakening the metallic characteristics of Mg-Mg bonds and strengthening their ionic characteristics, leading to increased stability of the interface structure.

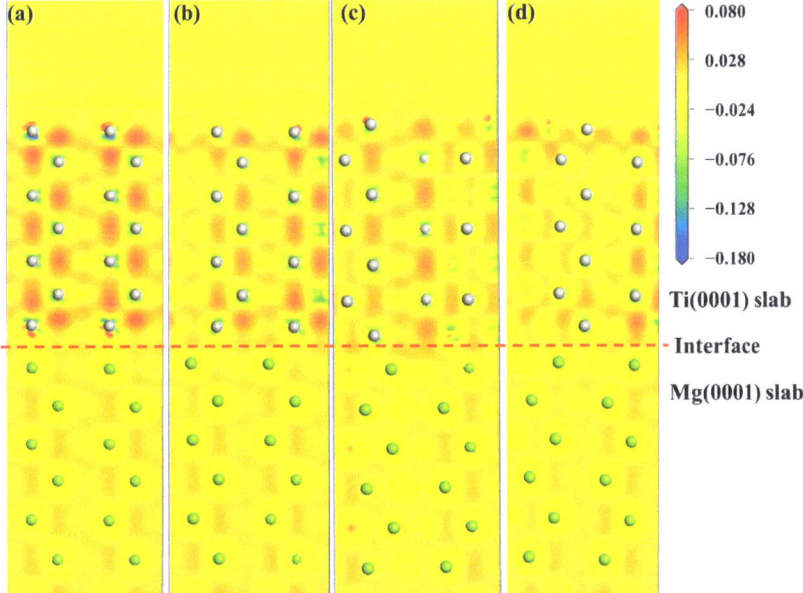

Figure 10. The charge density difference maps with different interface configurations for the Mg(0001)/Ti(0001) interface: (**a**) OT configuration, (**b**) MT configuration, (**c**) HCP1 configuration, and (**d**) HCP2 configuration, and the dashed lines indicate the Mg/Ti interface.

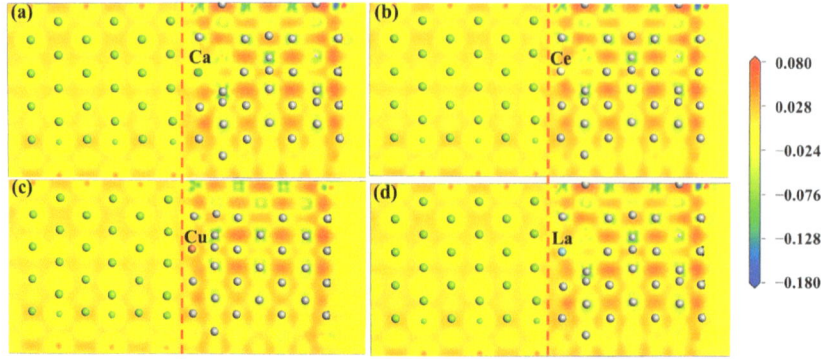

**Figure 11.** The charge density difference maps of Mg(0001)/Ti(0001) interface with different alloy elements doping the first layer of Ti atoms: (**a**) doping Ca atom, (**b**) doping Ce atom, (**c**) doping Cu atom, and (**d**) doping La atom, and the dashed lines indicate the Mg/Ti interface.

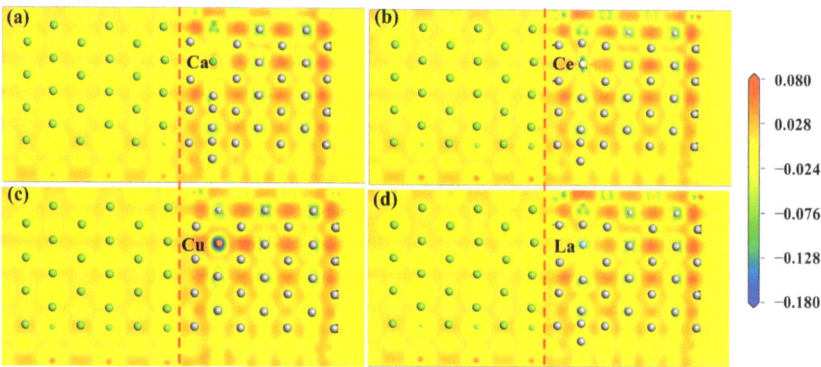

**Figure 12.** The charge density difference maps of Mg(0001)/Ti(0001) interface with different alloy elements doping the sub-surface layer of Ti atoms, (**a**) doping Ca atom, (**b**) doping Ce atom, (**c**) doping Cu atom, and (**d**) doping La atom, and the dashed lines indicate the Mg/Ti interface.

## 3. Computational Method Details

The first-principles calculations of the bulk and surface properties of Mg and Ti, as well as interface properties of Mg/Ti composites, were conducted using the density functional theory (DFT) within the framework of the Cambridge Serial Total Energy Package Code (CASTEP) [73]. Additionally, the segregation behavior of alloying elements Si, Ca, Sc, V, Cr, Mn, Fe, Cu, Zn, Y, Zr, Nb, Mo, Sn, La, Ce, Nd, and Gd at the interfaces was investigated systematically [65,74]. The interaction between valence electrons and ion cores was characterized using ultrasoft pseudopotentials (USPPs) [75]. For Mg, Ti, and the aforementioned alloying elements, their respective valence electron configurations were as: $2p^63s^2$, $3s^23p^63d^24s^2$, $3s^23p^2$, $3s^23p^64s^2$, $3s^23p^63d^14s^2$, $3s^23p^63d^34s^2$, $3s^23p^63d^54s^1$, $3d^54s^2$, $3d^64s^2$, $3d^{10}4s^1$, $3d^{10}4s^2$, $4d^15s^2$, $4s^24p^64d^25s^2$, $4s^24p^64d^45s^1$, $4s^24p^64d^55s^1$, $5s^25p^2$, $5s^25p^65d^16s^2$, $4f^15s^25p^65d^16s^2$, $4f^45s^25p^66s^2$ and $4f^75s^25p^65d^16s^2$, respectively. To achieve convergence and ensure computational accuracy, the maximum kinetic energy cutoff for the expansion of plane waves in reciprocal space was established at 450 eV. For bulk Mg and Ti, a $9 \times 9 \times 9$ grid of $k$ points was chosen for sampling the first Brillouin zone (BZ). For the Mg(0001) and Ti(0001) surfaces, the $k$ point was set as $7 \times 7 \times 1$ to ensure the convergence. The Mg/Ti interface models with different atomic stacking sequences were built using a

2 × 2 supercell model to guarantee periodic boundary conditions, which contained 56 Mg and 56 Ti atoms, and the interface models had 4 × 2 × 1 $k$ points. Moreover, the Mg(0001) and Ti(0001) surface slab models with a 2 × 2 supercell model consisting of seven atomic layers were adopted to establish the Mg(0001)/Ti(0001) interface models with different atomic stacking sequences according to our previous work [76]. Additionally, a vacuum region of 15 Å was employed to eliminate interactions between atoms at the interface. In addition, to achieve equilibrium in the bulk, surface, and interface structures, the Broyden–Fletcher–Goldfarb–Shanno (BFGS) algorithm was employed [77,78]. Additionally, this was a quasi-Newton method, which iteratively solves for the minimum point of an objective function by gradually constructing an approximation of the inverse of the Hessian matrix. The exchange-correlation function was modeled using the Perdew–Burke–Ernzerhof (PBE) within a generalized gradient approximation (GGA) [79] to calculate the bulk, surface, and interface properties. The convergence criteria for the total energy, atomic forces, and displacements in each crystal and interface structure were established at $1 \times 10^{-6}$ eV, 0.01 eV/Å, and 0.001 Å, respectively.

## 4. Conclusions

This study utilizes first-principles calculations based on density functional theory to explore the interface stability and the interfacial segregation behavior of alloying elements at the interface of the Mg/Ti interface. Through an in-depth analysis of interface electronic properties, the stability of the interface and the segregation behavior of elements at the interface are examined. The main conclusions of this work are as follows:

(1) The calculated phonon spectra of Mg and Ti indicate that both are dynamically stable phases. Additionally, criteria for mechanical stability also suggest that they are mechanically stable phases. The calculated elastic properties results show that Ti exhibits the largest $C_{11}$ value of approximately 205.9 GPa and Young's modulus of around 153.4 GPa, indicating that Ti can effectively enhance the modulus of Mg alloys.

(2) First-principles calculations determined that the optimal interface distance for the Mg/Ti interface configurations is approximately 2.5 Å. They are using seven-layer Mg(0001) surface and seven-layer Ti(0001) surface slab models to build Mg(0001)/Ti(0001) interface configurations with OT, MT, HCP1, and HCP2 atomic stacking interface configurations. Based on the results of interface adhesion work and electronic structure information, it can be concluded that the Mg(0001)/Ti(0001) interface with HCP2 configuration has the best stability.

(3) The segregation calculations for eighteen alloying elements near the Mg(0001)/Ti(0001) interface indicate that Gd atoms, when doped into the first layer of Ti atoms, result in the lowest heat of segregation of $-5.83$ eV, suggesting that Gd is the most prone to segregation. Also, alloying elements such as Si, Sn, and Nd tend to segregate at the interface. Conversely, alloying elements like Ca, La, Cr, and V are less likely to segregate. These findings are further supported by electronic structure information.

**Author Contributions:** Conceptualization, Y.Z. (Yunxuan Zhou) and J.T.; methodology, Y.Z. (Yunxuan Zhou); software, Y.Z. (Yunxuan Zhou) and J.T.; validation, T.C., Y.Z. (Yunxuan Zhou), S.T. and Y.Z. (Yulin Zhang); formal analysis, S.T. and Y.Z. (Yulin Zhang); investigation, Y.Z. (Yunxuan Zhou) and H.L.; writing—original draft preparation, Y.Z. (Yunxuan Zhou); writing—review and editing, Y.Z. (Yunxuan Zhou), T.C., Y.Z. (Yulin Zhang) and J.T.; supervision, J.T., B.W., X.C. and F.P.; funding acquisition, J.T. and F.P. All authors have read and agreed to the published version of the manuscript.

**Funding:** This research was funded by the National Key Research and Development Program of China (2022YFB3709300) and the National Natural Science Foundation of China (Grant No. U2167213).

**Institutional Review Board Statement:** Not applicable.

**Informed Consent Statement:** Not applicable.

**Data Availability Statement:** Data are contained within the article.

**Acknowledgments:** The authors thank the Joint Lab for Electron Microscopy of Chongqing University and the Analytical and Testing Center of Chongqing University.

**Conflicts of Interest:** The authors declare no conflict of interest.

## References

1. Pollock, T.M. Weight loss with magnesium alloys. *Science* **2010**, *328*, 986–987. [CrossRef] [PubMed]
2. Esmaily, M.; Svensson, J.E.; Fajardo, S.; Birbilis, N.; Frankel, G.S.; Virtanen, S.; Arrabal, R.; Thomas, S.; Johansson, L.G. Fundamentals and advances in magnesium alloy corrosion. *Prog. Mater. Sci.* **2017**, *89*, 92–193. [CrossRef]
3. Ding, Z.; Li, Y.; Yang, H.; Lu, Y.; Tan, J.; Li, J.; Li, Q.; Chen, Y.A.; Shaw, L.L.; Pan, F. Tailoring MgH$_2$ for hydrogen storage through nanoengineering and catalysis. *J. Magnes. Alloys* **2022**, *10*, 2946–2967. [CrossRef]
4. Wang, C.; Ning, H.; Liu, S.; You, J.; Wang, T.; Jia, H.-J.; Zha, M.; Wang, H.-Y. Enhanced ductility and strength of Mg-1Zn-1Sn-0.3Y-0.2Ca alloy achieved by novel micro-texture design. *Scr. Mater.* **2021**, *204*, 114119. [CrossRef]
5. Saxena, A.; Raman, R.K.S. Role of surface preparation in corrosion resistance due to silane coatings on a magnesium alloy. *Molecules* **2021**, *26*, 6663. [CrossRef] [PubMed]
6. Ding, Z.; Li, H.; Shaw, L. New insights into the solid-state hydrogen storage of nanostructured LiBH$_4$-MgH$_2$ system. *Chem. Eng. J.* **2020**, *385*, 123856. [CrossRef]
7. Zhou, B.; Li, Y.; Wang, L.; Jia, H.; Zeng, X. The role of grain boundary plane in slip transfer during deformation of magnesium alloys. *Acta Mater.* **2022**, *227*, 117662. [CrossRef]
8. Yan, C.; Xin, Y.; Chen, X.B.; Xu, D.; Chu, P.K.; Liu, C.; Guan, B.; Huang, X.; Liu, Q. Evading strength-corrosion tradeoff in Mg alloys via dense ultrafine twins. *Nat. Commun.* **2021**, *12*, 4616. [CrossRef]
9. Gnedenkov, A.S.; Filonina, V.S.; Sinebryukhov, S.L.; Gnedenkov, S.V. A superior corrosion protection of Mg alloy via smart nontoxic hybrid inhibitor-containing coatings. *Molecules* **2023**, *28*, 2538. [CrossRef]
10. Xu, Y.H.; Zhou, Y.; Li, Y.C.; Wu, P.K.; Ding, Z. Recent advances in the preparation methods of magnesium-based hydrogen storage materials. *Molecules* **2024**, *29*, 2451. [CrossRef]
11. Wang, W.Y.; Tang, B.; Shang, S.L.; Wang, J.W.; Li, S.L.; Wang, Y.; Zhou, J.; Wei, S.Y.; Wang, J. Local lattice distortion mediated formation of stacking faults in Mg alloys. *Acta Mater.* **2019**, *170*, 231–239. [CrossRef]
12. Song, J.; She, J.; Chen, D.; Pan, F. Latest research advances on magnesium and magnesium alloys worldwide. *J. Magnes. Alloys* **2020**, *8*, 1–41. [CrossRef]
13. Zhang, Z.; Zhang, J.; Xie, J.; Liu, S.; He, Y.; Guan, K.; Wu, R. Developing a low-alloyed fine-grained Mg alloy with high strength-ductility based on dislocation evolution and grain boundary segregation. *Scr. Mater.* **2022**, *209*, 114414. [CrossRef]
14. Zhang, C.; Feng, Z.; Zhang, Y.; Xia, Z.; Hakimi, N.; Li, T.; Xue, B.; Tan, J. Structural evolution of MgO layer in Mg-based composites reinforced by Metallic Glasses during the SPS sintering process. *Vacuum* **2023**, *214*, 112141. [CrossRef]
15. Chen, W.; Yu, W.; Ma, C.; Ma, G.; Zhang, L.; Wang, H. A review of novel ternary nano-layered MAX phases reinforced AZ91D magnesium composite. *J. Magnes. Alloys* **2022**, *10*, 1457–1475. [CrossRef]
16. Harte, A.; Griffiths, M.; Preuss, M. The characterisation of second phases in the Zr-Nb and Zr-Nb-Sn-Fe alloys: A critical review. *J. Nucl. Mater.* **2018**, *505*, 227–239. [CrossRef]
17. Vijayakumar, P.; Pazhanivel, K.; Ramadoss, N.; Ganeshkumar, A.; Muruganantham, K.; Arivanandhan, M. Synthesis and characterization of AZ91D/SiC/BN hybrid magnesium metal matrix composites. *Silicon* **2022**, *14*, 10861–10871. [CrossRef]
18. Huang, S.-J.; Subramani, M.; Borodianskiy, K. Strength and ductility enhancement of AZ61/Al$_2$O$_3$/SiC hybrid composite by ECAP processing. *Mater. Today Commun.* **2022**, *31*, 103261. [CrossRef]
19. Luo, X.; Liu, J.; Zhang, L.; He, X.; Zhao, K.; An, L. Deformation and failure behavior of heterogeneous Mg/SiC nanocomposite under compression. *J. Magnes. Alloys* **2022**, *10*, 3433–3446. [CrossRef]
20. Ding, C.; Hu, X.; Shi, H.; Gan, W.; Wu, K.; Wang, X. Development and strengthening mechanisms of a hybrid CNTs@SiCp/Mg-6Zn composite fabricated by a novel method. *J. Magnes. Alloys* **2021**, *9*, 1363–1372. [CrossRef]
21. Yang, H.; Chen, X.; Huang, G.; Song, J.; She, J.; Tan, J.; Zheng, K.; Jin, Y.; Jiang, B.; Pan, F. Microstructures and mechanical properties of titanium-reinforced magnesium matrix composites: Review and perspective. *J. Magnes. Alloys* **2022**, *10*, 2311–2333. [CrossRef]
22. Pérez, P.; Garcés, G.; Adeva, P. Mechanical properties of a Mg–10 (vol.%)Ti composite. *Compos. Sci. Technol.* **2004**, *64*, 145–151. [CrossRef]
23. Wu, B.; Li, J.; Ye, J.; Tan, J.; Liu, L.; Song, J.; Chen, X.; Pan, F. Work hardening behavior of Ti particle reinforced AZ91 composite prepared by spark plasma sintering. *Vacuum* **2021**, *183*, 109833. [CrossRef]
24. Bao, L.; Duan, Y.; Shi, R.; Liu, X.; Zheng, K. Adhesion strength, interfacial bonding, and fracture mechanism of the Mg/Ti$_2$AlC interface from first-principles calculation. *J. Mater. Res. Technol.* **2022**, *20*, 3195–3207. [CrossRef]
25. Hu, J.; Xiao, Z.; Wang, Q.; Shen, Z.; Li, X.; Huang, J. First-principles calculations on interfacial properties and fracture behavior of the Mg(1-101)||TiC(1-11) interfaces. *Mater. Today Commun.* **2021**, *27*, 102399. [CrossRef]
26. Yang, T.; Chen, X.; Li, W.; Han, X.; Liu, P. First-principles calculations to investigate the interfacial energy and electronic properties of Mg/AlN interface. *J. Phys. Chem. Solids* **2022**, *167*, 110705. [CrossRef]

27. Yang, S.-Q.; Du, J.; Zhao, Y.-J. First-principles study of ZnO/Mg heterogeneous nucleation interfaces. *Mater. Res. Express* **2018**, *5*, 036519. [CrossRef]
28. Wang, F.; Li, K.; Zhou, N.G. First-principles calculations on Mg/Al$_2$CO interfaces. *Appl. Surf. Sci.* **2013**, *285*, 879–884. [CrossRef]
29. Li, X.; Hui, Q.; Shao, D.; Chen, J.; Wang, P.; Jia, Z.; Li, C.; Chen, Z.; Cheng, N. First-principles study on the stability and electronic structure of Mg/ZrB$_2$ interfaces. *Sci. China Mater.* **2016**, *59*, 28–37. [CrossRef]
30. Wang, H.-L.; Tang, J.-J.; Zhao, Y.-J.; Du, J. First-principles study of Mg/Al$_2$MgC$_2$ heterogeneous nucleation interfaces. *Appl. Surf. Sci.* **2015**, *355*, 1091–1097. [CrossRef]
31. Liu, R.; Yin, X.; Feng, K.; Xu, R. First-principles calculations on Mg/TiB$_2$ interfaces. *Comput. Mater. Sci.* **2018**, *149*, 373–378. [CrossRef]
32. Li, K.; Sun, Z.G.; Wang, F.; Zhou, N.G.; Hu, X.W. First-principles calculations on Mg/Al$_4$C$_3$ interfaces. *Appl. Surf. Sci.* **2013**, *270*, 584–589. [CrossRef]
33. Wang, F.; Bai, G.; Guo, Q.; Hou, H.; Zhao, Y.; Zhang, Y. Stability of Mg$_2$Sn(001)/Mg(0001)/MgZn(001) interface doped with transition elements. *Comput. Mater. Sci.* **2023**, *224*, 112154. [CrossRef]
34. Li, X.; Xie, H.; Yang, B.; Li, S. Elastic and thermodynamic properties prediction of Mg$_2$Sn and MgTe by first-principle calculation and quasi-harmonic Debye model. *J. Electron. Mater.* **2019**, *49*, 464–471. [CrossRef]
35. Song, Y.; Zhan, S.; Nie, B.; Qi, H.; Liu, F.; Fan, T.; Chen, D. First-Principles Investigations on Structural Stability, Elastic Properties and Electronic Structure of Mg$_{32}$(Al,Zn)$_{49}$ Phase and MgZn$_2$ Phase. *Crystals* **2022**, *12*, 683. [CrossRef]
36. Huang, Z.W.; Zhao, Y.H.; Hou, H.; Han, P.D. Electronic structural, elastic properties and thermodynamics of Mg$_{17}$Al$_{12}$, Mg$_2$Si and Al$_2$Y phases from first-principles calculations. *Phys. B Condens. Matter* **2012**, *407*, 1075–1081. [CrossRef]
37. Bao, L.; Yao, Z.; Zhang, Y.; Wang, C.; Zheng, K.; Shi, R.; Liu, X.; Pan, F. First-principles investigation of adhesion strength and interfacial bonding in Mg/X (X = Ti, Zr, Hf, V, Nd, Cr, Mo, Mn, and Fe) interface. *J. Magnes. Alloys* **2024**. [CrossRef]
38. Ganeshan, S.; Shang, S.L.; Wang, Y.; Liu, Z.K. Effect of alloying elements on the elastic properties of Mg from first-principles calculations. *Acta Mater.* **2009**, *57*, 3876–3884. [CrossRef]
39. Nie, Y.; Xie, Y. Ab initio thermodynamics of the hcp metals Mg, Ti, and Zr. *Phys. Rev. B* **2007**, *75*, 174117. [CrossRef]
40. Liu, T.; Chong, X.-Y.; Yu, W.; Zhou, Y.-X.; Huang, H.-G.; Zhou, R.-F.; Feng, J. Changes of alloying elements on elasticity and solid solution strengthening of α-Ti alloys: A comprehensive high-throughput first-principles calculations. *Rare Metals* **2022**, *41*, 2719–2731. [CrossRef]
41. Ahuja, R.; Wills, J.M.; Johansson, B.; Eriksson, O. Crystal structures of Ti, Zr, and Hf under compression: Theory. *Phys. Rev. B* **1993**, *48*, 16269–16279. [CrossRef]
42. Becerra, A.; Pekguleryuz, M. Effects of lithium, indium, and zinc on the lattice parameters of magnesium. *J. Mater. Res.* **2011**, *23*, 3379–3386. [CrossRef]
43. Chen, L.; Lü, S.; Guo, W.; Li, J.; Wu, S. High thermal conductivity of highly alloyed Mg-Zn-Cu alloy and its mechanism. *J. Alloys Compd.* **2022**, *918*, 165614. [CrossRef]
44. JHan, J.; Wang, C.P.; Liu, X.J.; Wang, Y.; Liu, Z.K. First-principles calculation of structural, mechanical, magnetic and thermodynamic properties for gamma-M$_{23}$C$_6$ (M = Fe, Cr) compounds. *J. Phys.-Condens. Matter* **2012**, *24*, 505503.
45. Ivanovskii, A.L. Mechanical and electronic properties of diborides of transition 3d–5d metals from first principles: Toward search of novel ultra-incompressible and superhard materials. *Progress Mater. Sci.* **2012**, *57*, 184–228. [CrossRef]
46. Wu, Z.J.; Zhao, E.J.; Xiang, H.P.; Hao, X.F.; Liu, X.J.; Meng, J. Crystal structures and elastic properties of superhard IrN$_2$ and IrN$_3$ from first principles. *Phys. Rev. B* **2007**, *76*, 054115. [CrossRef]
47. Bao, L.; Kong, Z.; Qu, D.; Duan, Y. Insight of structural stability, elastic anisotropies and thermal conductivities of Y, Sc doped Mg$_2$Pb from first-principles calculations. *Chem. Phys. Lett.* **2020**, *756*, 137833. [CrossRef]
48. Cheng, J.; Guo, T.T.; Barnett, M.R. Influence of temperature on twinning dominated pop-ins during nanoindentation of a magnesium single crystal. *J. Magnes. Alloys* **2022**, *10*, 169–179. [CrossRef]
49. Khokhlova, J.A.; Khokhlov, M.A. 3d-visualization of magnesium strengthening mechanisms for a description of experimentally obtained data of alloying effect in Mg-Ga system. *J. Magnes. Alloys* **2020**, *8*, 546–551. [CrossRef]
50. Tu, T.; Chen, X.H.; Zhao, C.Y.; Yuan, Y.; Pan, F.S. A simultaneous increase of elastic modulus and ductility by Al and Li additions in Mg-Gd-Zn-Zr-Ag alloy. *Mater. Sci. Eng. A* **2020**, *771*, 138576. [CrossRef]
51. Jang, H.S.; Seol, D.; Lee, B.J. Modified embedded-atom method interatomic potentials for Mg-Al-Ca and Mg-Al-Zn ternary systems. *J. Magnes. Alloys* **2021**, *9*, 317–335. [CrossRef]
52. Song, X.; Fu, X.; Wang, M. First–principles study of β′ phase in Mg–RE alloys. *Int. J. Mech. Sci.* **2023**, *243*, 108045. [CrossRef]
53. Wang, M.; Zhou, Y.; Tian, W.; Li, J.; Chen, H.; Tan, J.; Chen, X. First-principles study the mechanical, electronic, and thermodynamic properties of Mg-Al-Mn ternary compounds. *Vacuum* **2023**, *213*, 112140. [CrossRef]
54. Ranganathan, S.I.; Ostojastarzewski, M. Universal elastic anisotropy index. *Phys. Rev. Lett.* **2008**, *101*, 055504. [CrossRef] [PubMed]
55. Dai, J.H.; Xie, R.W.; Chen, Y.Y.; Song, Y. First principles study on stability and hydrogen adsorption properties of Mg/Ti interface. *Phys. Chem. Chem. Phys.* **2015**, *17*, 16594–16600. [CrossRef] [PubMed]
56. Yang, S.-Q.; Li, C.-B.; Luo, G.; Du, J.; Zhao, Y.-J. Mg adsorption on MgAl$_2$O$_4$ surfaces and the effect of additive Ca: A combined experimental and theoretical study. *J. Alloys Compd.* **2021**, *861*, 158564. [CrossRef]

57. Ju, H.; Ning, H.; Meng, Z.-Y.; Wang, C.; Wang, H.-Y. First-principles study on the segregation behavior of solute atoms at {101$\bar{\ }$2} and {101$\bar{\ }$1} twin boundaries of Mg. *J. Mater. Res. Technol.* **2023**, *24*, 8558–8571. [CrossRef]
58. Jia, Z.; Xing, Y.; Ning, Y.; Ding, L.; Ehlers, F.J.H.; Hao, L.; Liu, Q. Density gradient segregation of Cu at the $Si_2Hf/Al$ interface in an Al-Si-Cu-Hf alloy. *Scr. Mater.* **2023**, *222*, 115022. [CrossRef]
59. Jiao, Z.; Liu, Q.-J.; Liu, F.-S.; Tang, B. Structural and electronic properties of low-index surfaces of $NbAl_3$ intermetallic with first-principles calculations. *Appl. Surf. Sci.* **2017**, *419*, 811–816. [CrossRef]
60. Chen, Y.; Dai, J.; Song, Y. Stability and hydrogen adsorption properties of $Mg/Mg_2Ni$ interface: A first principles study. *Int. J. Hydrogen Energy* **2018**, *43*, 16598–16608. [CrossRef]
61. Liu, G.; Huang, Z.; Gao, W.; Sun, B.; Yang, Y.; Zhao, D.; Yan, M.; Fu, Y.-d. The effect of impurities on the adhesion behavior of TiN(111)/α-Ti(0001) semi-coherent interface: A first-principles investigation. *Surf. Interfaces* **2022**, *35*, 102488. [CrossRef]
62. Zhao, C.; Xing, X.; Guo, J.; Shi, Z.; Zhou, Y.; Ren, X.; Yang, Q. Microstructure and wear resistance of (Nb,Ti)C carbide reinforced Fe matrix coating with different Ti contents and interfacial properties of (Nb,Ti)C/α-Fe. *Appl. Surf. Sci.* **2019**, *494*, 600–609. [CrossRef]
63. Feng, Y.; Chen, X.; Hao, Y.; Chen, B. Characterization and energy calculation of the S/Al interface of Al–Cu–Mg alloys: Experimental and first-principles calculations. *Vacuum* **2022**, *202*, 111131. [CrossRef]
64. Chen, L.; Li, Y.; Xiao, B.; Zheng, Q.; Yi, D.; Li, X.; Gao, Y. A hierarchical high-throughput first principles investigation on the adhesion work, interfacial energy and tensile strength of $NiTi_2(100)/α-Al_2O_3(0001)$ interfaces. *J. Mater. Res. Technol.* **2021**, *14*, 2932–2944. [CrossRef]
65. Gao, Y.; Liu, X.; Wei, L.; Zhang, X.; Chen, M. The segregation behavior of elements at the Ti/TiFe coherent interface: First-principles calculation. *Surf. Interfaces* **2022**, *34*, 102321. [CrossRef]
66. Wang, G.; Chong, X.; Li, Z.; Feng, J.; Jiang, Y. Strain-stiffening of chemical bonding enhance strength and fracture toughness of the interface of $Fe_2B$/Fe in situ composite. *Mater. Charact.* **2024**, *207*, 113575. [CrossRef]
67. Ouadah, O.; Merad, G.; Abdelkader, H.S. Energetic segregation of B, C, N, O at the γ-TiAl/$α_2$-$Ti_3$Al interface via DFT approach. *Vacuum* **2021**, *186*, 110045. [CrossRef]
68. Rong, J.; Wang, X.; Zhang, Y.; Feng, J.; Zhong, Y.; Yu, X.; Zhan, Z. $Al_2O_3$/FeAl interfacial behaviors by yttrium doping in high temperature oxidation. *Ceram. Int.* **2019**, *45*, 22273–22280. [CrossRef]
69. Li, R.; Chen, Q.; Ouyang, L.; Zhang, Y.; Nie, B.; Ding, Y. Insight into the strengthening mechanism of α-$Al_2O_3$/γ-Fe ceramic-metal interface doped with Cr, Ni, Mg, and Ti. *Ceram. Int.* **2021**, *47*, 22810–22820. [CrossRef]
70. Garrett, A.M.; Race, C.P. Segregation of Ni and Si to coherent bcc Fe-Cu interfaces from density functional theory. *J. Nucl. Mater.* **2021**, *556*, 153185. [CrossRef]
71. Wang, J.; Enomoto, M.; Shang, C. First-principles study on the interfacial segregation at coherent Cu precipitate/Fe matrix interface. *Scr. Mater.* **2020**, *185*, 42–46. [CrossRef]
72. Kim, K.; Zhou, B.-C.; Wolverton, C. Interfacial stability of θ′/Al in Al-Cu alloys. *Scr. Mater.* **2019**, *159*, 99–103. [CrossRef]
73. Segall, M.D.; Lindan, P.J.D.; Probert, M.J.; Pickard, C.J.; Hasnip, P.J.; Clark, S.J.; Payne, M.C. First-principles simulation: Ideas, illustrations and the CASTEP code. *J. Phys. Condens. Matter* **2002**, *14*, 2717–2744. [CrossRef]
74. Biswas, A.; Siegel, D.J.; Seidman, D.N. Simultaneous segregation at coherent and semicoherent heterophase interfaces. *Phys. Rev. Lett.* **2010**, *105*, 076102. [CrossRef]
75. Vanderbilt, D. Soft self-consistent pseudopotentials in a generalized eigenvalue formalism. *Phys. Rev. B Condens. Matter* **1990**, *41*, 7892–7895. [CrossRef] [PubMed]
76. Zhou, Y.; Tian, W.; Dong, Q.; Wang, H.; Tan, J.; Chen, X.; Zheng, K.; Pan, F. A first-principles study on the adhesion strength, interfacial stability, and electronic properties of $Mg/Mg_2Y$ interface. *Acta Metall. Sin. (Engl. Lett.)* **2024**, *37*, 537–550. [CrossRef]
77. Fischer, T.H.; Almlof, J. General methods for geometry and wave function optimization. *J. Chem. Phys.* **1992**, *96*, 9768–9774. [CrossRef]
78. Pfrommer, B.G.; CôtéSteven, M.; Louie, G.; Cohen, M.L. Relaxation of crystals with the Quasi-Newton method. *J. Comput. Phys.* **1997**, *131*, 233–240. [CrossRef]
79. Perdew, J.P.; Burke, K.; Ernzerhof, M. Generalized gradient approximation made simple. *Phys. Rev. Lett.* **1997**, *78*, 3865–3868. [CrossRef]

**Disclaimer/Publisher's Note:** The statements, opinions and data contained in all publications are solely those of the individual author(s) and contributor(s) and not of MDPI and/or the editor(s). MDPI and/or the editor(s) disclaim responsibility for any injury to people or property resulting from any ideas, methods, instructions or products referred to in the content.

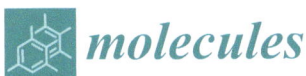

*Review*

# Comparison of Construction Strategies of Solid Electrolyte Interface (SEI) in Li Battery and Mg Battery—A Review

Zhongting Wang [1], Rongrui Deng [2], Yumei Wang [2,*] and Fusheng Pan [1]

[1] National Engineering Research Center for Magnesium Alloys, College of Materials Science and Engineering, Chongqing University, Chongqing 400044, China; wang.zhongting@cqu.edu.cn (Z.W.); fspan@cqu.edu.cn (F.P.)

[2] National University of Singapore (Chongqing) Research Institute, Chongqing 401123, China; rongrui.deng@nusricq.cn

* Correspondence: yumei.wang@nusricq.cn

**Abstract:** The solid electrolyte interface (SEI) plays a critical role in determining the performance, stability, and longevity of batteries. This review comprehensively compares the construction strategies of the SEI in Li and Mg batteries, focusing on the differences and similarities in their formation, composition, and functionality. The SEI in Li batteries is well-studied, with established strategies that leverage organic and inorganic components to enhance ion diffusion and mitigate side reactions. In contrast, the development of the SEI in Mg batteries is still in its initial stages, facing significant challenges such as severe passivation and slower ion kinetics due to the divalent nature of magnesium ions. This review highlights various approaches to engineering SEIs in both battery systems, including electrolyte optimization, additives, and surface modifications. Furthermore, it discusses the impact of these strategies on electrochemical performance, cycle life, and safety. The comparison provides insights into the underlying mechanisms, challenges, and future directions for SEI research.

**Keywords:** solid electrolyte interface (SEI); lithium-ion battery; magnesium-ion battery

## 1. Introduction

Renewable energy has been rapidly adopted in recent years to relieve the emissions of $CO_2$ all over the world. However, renewable energy heavily depends on natural resources, such as sunlight, wind, water and so on, which are unpredictable and out of human control. Therefore, renewable energy is stored and then used in a controlled manner. Electrochemical energy storage systems, which are based on storing chemical energy and converting to electrical energy when needed, are the most traditional energy storage devices for power generation. Rechargeable batteries are one of the oldest and also one of the most widely used electrochemical energy storage systems.

Lithium-ion batteries have dominated the commercial battery market since the 1990s, including in aerospace, transport and electronics, due to their high gravimetric and volumetric energy density. Other than lithium-ion batteries, next-generation rechargeable battery technologies are also in development. Besides alkali metal-ion batteries, other metals are also considered as anodes in rechargeable batteries. For example, magnesium has a very high theoretical volumetric energy density—around 50% higher than that of lithium. Moreover, magnesium anodes do not exhibit dendrite formation, albeit only in certain nonaqueous solvents and at certain current densities. This allows magnesium metal to be used at the anode with around a five times higher volumetric energy density than a graphite electrode. The magnesium's relative abundance and ease of mining make magnesium-ion batteries good candidates for large-scale energy storage [1].

The working principle of these batteries is similar. As shown in Figure 1, during the discharge process, the oxidation and reduction reactions happen on the anode and cathode, respectively, while the metal ions move from the anode to the cathode through electrolytes (vice versa during the charge process) [2,3]. The electrode/electrolyte interface is obviously an important electrochemical juncture that determines the behaviors of metal ions and electrons. Although the electrolytes in batteries are designed to be stable with a wide electrochemical window, the kinetic stability between electrolytes and electrodes is attained after a stable solid electrolyte interface (SEI) forms. The SEI is the product, where trace amounts of electrolyte decompose and react with electrodes. An ideal SEI film should inhibit further electrolyte degradation and electron transport while facilitating ion transport.

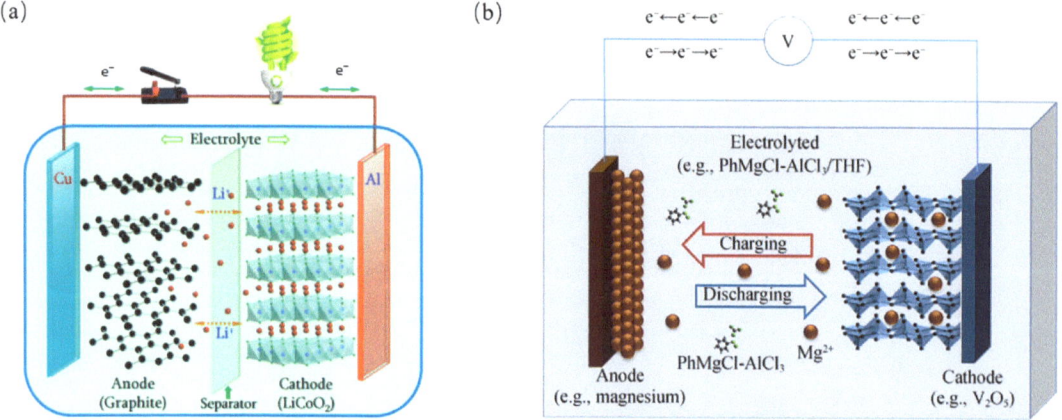

**Figure 1.** Working principle of (**a**) Lithium-ion battery (**b**) Magnesium-ion battery [2,3].

In recent decades, many researchers have spent huge amounts of time trying to figure out the exact formation, structure and functional mechanisms of the SEI. However, these questions remain the most ambiguous issues in battery science. The thickness of the SEI is around 10–15 nm, containing both organic and inorganic species, which is the result of a delicate balance between electrolyte decomposition and passivation. The thickness is controlled by several factors, including the composition of the electrolyte, the applied current density, and the anode surface properties. A thinner SEI might not provide sufficient protection against side reactions, leading to reduced cycling stability, while a thicker SEI could impede ion transport, adversely affecting battery performance [4,5]. Therefore, this range is optimal for maintaining a balance between protection and ion conductivity. In addition, the formation and growth of the SEI occurs during the charging/discharging processes. These characteristics make it very hard to investigate SEIs using traditional real-time in situ characterization technology. To further improve the capacity of current commercial batteries and the development of next-generation batteries, the design of the SEI is an unavoidable challenge. Specially, the Li metal battery is considered the 'holy grail' of batteries due to its extremely high capacity. One of the greatest obstacles of Li metal batteries is that it is difficult to construct a stable SEI film on an Li metal surface, which not only degrades the capacity after charging/discharging cycles but also causes the hazards of flammability and explosiveness. Moreover, in other battery systems, such as magnesium-ion batteries, the ideal anode materials are also the corresponding metals. Therefore, these batteries also face the same challenge: a stable and ion-conductive SEI film.

However, although the properties of alkali elements and alkaline elements are very similar, the slight difference makes a significant difference to the interface configuration. Since dendrite is the main reason for fires and explosions, the focus of SEI configuration in lithium-ion batteries (LIBs) is not to stabilize the interface but to also suppress the formation of dendrite. For sodium-ion batteries (NIBs), although sodium is a monovalent ion like lithium, its larger ionic radius leads to greater volume changes during cycling. This can cause the SEI in NIBs to crack and reform, making it less stable over time. The

SEI tends to be thicker and less uniform compared to LIBs, and while $Na_2CO_3$ and NaF are formed similarly to their lithium counterparts, the mechanical stresses in NIBs due to the size of $Na^+$ present additional challenges. Similar to NIBs, the SEI in potassium-ion batteries (KIBs) forms through electrolyte decomposition, but the larger size of potassium ions can complicate the formation mechanism and composition. The stability and ionic conductivity of the SEI are often lower than those in LIBs and NIBs, potentially limiting the long-term performance of KIBs. On the other hand, now, the passive film on the anode is the main bottleneck in magnesium-ion batteries (MIBs); hence, the SEI configuration in MIBs mainly focuses on constructing a stable interface with high ionic conductivity. Calcium-ion batteries (CIBs) face similar challenges: the SEI should provide ionic conductivity and prevent the direct reaction of the calcium metal with the electrolyte, which can lead to unwanted side reactions and decreased battery efficiency. Hence, we find that the SEI functions of alkali metal-ion batteries and alkaline earth metal-ion batteries are not the same, so we selected the SEIs of lithium-ion batteries and magnesium-ion batteries as representatives for discussion.

This review will summarize SEI formation and the influence on the electrode/electrolyte interfaces, as well as compare the different configurations between LIBs and MIBs. Finally, perspectives on the investigation of SEI films are also discussed, including computer simulations and experiments.

## 2. The Formation Mechanism of SEIs

In 1970, Dey [6] first observed the passive film on the Li metal surface, and Peled [7] first proposed the concept of the solid electrolyte interface (SEI) in 1979. In 1985, Muller [8] firstly identified the existence of $Li_2Co_3$ and polymers in SEIs by X-ray diffraction, which illustrates the presence of both inorganic and organic components in SEIs. In 1990, Dahn [9] reported the gradual formation of an SEI on graphite anodes. In 1995, Kanamura [10] found that a thin, dense LiF film is attached on the Li anode surface, and another porous composite layer is above this film. This study inspired the design of components for artificial SEI films. In 1997, Peled [11] developed the mosaic model for the SEI, which considers the grain boundaries. In 1999, Aurbach [12] combined ex situ Fourier-transform infrared spectroscopy (FTIR) and in situ atomic force microscopy (AFM) to investigate the formation process of the SEI. In the 21st century, researchers began to use computer simulations and advanced characterization techniques to accelerate the study of SEIs. In 2001, Balbuena [13] utilized density functional theory to study the reduction mechanism of electrolytes on anodes, which also illustrated the formation mechanism of the SEI. In 2010, Xu [14] quantitatively measured the energy barrier for Li ions to pass through the SEI. In 2017, Cui [15] observed mosaic structure of the SEI film by cryo-electron microscopy. In 2022, Song [16] investigated the chemical composition of the SEI by time-of-flight secondary ion mass spectrometry (TOF-SIMS).

At present, molecular orbital theory is the general explanation of the SEI formation mechanism in LIBs, as shown in Figure 2 [17,18]. The theory explains that when the lowest unoccupied molecular orbital (LUMO) of the electrolyte is lower than the electrochemical potential of the anode ($\mu_A$), the electrolyte will gain electrons from the anode and is reduced, forming an SEI film on the anode surface. On the other hand, when the highest occupied molecular orbital (HOMO) of the electrolyte is higher than the electrochemical potential of the cathode ($\mu_C$), the electrolyte will lose electrons and is oxidized, forming a CEI (cathode electrolyte interface) film on the cathode surface. The SEI film then will expand the electrochemical window of the electrolyte, hindering further reactions and preventing the decomposition of the organic electrolyte.

It is believed that the formation mechanism of the SEI in Mg ions also follows Peled's model, in which the SEI is considered to be an inorganic/organic nanocomposite material, and the ion transport through the bulk inorganic part is the rate-determining step [19]. However, the low ionic conductivity of inorganic compounds, such as MgO, $MgF_2$, and MgS, and the Pilling–Bedworth (P–B) ratios (ratio of the volume of the elementary cell of a compound and the elementary Mg cell) are dissimilar, pointing toward the formation of a porous surface layer on the Mg. In a recent study, anion adsorption from the electrolyte on the surface of such Mg-SEIs was suggested, which fully blocks the cation transport [20].

Two scenarios of continuous SEI growth on Mg are thus considered, as shown in Figure 1. In the first scenario, the growth proceeds because of the electronic conductivity and/or reactive radical existence in the thin film formed upon initial Mg contact with the electrolyte [21]. In the second, long-term growth occurs due to the decomposition of the anion and/or solvent molecules, which arrive at the Mg/SEI interface by diffusion through the SEI pores [22,23]. Electronic tunneling is disregarded as the SEI thickness is expected to be higher than several nm after a longer cell rest time. In both cases, the amount of SEI material typically increases over time [23].

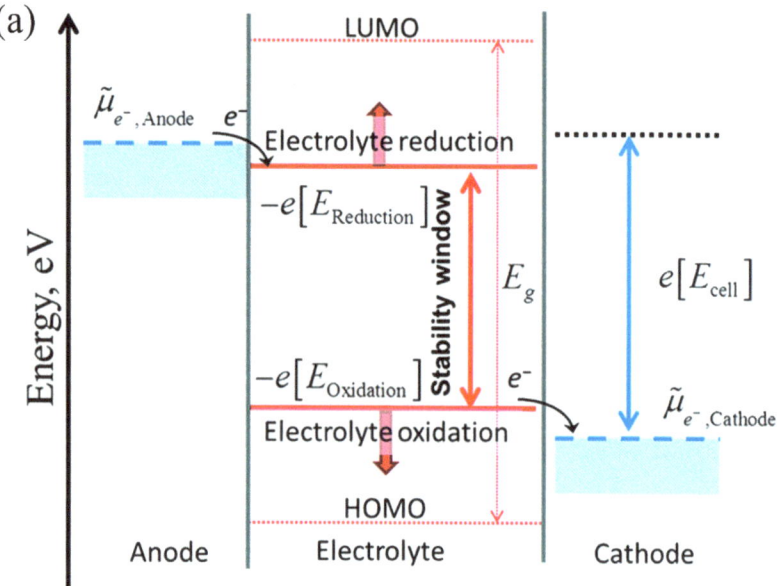

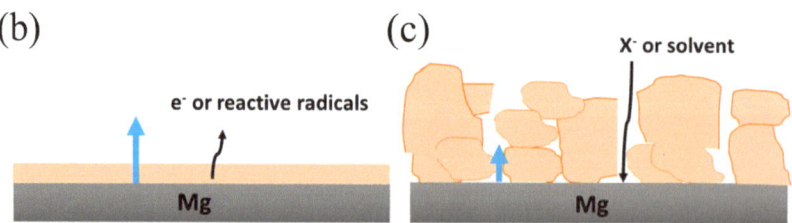

**Figure 2.** (**a**) Schematic illustration of the positive and negative potential limits of electrolyte stability, and the energy levels of LUMO and HOMO [17,18]. The red arrow represents stability window, the pink arrow represents the energy difference between LUMO and HOMO, the blue arrow represents the electrochemical potential difference between cathode and anode. Mechanisms of SEI growth on Mg electrode: (**b**) dense film growth by electronic or magnesium interstitial conduction and (**c**) porous film growth by anion or solvent diffusion through the pores. In both cases, growth occurs at the metal/SEI interface [24].

## 3. SEI in Li-Ion Batteries

Researchers have illustrated that the initial SEI forms during the charging process in the early cycles. At the early stage, the SEI hinders the transportation of solvent molecules and lithium salt. Therefore, the SEI continues to grow at this stage.

The well-known single-electron reduction reaction, which explains the organic by-products, happens at this stage. During the reaction, the nucleophilic interactions between radical anions formed by electron addition to the carbonate molecules, assisted by the vicinity of lithium ions and carbonyl group, occurs and generates lithium salts of semi-carbonates or alkyl carbonates [25]. It is found that ethylene and propylene are the gaseous side-reaction products in the reduction, attributed to the decomposition of ethylene carbonate (EC) and propylene carbonate (PC), respectively, while alkanes are the reduction side-reaction product of linear carbonates through the single-electron reaction mechanism [26–32]. Besides this mechanism, Collins proposed the two-electron reaction mechanism, which also explains the alkyl carbonates and gaseous side-reaction products [33]. Besides the lithium alkyl carbonates mentioned above, oxalates and succinates are also SEI components in the SEI in EC/PC or EC/DMC electrolytes, where DMC is the abbreviation for dimethyl carbonate [34,35]. Moreover, acetals and ortho-esters are also found in the SEI by NMR through various formative mechanisms [36].

On the other hand, the typical inorganic products, including LiF, LiCl and $Li_2O$, precipitate on the electrode surface through a reduction reaction [19]. Low-abundance $CO_2$ is also detected during the formation of the SEI [37]. CO instead of $CO_2$ is also reported as a by-product [38–41]. $Li_2CO_3$ is also reported, due to the elimination of the reaction of $Li_2O$ with $CO_2$, in inefficient moisture elimination cells [42–44].

In addition to small molecules, polymers and oligomers are also involved in SEI composition [30,38,45,46]. Long-chain structures are reported in EC/DMC and PC electrolyte systems [47,48]. Compared with short-chain structures, polymer species could provide better protection function, and the branched polymer with carbonate/ethylene oxide units could assist the lithium ions in passing through the layer [49]. However, it is still ambiguous whether the polymer component and semi-carbonates are partially soluble, which affects the stability of the SEI [19].

After long cycles, the initial SEI would evolve and change gradually [50–52]. The unstable species growth at the initial stage in the SEI stops, and new stable products, such as inorganic compounds, tend to form [53,54]. The local dissolution or the uneven stress will also cause the mechanical breakdown of the SEI. In the case of fast-forming cracks, the electrolyte flows into the crack and immediately reacts with the fresh anode surface, forming a new thin protective film and preventing further local reactions. On the other hand, in the case of slow-forming cracks, the SEI becomes thinner and electrons pass through the thin region and reduce the electrolyte further [19].

Some models propose that inorganic species such as $Li_2O$, LiF and $Li_2CO_3$ tend to attach on the surface of electrode, while organic species tend to exist close to the electrolyte [55,56]. The study also shows that the inorganic section has higher conductivity than the organic section [55], which implies that during the evolution stage, the conductivity of the SEI tends to increase.

Gas is also detected during the evolution stage, which is believed to be one of the reasons for capacity fading [57]. The crossover reactions on the cathodic side can generate products like $CO_2$, which can diffuse inside the anode and destabilize the SEI, as well as be reduced into $Li_2CO_3$, leading the evolution of the SEI [58].

During the formation of the SEI, several factors affect the properties of the SEI layer, as shown in Figure 3 [19,59,60]. Firstly, the composition of the electrolyte is one of the key factors that determines the SEI's features [61]. For example, the weak interaction between solvents could prevent the exfoliation of graphite. EC, which is one of the most common solvents with low lithium binding energy, can participate in SEI formation, instead of co-intercalating into graphite [9,62–65]. On the other hand, PC, another commonly used solvent, tends to co-intercalate into graphite layers and make graphite exfoliate [66]. This phenomenon proved that the difference of a single methyl group between EC and PC would significantly change the SEI composition and affect the behavior of Li ions [67–69]. The functional groups of electrolyte molecules influence the precursor constituents and resultant reactivity. It is also found that increasing the lithium salt concentration in the electrolyte could weaken the Li$^+$ ion solvation sheath and consequently protect graphite against exfoliation [70]. Moreover, the solvents also affect the composition of the SEI. The PC-based electrolyte also promotes the formation of $Li_2CO_3$ in the SEI, while EC-based electrolytes promote the mixture of semi-carbonates, oxalates and oligoethers [71].

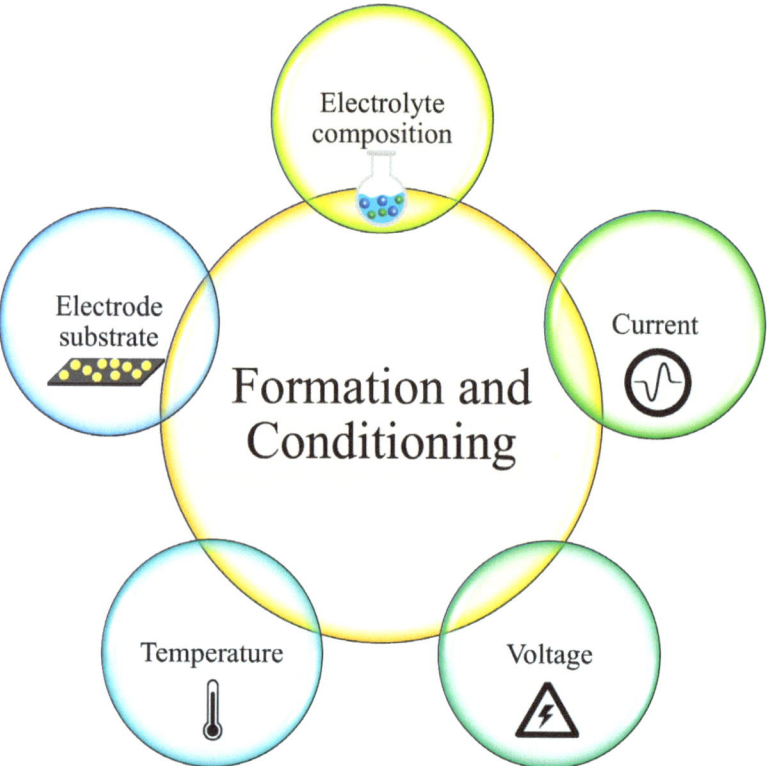

**Figure 3.** Factors affecting the formation of the SEI layer [19,59,60].

Besides the solvents, the type of lithium salt also affects the features of the SEI. $Li_2CO_3$ was the main SEI component in lithium bis(trifluoromethane)sulfonimide (LiTFSI) salt electrolytes, while the main component in LiBETI salt electrolytes was a mixture of $Li_2CO_3$ and semi-carbonates [27]. This is because the decomposition of anions varies significantly [72,73]. LiPF6 would cause the formation of $Li_xPF_y$ and $Li_xPF_yO_z$. LiBF$_4$ would lead the formation of $Li_xBF_y$. Lithium difluoro (oxalate) borate (LiDFOB) would form lithium oxalates, and LiFSI causes the formation of $Li_3N(SO_2)_2$ in the SEI [25].

As the substrate of the SEI, the electrode also an important factor for determining the SEI's features. The particle size, pore size, and degree of crystallinity of the electrode all affect the formation of the SEI, which influences the processes of industrial production [74–76]. The small particles provide more edge sites, which have higher energy and promote the formation of the SEI. Therefore, the thickness of the SEI is greater in the cross-sectional planes than the basal planes [77]. The oxygen groups on the graphite surface would reduce the potential and promote the formation of the SEI before the intercalation. These groups are also usually at the edge sites, where lithium needs to pass though before interaction. Therefore, the ratio of the edge planes to the basal planes determines the electrochemical performance of graphite in SEI formation [77,78]. Moreover, the components of the SEI at the edge are different from those of the SEI at the basal planes. More inorganic compounds like LiF are in the SEI at the edge sites, and more organic compounds are in the SEI at the basal planes [79].

Apart from the properties of the material, the external condition also affects SEI formation. The applied current rate, the current density, the state of charge and the temperature are the main external factors [51,78,80]. High current rates can accelerate the growth of the SEI and consequently cause significant capacity loss [81]. On the other hand, increasing the current density at the electrode then can relieve the capacity loss [19]. A high state of charge and overcharging will cause a change in SEI structure and capacity fade [51]. A high operation temperature will increase the thickness of the SEI and cause thermally unstable components to dissolve [82].

Normally, the intrinsic SEI has poor performance and causes capacity fade, especially in lithium metal batteries. Then, there are two ways to enhance the performance of the SEI. One is to enhance the inherent properties of the SEI, and the other is to construct an artificial SEI. To enhance the inherent properties of the SEI, modifications can be applied on the electrolyte and the electrode.

The modification of electrolytes is the most commonly used method to improve the intrinsic SEI [18]. The strategy of electrolyte modification is to change the $Li^+$ solvation structure. The anions then become more involved in the solvation structure, forming more contact ion pairs (CIPs) and aggregates (AGGs). Therefore, a more stable SEI is constructed, which can improve the columbic efficiency of the battery [83]. There are three methods to modify the electrolyte: modifying the solvent, modifying the lithium salts and adding additives.

The solvent affects the $Li^+$ solvent sheath structure, which in turn determines the SEI components and structure, as discussed previously. By adding 1,1,2,2-tetrafluoroethyl-2,2,3,3-tetrafluoropropyl ether (HFE) into a DME solvent, since HFE does not participate in the $Li^+$ solvent sheath structure when diluting the electrolyte, the decomposition of the anions in the sheath structure is promoted, resulting in the formation of inorganic-rich SEI, as shown in Figure 4a [84]. The development of all fluorinated electrolytes has wide LUMO-HOMO gaps in the solvent, and the formed LiF-rich SEI has a columbic efficiency of 97.1% [85]. The 1,1,2,2-tetrafluoro-3-methoxypropane (TFMP) solvent will induce the formation of a core–shell-like solvation structure of the electrolytes and exhibit more AGGs, as shown in Figure 4b [86]. This solvent will also effectively improve the ionic conductivity, reduce the solvation energy, and stabilize the SEI layer. Another fluorinated ether solvent, 1,1,1-trifluoro-2,3-dimethoxypropane (TFDMP), is also used and helps the electrolyte to achieve high ionic conductivity (7.4 mScm-1) and antioxidant properties (4.8 V) [87].

Lithium salts are another effective method to improve an SEI—for example, increasing the lithium salt concentration to form more CIPs and AGGs. It is reported that by increasing the concentration of LiFSI in the carbonate electrolyte, a stable LiF-rich SEI forms with high Coulomb efficiency (CE) (99.3%) [88]. $LiNO_3$, as the only lithium salt, combined with an FEC co-solvent can construct a stable $Li_3N$–LiF-rich SEI layer with a high CE of 98.31% [84].

Instead of changing solvent and salts, adding additives into mature electrolytes is a more convenient way to improve the intrinsic properties of electrolytes. Fluorinated additives are commonly used to form an LiF-rich SEI. The fluoroethylene carbonate (FEC) additives can produce an LiF-rich SEI, which promotes the uniform deposition of lithium ions [89]. However, HF gas is produced by the decomposition of FEC, which is detrimental to health [18]. Another fluorinated additive, LiDFOB, was synthesized and added into ether electrolytes. After adding LiDFOB, an LiF-rich SEI will form with an organic matrix due to the ring-opening polymerization of DOL. The organic–inorganic composite SEI endows LIBs with superior performance [90]. Surprisingly, protein can also be used as the additive. A natural protein from zein was added into electrolytes. As the result, a variety of polar functional groups, such as -COOH, -$NH_2$, and -OH, were introduced into the electrolyte, participated in the formation of the SEI, and formed an organic-rich SEI.

This organic-rich SEI can help lithium deposit more uniformly and repair the SEI crack induced by the volume change of the anode [91].

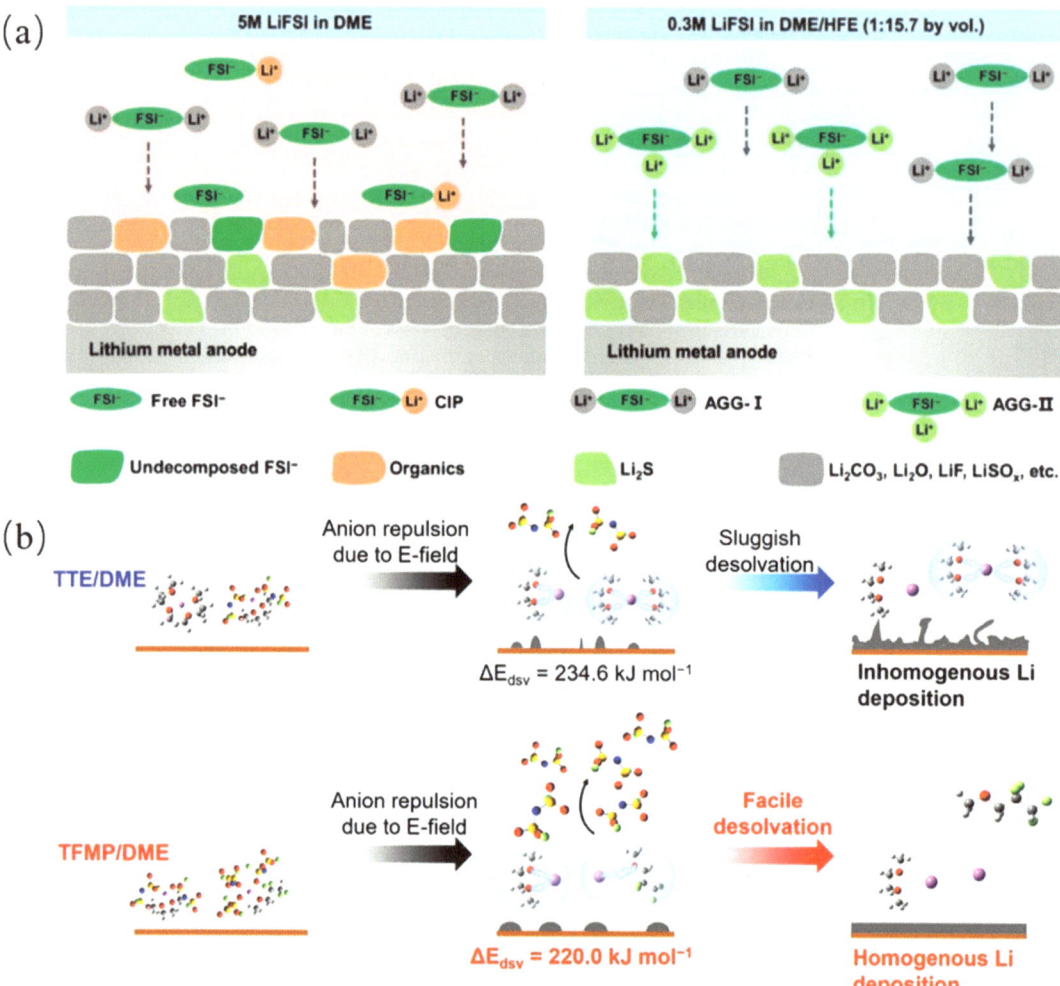

**Figure 4.** (**a**) Schematic diagram of solvent sheath structures of FSI$^-$ anion in 0.3 M LiFSI in DME/HFE and 5 M LiFSI in DME electrolytes and the generated component in SEI films [84]. (**b**) Desolvation mechanism and corresponding desolvation energy obtained from MD simulation and DFT calculation of 1 m LiFSI-TTE/DME localized high concentration electrolyte and 1 M LiFSI-TFMP/DME electrolyte [86].

Since one main reason for SEI breakup is due to the volume change of the electrode, modifying the electrode is another efficient way to enhance the inherent properties of the SEI. The fabrication of a lithium composite anode with no volume expansion by roll-to-roll can eliminate dendrite formation and help lithium ions uniformly deposit [92]. A sandwich structure anode is designed with high energy density, consisting of an insulating layer (a mixture of polyvinylidene fluorideco-hexafluoropropylene and LiNO$_3$), a mesoporous layer (a Cu-coated carbon fiber matrix), and a lithium-friendly layer (LiMg) in a roll-to-roll way. This sandwich anode can help lithium ions bottom-up deposit [93]. Also, 2D structured MXene nanosheets ($Ti_3C_2T_x$) were designed to promote the uniform growth of lithium. The fluorine end groups from MXene lead to a homogeneous distribution of LiF in the SEI [94]. Furthermore, 2D titanium carbonitride ($Ti_3CNT_x$) and 3D reduced graphene oxide (rGO) frameworks as Li scaffolds were designed to guide the formation of the SEI. The –F group of $Ti_3CNT_x$ promotes the decomposition of LiTFSI to promote the formation of an LiF-rich surface. The SEI layer has an ordered layered $Li_2O$ shell with internal LiF nanoparticles [95].

Enhancing SEI performance through material modification is more or less limited by the inherent properties of the material. Therefore, constructing an artificial SEI seems another good method to form an ideal interface.

The purpose of an artificial SEI is not only to protect the surface of electrode, but also to suppress dendrite growth. To achieve these goals, some general requirements of artificial SEIs need to be considered. First, the artificial SEI structure should be uniform. Otherwise, the SEI layer may cause nonuniform ion flux, resulting in nonuniform deposition and dendrites [96,97]. In addition, the SEI should be physically, chemically and electrochemically stable. Moreover, the SEI should have enough strength and toughness to withstand the plating/stripping and dendrite growth. Finally, the SEI needs to remain adherent and intact during cycling.

Three categories of artificial SEIs are designed based on the material types, including an inorganic SEI, an organic SEI and a composite SEI.

The effect of the lithium-ion diffusion rate on dendrite growth has previously been investigated [98,99]. Although the mechanism of the effect is not fully explained, the phenomenon is demonstrated by experiments and simulation. The diffusion control processes prefer dendritic lithium deposition, while reaction-controlled processes tend toward spherical lithium deposition. Therefore, improving ionic conductivity in SEIs can maintain lithium deposition under reaction-controlled conditions and lead to a dense lithium deposition morphology. Compared to organic compounds, inorganic compounds typically have higher ion conductivity. For example, inorganic components such as $Li_2S$ and $Li_3N$ have very high ionic conductivity, which can enhance the ion diffusion rate and promote spherical lithium deposition. In addition, inorganic compounds usually have better hardness. Hence, inorganic-rich components of the SEI have high mechanical strength, which can mechanically suppress the growth of dendrite.

$Li_3N$-based artificial SEI layers were constructed using the spontaneous reaction of lithium metal with zirconyl nitrate ($ZrO(NO_3)_2$); they consisted of $ZrO_2$, $Li_2O$, $Li_3N$, and $LiN_xO_y$, with abundant grain boundaries, as shown in Figure 5a [100]. Since the diffusion of Li ions along the grain boundaries is faster than that of the bulk phase [101], the SEI can provide a rapid pathway for Li ions. Based on magnetron co-sputtering technology, LiF nanocrystals could be embedded in an LiPON inorganic amorphous matrix. After the insertion of LiF, the artificial SEI has high ionic conductivity and stronger mechanical stability, as shown in Figure 5b [102]. Another artificial SEI protective layer with $Li_2S_2$ as the main component was constructed on the top layer of an array-structured Li foil, as shown in Figure 5c [103]. $Li_2S/Li_2S_2$ was homogeneously deposited on the top of Li foil via low-temperature selective vaporization $Li_2S_6$, while an $Li_2S$ layer with low electrical conductivity resulted in SEI deposition on the bottom layer of the Li foil. The uniform $Li_2S_2$ artificial SEI could protect the electrode–electrolyte interface and inhibit the growth of lithium dendrites, as well as provide a fast path for lithium-ion transport.

Although the inorganic SEI has high ionic conductivity and hardness, which is good for suppressing dendrite growth, the main disadvantage of inorganic compounds is the low flexibility, which leads to the failure of resisting the volume changes on the electrode during ion plating/stripping. On the other hand, organic polymeric components typically have high elasticity and flexibility, which can accommodate the volume changes of the electrode. Therefore, organic compounds are also considered to be used in artificial SEIs to achieve long-life batteries [73].

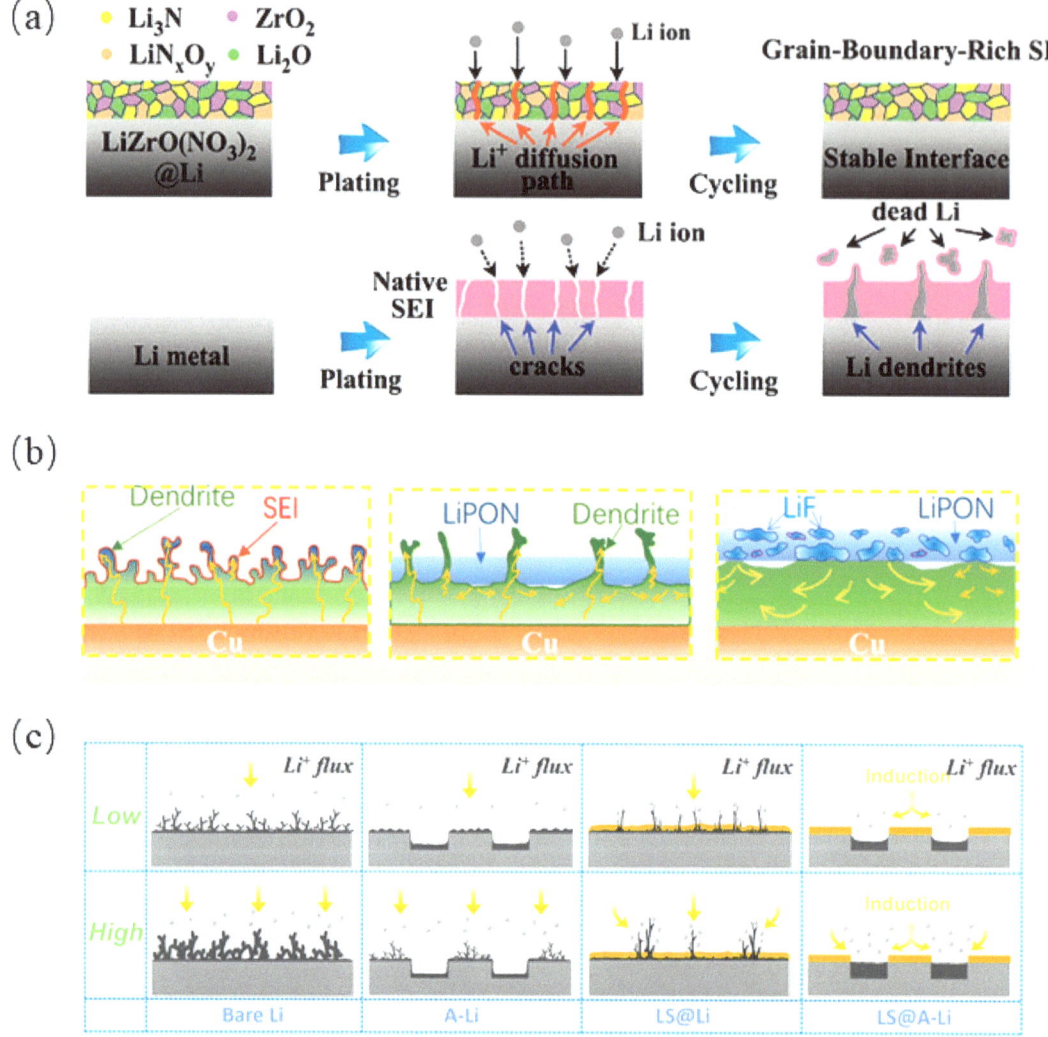

**Figure 5.** (a) Schematic illustration of Li stripping/plating behavior for the bare Li and LiZrO(NO$_3$)$_2$@Li anodes [100], (b) Schematic illustration of the lithium electrodeposition behavior in bare Cu, LiPON/Cu, and LiF–LiPON/Cu electrodes [102], (c) Schematic illustration of different Li deposition behavior of bare Li, A-Li, LS@Li, LS@A-Li at low and high current densities, respectively [103].

The preparation of organic lithium carboxylate SEI layers, which occurs through the in situ spontaneous reaction of lithium metal with carboxylic acid, has been reported [104]. Lithium carboxylate has a low Young's modulus and high flexibility, which enables it to accommodate the volume changes of the electrode. In addition, it is found that alginate-based SEI films can be formed by using alginic acid and lithium hydroxide [105]. Alginate has stable chemical properties and superior ion transport properties, which can reduce side reactions and enhance the cycling stability of batteries.

A dynamic SEI reinforced by an open-architecture metal–organic framework (OA-MOF) film has been proposed, which leverages the elastic volumetric changes of three-dimensional lithiophilic sites for self-regulation. The self-adjusting distribution of lithiophilic sites on vertically grown $Cu_2(BDC)_2$ nanosheets enables a uniform Li-ion flux, precise control over Li mass transport, and compact lithium deposition [106]. A robust artificial SEI film with biomimetic ionic channels and enhanced stability is proposed, incorporating a $ClO_4^-$-functionalized metal–organic framework (UiO-66-$ClO_4$) and a flexible lithiated Nafion (Li-Nafion) binder. The strong electronegativity and lithium affinity of $ClO_4^-$ groups, anchored within UiO-66 channels, establish a highly efficient single-ion conducting pathway, a high $Li^+$ transference number, and superior ionic conductivity. This structure effectively inhibits detrimental reactions between the lithium metal and the electrolyte, while regulating rapid and uniform $Li^+$ flux. Further reinforced by the flexible Li-Nafion binder, the UiO-66-$ClO_4$/Li-Nafion (UCLN) composite film exhibits remarkable mechanical strength, suppressing lithium dendrite formation and ensuring the long-term structural stability of the lithium metal anode during cycling [107]. Two frameworks functionalized with -$NH_2$ and -$CH_3$ groups have been utilized as fillers in polyethylene oxide (PEO) composite solid electrolytes, with their catalytic roles in lithium formation at the SEI interface being investigated. First-principles calculations elucidate the LiF-rich SEI formation mechanism, demonstrating that ZIFs-$NH_2$ significantly elongates the C–F bond in $TFSI^-$ compared to ZIFs-$CH_3$, thereby facilitating bond cleavage and enhancing LiF production [108].

However, most organic-based SEI films lack mechanical strength and have low ionic conductivity. Therefore, the pure organic SEI cannot meet the requirement for advanced batteries. As a result, the development of an organic–inorganic composite SEI, which combines the advantage of both materials to enhance SEI performance, is now attracting researchers' attention. It is reported that an organic–inorganic composite SEI with both mechanical strength and flexibility, based on reactive polymers as SEI precursors, has been synthesized [109]. This composite SEI consists of polymeric lithium salts in LiF and graphene oxide (GO) nanosheets, and it helps to inhibit dendrite growth, prevent electrolyte decomposition, and promote efficient lithium deposition. Another organic–inorganic composite SEI is reported to have been synthesized via the in situ polymerization of precursors composed of poly(ethylene glycol) diacrylate (PEGDA) and LiDFOB, as shown in Figure 6a [110]. PEGDA can provide good mechanical strength, and the decomposition of LiDFOB provides a good $Li^+$ transport pathway and better chemical stability. The high mechanical strength and good flexibility help the SEI accommodate volume changes during cycling.

In addition, anion migration blocks the transport of cation ions, which causes the slow diffusion of cation ions and the depletion of the anions, resulting in a strong electric field that promotes dendrite growth. A single-ion conducting artificial SEI with a 3D crosslinked network has been prepared by using pentaerythritol tetrakis (2-mercaptoacetate) (PETMP) and lithium bis(allylmalonato)borate (LiBAMB) in a thiol–ene click reaction [111]. The migration of the anion was limited due to the covalent binding of the BAMB anion. Therefore, only lithium ions can be transported in the 3D cross-linked network. Furthermore, the weak electrostatic interaction between the off-domain $sp^3$ boron anions and the lithium ion improves the conductivity of the SEI. Another single-ion conducting SEI was prepared by using $Li_{6.4}La_3Zr_{1.4}Ta_{0.6}O_{12}$ (LLZTO) as the base layer and Li-Nafion as the top layer, as shown in Figure 6b [112]. Moreover, LLZTO has high mechanical strength and Li-Nafion has high elasticity, which inhibits dendrite formation.

The SEI on the graphite anode and metallic Li anode attracts the majority of the attention. Graphite was the first commercialized and widely used anode in Li-ion batteries, while in pursuit of high capacity, researchers are increasingly focusing on metallic lithium anodes. The co-intercalation of lithium ions and solvent molecules leads to the exfoliation of the graphite anode. The failure mechanism requires the SEI on graphite to adjust the volume change as well as block the intercalation of solvent molecules. However, the capacity of the graphite anode limits further improvement. The study of the SEI on graphite focuses on explaining the failure mechanism rather than the applications. On the contrary, metallic lithium metal is believed to be the ideal anode. The main concern hindering its commercial application is dendrite growth. Although the formation mechanism of the SEI on lithium is also discussed, the ultimate goal is to construct a stable SEI on a metallic lithium anode that suppresses the growth of dendrite and eliminates fire hazards.

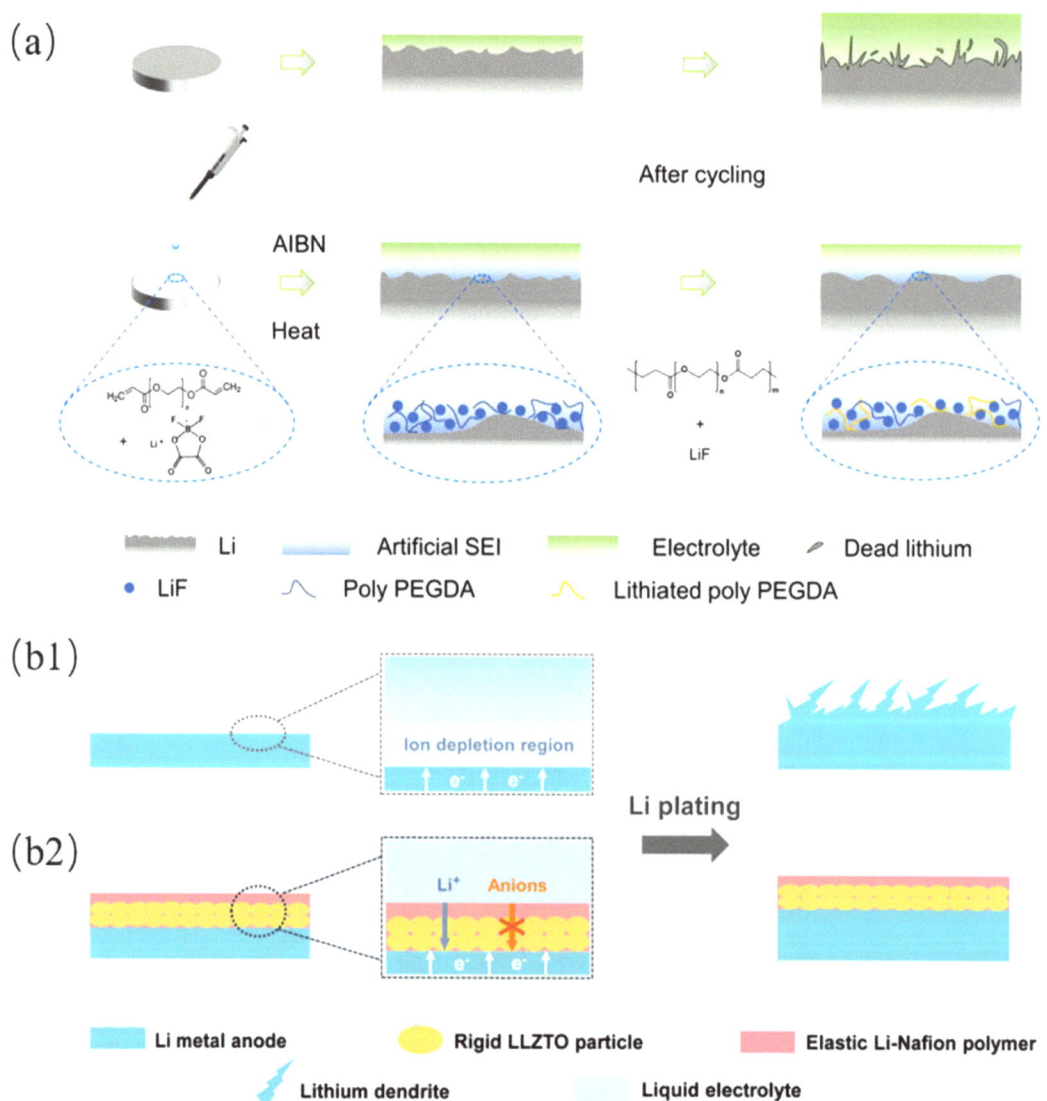

**Figure 6.** (**a**) Schematic illustration of organic-inorganic composite SEI preparation through in-situ polymerization and the corresponding Li deposition behaviors of bare Li and modified Li [110]. (**b1**) Schematic illustrations of different Li deposition patterns. (**b1**) The space charge region induced by anion depletion will impose a strong electric field at the vicinity of bare Li, leading to dendritic Li deposits. (**b2**) After incorporating the single-ion-conducting LLZTO/Li-Nafion coating composed of rigid LLZTO and elastic Li-Nafion, a uniform and compact Li plating behavior can be obtained [112].

## 4. SEI in Mg-Ion Batteries

Mg metal is probably the most promising anode material due to its low standard potential (−2.37 vs. SHE) and dendrite-free characteristic [113,114]. However, the formation of a passivating surface film rather than an $Mg^{2+}$ conducting SEI on the Mg anode surface, which hinders the transport of $Mg^{2+}$ ions, has always restricted the development of MIBs [115]. Thus, constructing an SEI with high ion conductivity becomes one of the most critical bottlenecks hindering the development of magnesium-ion batteries. Similar to lithium-ion batteries, electrolyte modification and artificial SEI construction are considered to help in the construction of a stable SEI.

In 2000, the first prototype electrolyte for an MIB was developed based on a Grignard reagent. The chemical formula can be expressed as RMgX (R may be alkyl or aryl; X is Cl, Br, or other halides). This electrolyte allows for reversible Mg deposition-stripping while preventing the formation of a passivation film [116]. However, due to the presence of halides, Grignard reagents are corrosive, particularly to current collectors [117,118], which leads to stability issues over time. In addition, Grignard-based electrolytes typically have a limited electrochemical stability window, which restricts their use with high-voltage cathodes. Moreover, Grignard-based electrolytes are highly sensitive to air and moisture, which makes handling and manufacturing challenging. Researchers continue to work hard to overcome these disadvantages, which limit the overall energy density of the battery [119,120].

To address the interfacial passivation of Mg metal anodes in electrolytes, researchers focus on changing salts and adding additives into the electrolytes. Mg salt (MgFPA), which has an Al(III)-centered anion $Al(O_2C_2(CF_3)_4)_2$, abbreviated as FPA, with a large radius could induce solvent coordination [121]. The LUMO energy level of the FPA anion was decreased after the coordination between the FPA anion and the THF solvent molecule. As a result, a thin and stable SEI with superior $Mg^{2+}$ conductivity was formed on the Mg metal anode in the MgFPA/Tetrahydrofuran electrolyte. From the same research group, another electrolyte consisting of Li $[B(hfip)_4]$/DME (LBhfip/DME) (hfip=OC(H)(CF$_3$)$_2$) was also synthesized [122]. In the initial cycling process, $Mg^{2+}$ would be introduced into LBhfip/DME, forming a hybrid $Li^+/Mg^{2+}$ electrolyte, which could conduct $Mg^{2+}$ in subsequent cycles. Moreover, an Li-containing SEI was formed on the Mg metal anode, which could not only effectively conduct $Mg^{2+}$ but also prevent the continuous corrosion of the Mg metal anode by liquid electrolytes. A stable SEI formed on the Mg metal surface by adding an $Mg(BH_4)_2$ additive to the Mg $[B(hfip)_4]_2$/DME electrolyte. In this electrolyte system, the $Mg(BH_4)_2$ additive could remove the passivation layer on the Mg metal surface and then enhance the Mg storage performance [123].

Introducing a non-passivating anionic additive—reduced perylene diimide ethylenediamine (rPDI)—into the electrolyte enables the rapid and reversible deposition/dissolution of Mg within a simple non-nucleophilic electrolyte system. The rPDI additive demonstrates higher adsorption energy on the Mg surface compared to TFSI salt, while PDI preferentially adsorbs onto the Mg surface. Acting as a protective anion, it prevents TFSI decomposition and Mg anode passivation by forming a solid electrolyte interface (SEI) layer on the surface of the Mg anode that facilitates $Mg^{2+}$ conduction, which provides a straightforward and effective strategy for integrating magnesium anodes with diverse organic and conversion materials in non-nucleophilic electrolyte environments [124]. An ideal solvent system for developing high-performance MIBs must simultaneously exhibit high solubility for magnesium salts and provide effective protection for magnesium metal. Meeting these criteria with a single solvent proves challenging. Diethyl malonate (DEM) is frequently utilized to enhance the dissociation of magnesium salts through multidentate coordination with $Mg^{2+}$ cations, which facilitates ion dissociation and migration under an electric field. In contrast, cyclic ethers aid in the formation of protective films on metal anodes via ring-opening reactions. By harnessing the advantages of both types of solvents, a solution composed of non-nucleophilic $Mg(TFSI)_2$-$MgCl_2$ in DME, dispersed within a non-fluorinated, weakly coordinating solvent such as THF, can effectively prevent the decomposition of DME while establishing a stable SEI. The dimethyl ether solvation shell, characterized by its migratory components, is surrounded by weakly coordinated cyclic ethers, which facilitates SEI formation without inducing ion binding. Compared to DME alone, the mixed solvent system exhibits a slightly reduced solvation capacity, thereby ensuring compatibility with $Mg^{2+}$ without compromising coordination efficiency [125].

To avoid the issues associated with Grignard-based liquid electrolytes, many new liquid electrolytes have been proposed, such as organoborate-based electrolytes, borohydride-based electrolytes, nitrogen-containing electrolytes, magnesium aluminate chloride complex electrolytes, $Mg(TFSI)_2$-based electrolytes, and ionic liquid electrolytes [116,126]. However, there is still no mature electrolyte system for Mg-ion batteries.

Hence, constructing the artificial SEI on the anode surface can bypass the issues inherent in the electrolyte. An artificial SEI layer can be formed on the surface of the magnesium anode through a displacement reaction involving $ZnCl_2$ and metallic Mg. Due to the higher equilibrium electrode potential of zinc compared to magnesium ($E_{Zn^{2+}/Zn} = -0.763$ V vs. SHE, $E_{Mg^{2+}/Mg} = -2.3$ V vs. SHE), $ZnCl_2$ readily undergoes a substitution reaction with metallic Mg ($ZnCl_2 + Mg \rightarrow MgCl_2 + Zn$). This reaction is exothermic ($\Delta H_{rxn} = -102$ kJ/mol), indicating its spontaneity. As the reaction proceeds, an SEI layer incorporating an $MgZn_2$ alloy is formed. This alloy induces a significant number of tilted grain boundaries on the magnesium surface, which symmetrically lowers the reaction barriers for both anode and cathode processes, thereby enhancing the exchange current density [127].

Similarly, inorganic, organic and composite SEIs are all investigated by researchers. SEIs containing magnesium fluoride ($MgF_2$), which control the reaction of the Mg metal surface with hydrofluoric acid (HF), can not only suppress the side reaction with the electrolyte but also allow for the generation of $Mg^{2+}$ transport between electrodes and electrolytes, as shown in Figure 7a [128]. Another artificial interface composed of Mg powder, $Mg(CF_3SO_3)_2$, polyacrylonitrile (PAN), and carbon black is compatible even within the carbonate-based electrolyte [129]. Figure 7b illustrates that this artificial interface delivers a moderate ionic conductivity and a low electronic conductivity, which could promote Mg stripping/plating reversibility and prevent electrolyte reduction. Moreover, a 3D SEI with $Mg_3Bi_2$ scaffolds on the Mg anode surface is designed to avoid continuous passivation and to mitigate the degradation of the SEI [130]. Bi is a good candidate of anodes due to its excellent electrochemical properties, despite its price [131]. The 3D $Mg_3Bi_2$ scaffolds possess large specific surface areas, thereby greatly reducing the current density, and the continuous passivation is avoided. Another Bi-based artificial protecting layer on Mg metal anodes was designed via a facile solution strategy [132,133]. In $Mg(TFSI)_2$-based electrolytes, this artificial layer could avoid parasitic reactions, while in APC electrolytes, this protective layer could facilitate Mg-atom adsorption and diffusion. An Sb-based artificial interface layer mainly containing $MgCl_2$ and $Mg_3Sb_2$ endows the significantly improved interfacial kinetics and electrochemical performance of the Mg anode, which significantly reduces overpotential and enables swift $Mg^{2+}$ migration, as shown in Figure 7c [134]. By simply soaking Mg foil in a tetraethylene glycol dimethyl ether solution containing LiTFSI and $AlCl_3$, an artificial SEI is constructed, which could mitigate Mg passivation in $Mg(TFSI)_2$/DME electrolytes. This approach is also extended to $Mg(ClO_4)_2$/DME and $Mg(TFSI)_2$/PC electrolytes to achieve reversible Mg plating and stripping, which also ensures the interfacial resistance of the cells, with the SEI protected by Mg two orders of magnitude lower than bare Mg [135]. An artificial SEI coating composed of $MgBr_2$, $MgI_2$, and Sb on the Mg surface through an off-site displacement reaction can enhance the reversible deposition and dissolution of $Mg^{2+}$, significantly reduce overpotential, and achieve superior specific capacity retention with lower polarization across the entire battery. Calculations reveal that the diffusion energy barriers for $Mg^{2+}$ in Sb, $MgBr_2$, and $MgI_2$ are 1.72 eV, 0.41 eV, and 0.18 eV, respectively, indicating that the SEI layer effectively facilitates ion conduction [136].

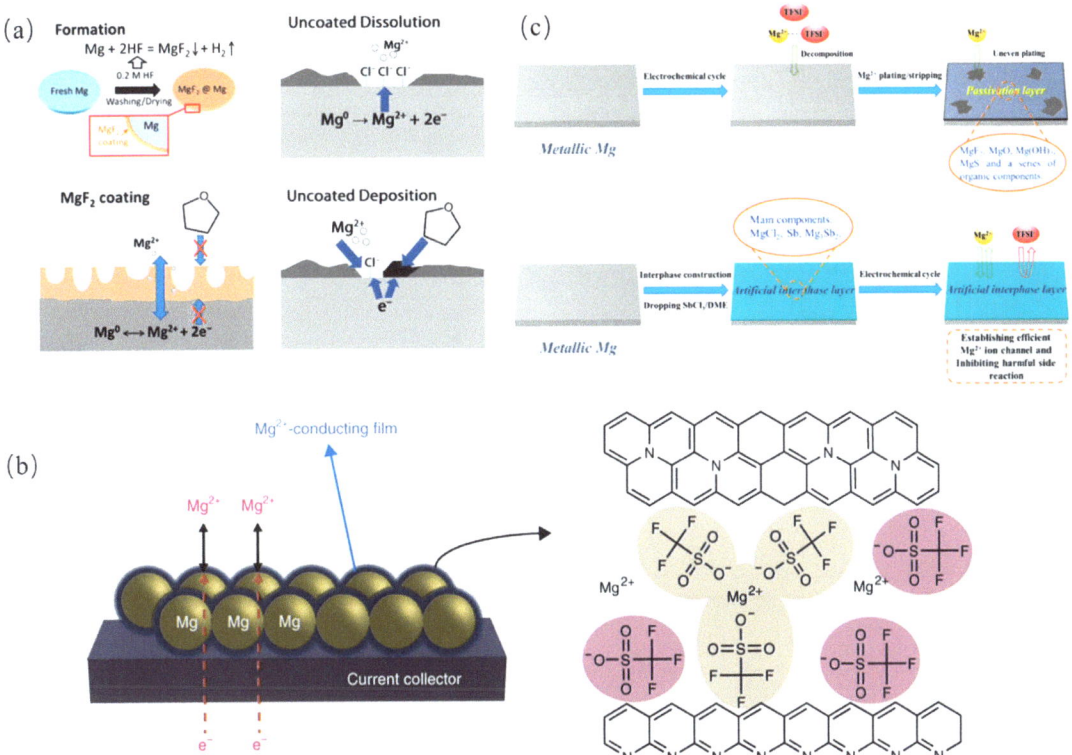

**Figure 7.** (**a**) Schematic illustration of the formation process of the MgF$_2$ surface coating and surface chemistry of coated/uncoated Mg anode [128]. (**b**) Schematic of a Mg powder electrode coated with the artificial Mg$^{2+}$-conducting interface, and the proposed structure for the artificial Mg$^{2+}$-conducting interface [129]. (**c**) Schematic diagrams of electrochemical behavior of pristine Mg anode and modified Mg anode [134].

An organic SEI is designed using the dynamic self-assembly coordination of phytic acid (PA) with Mg$^{2+}$. Figure 8a shows that the 3D porous channel structure of the PA skeleton could regulate ion flux and efficiently homogenize the distribution of Mg$^{2+}$ [137]. Through the drip-coating method, a polymer-alloy composite SEI is constructed on the Mg surface, with a polymerized tetrahydrofuran (PTHF) network cross-linked with Mg-Cl and Sn-Cl complexes and a metallic layer with Sn and Mg-Sn domains from top to bottom. The upper PTHF network with rich Mg-Cl moieties facilitates fast Mg-ion transport and its flux homogenization, while the lower Sn-based magnesophilic domains provide abundant Mg deposition sites with low nucleation and migration barriers, ensuring uniform Mg plating and stripping [138]. Using a solvent-assisted additive displacement strategy, another composite SEI with a low surface composed of an MgCl$_2$-rich top layer and an organosilicon-dominated bottom layer is designed, which can withstand long-term anode cycling and permanently protect the Mg anode against passivation in conventional electrolytes, as shown in Figure 8b [139]. An SEI composed of amorphous an MgCl$_2$@polymer on the Mg-metal surface is prepared by the in situ chemical reaction of metallic Mg with H$_3$PO$_4$ and SiCl$_4$ in sequence, which can effectively inhibit electrolyte decomposition and facilitate Mg$^{2+}$ transport [136]. Incorporating Aquivion and SPEEK polymers into polyacrylonitrile (PAN) can also create an organic artificial SEI on Mg metal foil. Unlike inorganic SEI layers, this polymer/ionic organic SEI layer mitigates severe surface reactions that lead to the formation of macroscopic pores and localized coating failures during cell operation. Consequently, the Mg-S battery constructed using this approach exhibits high initial-cycle Coulombic efficiency and maintains a high discharge capacity over cycling [136].

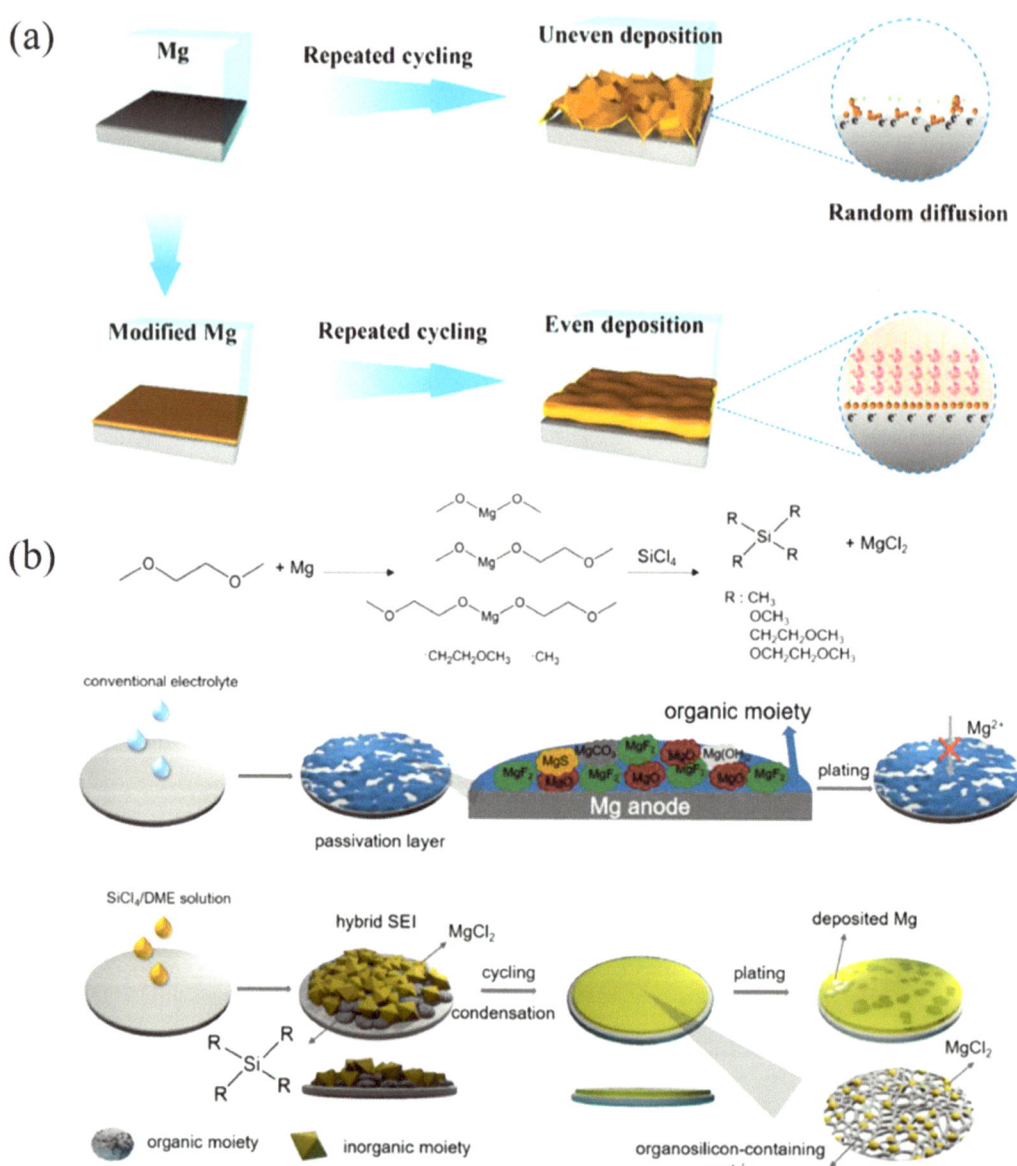

**Figure 8.** (**a**) Scheme illustrations for interface reactions with and without PA artificial SEI layers on the Mg surface [137]. (**b**) Possible mechanism on the solvent-assisted additive displacement strategy and the formation of inorganic/organic hybrid SEI after the contact of Mg surface with $SiCl_4$/DME solution. Schematic diagrams of SEI evolution and Mg deposition manner based on bare Mg electrode and Mg-Si electrode in conventional electrolyte [139].

Moreover, the Mg-Li alloy exhibits unique SEI characteristics in magnesium-based battery systems. Due to the electrochemical differences between magnesium and lithium, the alloying process on the electrode surface leads to the formation of a more stable SEI layer. Compared to pure magnesium electrodes, the SEI layer on Mg-Li alloys typically shows enhanced stability and ionic conductivity. This is primarily because the SEI layer contains lithium/magnesium compounds, which effectively prevent further side reactions between magnesium ions and the electrolyte, thereby reducing corrosion and improving the cycling stability. Furthermore, the incorporation of lithium modifies the interfacial structure of the magnesium electrode, facilitating the reversible insertion and extraction of magnesium ions and ultimately enhancing the overall electrochemical performance. A robust SEI layer that develops on the surface of the Li-Mg alloy anode can effectively mitigate the side reactions and preserve surface smoothness throughout cycling. The Li-deficient Li-Mg alloy forms a porous skeletal structure that facilitates both electron and Li-ion conduction, ensuring the structural integrity of the anode during the Li/Mg stripping/plating process [140]. A magnesium-lithium alloy has been identified as a passivation-free anode, effectively preventing passivation reactions through a substitution mechanism between lithium in the alloy and magnesium ions in the electrolyte. This alloy anode demonstrates significantly enhanced interfacial reaction kinetics, with an impedance reduction of five orders of magnitude compared to that of a magnesium anode [141,142].

In summary, the SEI construction strategies can be classified as solvent shell structure alteration, electrolyte additives, electrode modification, artificial SEI, in situ SEI formation via spontaneous reactions, etc. The characteristics of each method are summarized in Table 1. The challenges of the construction strategies limit their wide utilizations and become the focus of the SEI research.

Table 1. The characteristics of SEI construction strategies.

| Method | Description | Key Advantages | Challenges | Impact on SEI Performance |
|---|---|---|---|---|
| Solvent Shell Structure Alteration [22,23] | Altering solvent shell structures around ions in the electrolyte to form a more stable SEI | Improved control over SEI composition | Requires precise solvent system design to balance ion transport and SEI stability | Alters SEI formation by controlling ion solvation, leading to more uniform and protective SEI layers |
| Electrolyte Additives [89,90] | Introducing additives to the electrolyte to enhance SEI formation | Low-cost, easily adaptable | Additives may decompose, leading to impurities or unwanted reactions | Enhances stability and conductivity by promoting favorable SEI compounds |
| Electrode Modification [18,115] | Interlayer the electrodes to reduce the volume change of the electrode | Enhances electrode stability | Requires complex processing | Produces a stable, uniform SEI by modifying the electrode surface to encourage better electrolyte interaction |
| Artificial SEI [135,139] | Pre-fabricated SEI films applied to the electrode to control initial SEI formation | Highly tunable and can be designed for specific ion transport properties | Complicated fabrication process | Artificial SEIs can be customized for high stability and conductivity, suppressing dendrites and improving performance |
| In situ SEI Formation via Spontaneous Reactions [136] | SEI forms spontaneously during cycling from electrolyte decomposition | Simple process, naturally conforms to electrode surface | Often uncontrolled and result in non-uniform SEI | In-situ formed SEI layers may be thicker and less uniform, resulting in slower ion transport |

## 5. Summary and Perspectives

This review aims to clarify the basic understanding of the electrochemical processes, influencing factors, and multiple approaches to constructing a stable SEI. The basic formation mechanism of SEIs is now explained well by molecular orbital theory, while the explanation of redox reaction processes remains ambiguous. The intrinsic properties of electrolytes and electrodes, as well as external factors such as temperature and current density, affect formation and evolution, which also signals to researchers to construct SEIs with good stability and ionic conductivity by modifying electrolytes and electrodes or controlling experimental conditions. The SEI in two battery systems—Li-ion batteries and Mg-ion batteries—is reviewed in detail.

The research history of Li-ion batteries is much longer than that of Mg-ion batteries. Most of the SEI construction ideas in Mg-ion batteries come from the work of Li-ion batteries, which makes the SEI construction strategies in the two battery systems very similar, including electrolyte modification and artificial SEI construction. There are two methods widely used in both Li-ion batteries and Mg-ion batteries. Electrolyte modification not only helps in constructing an ideal SEI but also improves the intrinsic property of the electrolyte. Since the electrolyte system in Li-ion batteries is quite mature, the focus of electrolyte modification is on the additive. On the contrary, in Mg-ion batteries, there is still no satisfactory electrolyte, and the focus shifts to developing an ideal electrolyte system rather than additives. On the other hand, in situ artificial SEI construction attracts more and more attention due to its good adhesion and customization, despite the high cost and mass production problem, which hinders commercial applications.

However, the functionality of SEI construction in the two batteries is different, which causes the strategic focus to differ. The main purpose of the SEI in an Li-ion battery is suppressing dendrite growth, while in an magnesium-ion battery, the focus of SEI construction is to suppress the passivation film and improve ion transport. Therefore, when constructing the SEI in an Li-ion battery, the stiffness of the SEI is a primary concern. It is preferred to construct inorganic compounds and ceramics in the SEI. On the contrary, when constructing the SEI in an Mg-ion battery, the key point is to improve the ionic conductivity of the interface. Since the Mg anode is believed to be a dendrite-free anode and simple Mg salts have lower ionic conductivity than their Li salt counterparts, polymer and other organic compounds are used to construct the SEI. Another difference is that Mg alloys are considered not only as anodes but also as components of the SEI due to good conductivity and stability, while few Li alloys are discussed in the literature. In summary, the SEI construction strategies and technologies are quite similar in the two battery systems. The different concerns and requirements lead to different choices of materials and compositions of SEIs.

Although considerable research has been conducted, there is still no satisfactory way to construct a mature SEI due to the following challenges. The understanding of SEI formation, in terms of the reaction kinetics and mechanisms, composition, and role in battery performance is insufficient. Moreover, a deeper understanding of the fluctuating local current density distribution regarding ion deposition nucleation and further growth is lacking. The characterization technologies, especially the in situ characterization, still has many shortcomings, which hinders its wide application in the study of the SEI. For example, the current distribution and electric field gradient in an in situ electrochemical cell are different from those in coin batteries or commercial batteries. In situ electrochemical cells are limited by their electrolyte volume, which cannot measure the size effect of the electrodes on the electric field distribution in the electrolyte. Hence, in situ characterization currently has difficulty directly reflecting the same process in coin batteries and commercial batteries.

On the other hand, these issues also guide us in overcoming the challenges. Several future research directions may be proposed as follows.

QC/AIMD/DFT calculations should be promising methods for SEI modeling. With the optimization of computing software and the improvements in computing capability, the multi-scale and full-scale modeling of SEIs have been gradually implemented. The influence of geometry on local current density and deposition behavior can be further investigated. The current is affected by the uneven geometry, causing inconsistent current density, which significantly impacts deposition behavior. Thus, quantitatively analyzing the current at the interface is essential to understanding deposition behavior.

New advanced in situ characterization methods can be further developed. The size of current in situ electrochemical cells limits the full understanding of the performance of materials. Local performance or behavior can even mislead our understanding. The study of the impact of multi-physics coupling on material performance is also limited by the current in situ characterization hardware. Advanced in situ characterization methods can ensure the accuracy of experimental results and provide new insights into the SEI working mechanism.

In this review, we address the issues related to the SEIs of LIBs and MIBs. Meanwhile, the factors affecting SEI construction are explained. The strategies for constructing the SEI on the anode are also discussed through case studies. In view of the interfacial complexity, only small aspects of these issues have been solved under specific conditions. Many phenomena remain unresolved and not yet fully understood. The treatment of the interface and the characterization of the SEI can provide adequate explanations and help construct better SEIs in batteries.

**Funding:** This research was funded by [Chongqing Postdoctoral Research Special Funding] grant number [2021XM2002], [Natural Science Foundation of Chongqing] grant number [cstc2021jcyj-msxmX0086], and [Chongqing Innovative Project for oversea-experience researchers] grant number [cx2023037].

**Conflicts of Interest:** The authors declare no conflicts of interest.

# References

1. Ding, Z.; Li, H.; Shaw, L. New insights into the solid-state hydrogen storage of nanostructured LiBH$_4$-MgH$_2$ system. *Chem. Eng. J.* **2020**, *385*, 123856. [CrossRef]
2. Guo, Q.; Zeng, W.; Liu, S.-L.; Li, Y.-Q.; Xu, J.-Y.; Wang, J.-X.; Wang, Y. Recent developments on anode materials for magnesium-ion batteries: A review. *Rare Met.* **2021**, *40*, 290–308. [CrossRef]
3. Liu, C.; Neale, Z.G.; Cao, G. Understanding electrochemical potentials of cathode materials in rechargeable batteries. *Mater. Today* **2016**, *19*, 109–123. [CrossRef]
4. Gao, Y.; Du, X.; Hou, Z.; Shen, X.; Mai, Y.-W.; Tarascon, J.-M.; Zhang, B. Unraveling the mechanical origin of stable solid electrolyte interphase. *Joule* **2021**, *5*, 1860–1872. [CrossRef]
5. Pokharel, J.; Cresce, A.; Pant, B.; Yang, M.Y.; Gurung, A.; He, W.; Baniya, A.; Lamsal, B.S.; Yang, Z.; Gent, S.; et al. Manipulating the diffusion energy barrier at the lithium metal electrolyte interface for dendrite-free long-life batteries. *Nat. Commun.* **2024**, *15*, 3085. [CrossRef] [PubMed]
6. Dey, A.N.; Sullivan, B.P. The Electrochemical Decomposition of Propylene Carbonate on Graphite. *J. Electrochem. Soc.* **1970**, *117*, 222. [CrossRef]
7. Peled, E. The Electrochemical Behavior of Alkali and Alkaline Earth Metals in Nonaqueous Battery Systems—The Solid Electrolyte Interphase Model. *J. Electrochem. Soc.* **1979**, *126*, 2047. [CrossRef]
8. Nazri, G.; Muller, R.H. In Situ X-ray Diffraction of Surface Layers on Lithium in Nonaqueous Electrolyte. *J. Electrochem. Soc.* **1985**, *132*, 1385. [CrossRef]
9. Fong, R.; von Sacken, U.; Dahn, J.R. Studies of Lithium Intercalation into Carbons Using Nonaqueous Electrochemical Cells. *J. Electrochem. Soc.* **1990**, *137*, 2009. [CrossRef]
10. Kanamura, K.; Tamura, H.; Shiraishi, S.; Takehara, Z.I. XPS Analysis of Lithium Surfaces Following Immersion in Various Solvents Containing LiBF4. *J. Electrochem. Soc.* **1995**, *142*, 340. [CrossRef]
11. Peled, E.; Golodnitsky, D.; Ardel, G. Advanced Model for Solid Electrolyte Interphase Electrodes in Liquid and Polymer Electrolytes. *J. Electrochem. Soc.* **1997**, *144*, L208. [CrossRef]
12. Aurbach, D.; Markovsky, B.; Levi, M.D.; Levi, E.; Schechter, A.; Moshkovich, M.; Cohen, Y. New insights into the interactions between electrode materials and electrolyte solutions for advanced nonaqueous batteries. *J. Power Sources* **1999**, *81–82*, 95–111. [CrossRef]
13. Wang, Y.; Nakamura, S.; Ue, M.; Balbuena, P.B. Theoretical Studies To Understand Surface Chemistry on Carbon Anodes for Lithium-Ion Batteries: Reduction Mechanisms of Ethylene Carbonate. *J. Am. Chem. Soc.* **2001**, *123*, 11708–11718. [CrossRef] [PubMed]
14. Xu, K.; von Cresce, A.; Lee, U. Differentiating Contributions to "Ion Transfer" Barrier from Interphasial Resistance and Li+ Desolvation at Electrolyte/Graphite Interface. *Langmuir* **2010**, *26*, 11538–11543. [CrossRef] [PubMed]
15. Li, Y.; Li, Y.; Pei, A.; Yan, K.; Sun, Y.; Wu, C.-L.; Joubert, L.-M.; Chin, R.; Koh, A.L.; Yu, Y.; et al. Atomic structure of sensitive battery materials and interfaces revealed by cryo–electron microscopy. *Science* **2017**, *358*, 506–510. [CrossRef]

16. Ma, C.; Xu, F.; Song, T. Dual-Layered Interfacial Evolution of Lithium Metal Anode: SEI Analysis via TOF-SIMS Technology. *ACS Appl. Mater. Interfaces* **2022**, *14*, 20197–20207. [CrossRef]
17. Peljo, P.; Girault, H.H. Electrochemical potential window of battery electrolytes: The HOMO–LUMO misconception. *Energy Environ. Sci.* **2018**, *11*, 2306–2309. [CrossRef]
18. Wu, Y.; Wang, C.; Wang, C.; Zhang, Y.; Liu, J.; Jin, Y.; Wang, H.; Zhang, Q. Recent progress in SEI engineering for boosting Li metal anodes. *Mater. Horiz.* **2024**, *11*, 388–407. [CrossRef]
19. Peled, E.; Menkin, S. Review—SEI: Past, Present and Future. *J. Electrochem. Soc.* **2017**, *164*, A1703–A1719. [CrossRef]
20. Gao, T.; Hou, S.; Huynh, K.; Wang, F.; Eidson, N.; Fan, X.; Han, F.; Luo, C.; Mao, M.; Li, X.; et al. Existence of Solid Electrolyte Interphase in Mg Batteries: Mg/S Chemistry as an Example. *ACS Appl. Mater. Interfaces* **2018**, *10*, 14767–14776. [CrossRef]
21. Soto, F.A.; Ma, Y.; Martinez de la Hoz, J.M.; Seminario, J.M.; Balbuena, P.B. Formation and Growth Mechanisms of Solid-Electrolyte Interphase Layers in Rechargeable Batteries. *Chem. Mater.* **2015**, *27*, 7990–8000. [CrossRef]
22. Single, F.; Latz, A.; Horstmann, B. Identifying the Mechanism of Continued Growth of the Solid-Electrolyte Interphase. *ChemSusChem* **2018**, *11*, 1950–1955. [CrossRef] [PubMed]
23. Horstmann, B.; Single, F.; Latz, A. Review on multi-scale models of solid-electrolyte interphase formation. *Curr. Opin. Electrochem.* **2019**, *13*, 61–69. [CrossRef]
24. Popovic, J. Solid Electrolyte Interphase Growth on Mg Metal Anode: Case Study of Glyme-Based Electrolytes. *Energy Technol.* **2021**, *9*, 2001056. [CrossRef]
25. Beheshti, S.H.; Javanbakht, M.; Omidvar, H.; Hosen, M.S.; Hubin, A.; Van Mierlo, J.; Berecibar, M. Development, retainment, and assessment of the graphite-electrolyte interphase in Li-ion batteries regarding the functionality of SEI-forming additives. *iScience* **2022**, *25*, 103862. [CrossRef]
26. Dedryvère, R.; Gireaud, L.; Grugeon, S.; Laruelle, S.; Tarascon, J.M.; Gonbeau, D. Characterization of Lithium Alkyl Carbonates by X-ray Photoelectron Spectroscopy: Experimental and Theoretical Study. *J. Phys. Chem. B* **2005**, *109*, 15868–15875. [CrossRef]
27. Dedryvère, R.; Leroy, S.; Martinez, H.; Blanchard, F.; Lemordant, D.; Gonbeau, D. XPS Valence Characterization of Lithium Salts as a Tool to Study Electrode/Electrolyte Interfaces of Li-Ion Batteries. *J. Phys. Chem. B* **2006**, *110*, 12986–12992. [CrossRef]
28. Nie, M.; Chalasani, D.; Abraham, D.P.; Chen, Y.; Bose, A.; Lucht, B.L. Lithium Ion Battery Graphite Solid Electrolyte Interphase Revealed by Microscopy and Spectroscopy. *J. Phys. Chem. C* **2013**, *117*, 1257–1267. [CrossRef]
29. Marom, R.; Haik, O.; Aurbach, D.; Halalay, I.C. Revisiting LiClO4 as an Electrolyte for Rechargeable Lithium-Ion Batteries. *J. Electrochem. Soc.* **2010**, *157*, A972. [CrossRef]
30. Tsubouchi, S.; Domi, Y.; Doi, T.; Ochida, M.; Nakagawa, H.; Yamanaka, T.; Abe, T.; Ogumi, Z. Spectroscopic Characterization of Surface Films Formed on Edge Plane Graphite in Ethylene Carbonate-Based Electrolytes Containing Film-Forming Additives. *J. Electrochem. Soc.* **2012**, *159*, A1786. [CrossRef]
31. Xu, K.; Zhuang, G.V.; Allen, J.L.; Lee, U.; Zhang, S.S.; Ross, P.N., Jr.; Jow, T.R. Syntheses and Characterization of Lithium Alkyl Mono- and Dicarbonates as Components of Surface Films in Li-Ion Batteries. *J. Phys. Chem. B* **2006**, *110*, 7708–7719. [CrossRef] [PubMed]
32. Zhuang, G.V.; Yang, H.; Ross, P.N.; Xu, K.; Jow, T.R. Lithium Methyl Carbonate as a Reaction Product of Metallic Lithium and Dimethyl Carbonate. *Electrochem. Solid-State Lett.* **2006**, *9*, A64. [CrossRef]
33. Collins, J.; Gourdin, G.; Foster, M.; Qu, D. Carbon surface functionalities and SEI formation during Li intercalation. *Carbon* **2015**, *92*, 193–244. [CrossRef]
34. Zhao, L.; Watanabe, I.; Doi, T.; Okada, S.; Yamaki, J.-I. TG-MS analysis of solid electrolyte interphase (SEI) on graphite negative-electrode in lithium-ion batteries. *J. Power Sources* **2006**, *161*, 1275–1280. [CrossRef]
35. Augustsson, A.; Herstedt, M.; Guo, J.H.; Edström, K.; Zhuang, G.V.; Ross, J.P.N.; Rubensson, J.E.; Nordgren, J. Solid electrolyte interphase on graphite Li-ion battery anodes studied by soft X-ray spectroscopy. *Phys. Chem. Chem. Phys.* **2004**, *6*, 4185–4189. [CrossRef]
36. Leifer, N.; Smart, M.C.; Prakash, G.K.S.; Gonzalez, L.; Sanchez, L.; Smith, K.A.; Bhalla, P.; Grey, C.P.; Greenbaum, S.G. 13C Solid State NMR Suggests Unusual Breakdown Products in SEI Formation on Lithium Ion Electrodes. *J. Electrochem. Soc.* **2011**, *158*, A471. [CrossRef]
37. Mantia, F.L.; Novák, P. Online Detection of Reductive $CO_2$ Development at Graphite Electrodes in the 1 M $LiPF_6$, EC:DMC Battery Electrolyte. *Electrochemical and Solid-State Letters* **2008**, *11*, A84. [CrossRef]
38. Xiao, A.; Yang, L.; Lucht, B.L.; Kang, S.-H.; Abraham, D.P. Examining the Solid Electrolyte Interphase on Binder-Free Graphite Electrodes. *J. Electrochem. Soc.* **2009**, *156*, A318. [CrossRef]
39. Onuki, M.; Kinoshita, S.; Sakata, Y.; Yanagidate, M.; Otake, Y.; Ue, M.; Deguchi, M. Identification of the Source of Evolved Gas in Li-Ion Batteries Using #2#1-labeled Solvents. *J. Electrochem. Soc.* **2008**, *155*, A794.
40. Mogi, R.; Inaba, M.; Iriyama, Y.; Abe, T.; Ogumi, Z. Study on the decomposition mechanism of alkyl carbonate on lithium metal by pyrolysis-gas chromatography-mass spectroscopy. *J. Power Sources* **2003**, *119–121*, 597–603. [CrossRef]
41. Kong, W.; Li, H.; Huang, X.; Chen, L. Gas evolution behaviors for several cathode materials in lithium-ion batteries. *J. Power Sources* **2005**, *142*, 285–291. [CrossRef]
42. Harilal, S.S.; Allain, J.P.; Hassanein, A.; Hendricks, M.R.; Nieto-Perez, M. Reactivity of lithium exposed graphite surface. *Appl. Surf. Sci.* **2009**, *255*, 8539–8543. [CrossRef]

43. Edström, K.; Herstedt, M.; Abraham, D.P. A new look at the solid electrolyte interphase on graphite anodes in Li-ion batteries. *J. Power Sources* **2006**, *153*, 380–384. [CrossRef]
44. Bryngelsson, H.; Stjerndahl, M.; Gustafsson, T.; Edström, K. How dynamic is the SEI? *J. Power Sources* **2007**, *174*, 970–975. [CrossRef]
45. Shu, J. Study of the Interface Between Li4Ti5O12 Electrodes and Standard Electrolyte Solutions in 0.0–5.0 V. *Electrochem. Solid-State Lett.* **2008**, *11*, A238. [CrossRef]
46. Ota, H.; Sakata, Y.; Inoue, A.; Yamaguchi, S. Analysis of Vinylene Carbonate Derived SEI Layers on Graphite Anode. *J. Electrochem. Soc.* **2004**, *151*, A1659. [CrossRef]
47. Tavassol, H.; Chan, M.K.Y.; Catarello, M.G.; Greeley, J.; Cahill, D.G.; Gewirth, A.A. Surface Coverage and SEI Induced Electrochemical Surface Stress Changes during Li Deposition in a Model System for Li-Ion Battery Anodes. *J. Electrochem. Soc.* **2013**, *160*, A888. [CrossRef]
48. Tavassol, H.; Buthker, J.W.; Ferguson, G.A.; Curtiss, L.A.; Gewirth, A.A. Solvent Oligomerization during SEI Formation on Model Systems for Li-Ion Battery Anodes. *J. Electrochem. Soc.* **2012**, *159*, A730. [CrossRef]
49. Shkrob, I.A.; Zhu, Y.; Marin, T.W.; Abraham, D. Reduction of Carbonate Electrolytes and the Formation of Solid-Electrolyte Interface (SEI) in Lithium-Ion Batteries. 1. Spectroscopic Observations of Radical Intermediates Generated in One-Electron Reduction of Carbonates. *J. Phys. Chem. C* **2013**, *117*, 19255–19269. [CrossRef]
50. Herstedt, M.; Abraham, D.P.; Kerr, J.B.; Edström, K. X-ray photoelectron spectroscopy of negative electrodes from high-power lithium-ion cells showing various levels of power fade. *Electrochim. Acta* **2004**, *49*, 5097–5110. [CrossRef]
51. Vetter, J.; Novák, P.; Wagner, M.R.; Veit, C.; Möller, K.C.; Besenhard, J.O.; Winter, M.; Wohlfahrt-Mehrens, M.; Vogler, C.; Hammouche, A. Ageing mechanisms in lithium-ion batteries. *J. Power Sources* **2005**, *147*, 269–281. [CrossRef]
52. Heiskanen, S.K.; Kim, J.; Lucht, B.L. Generation and Evolution of the Solid Electrolyte Interphase of Lithium-Ion Batteries. *Joule* **2019**, *3*, 2322–2333. [CrossRef]
53. Louli, A.J.; Ellis, L.D.; Dahn, J.R. Operando Pressure Measurements Reveal Solid Electrolyte Interphase Growth to Rank Li-Ion Cell Performance. *Joule* **2019**, *3*, 745–761. [CrossRef]
54. Nanda, J.; Yang, G.; Hou, T.; Voylov, D.N.; Li, X.; Ruther, R.E.; Naguib, M.; Persson, K.; Veith, G.M.; Sokolov, A.P. Unraveling the Nanoscale Heterogeneity of Solid Electrolyte Interphase Using Tip-Enhanced Raman Spectroscopy. *Joule* **2019**, *3*, 2001–2019. [CrossRef]
55. Lu, P.; Li, C.; Schneider, E.W.; Harris, S.J. Chemistry, Impedance, and Morphology Evolution in Solid Electrolyte Interphase Films during Formation in Lithium Ion Batteries. *J. Phys. Chem. C* **2014**, *118*, 896–903. [CrossRef]
56. Takenaka, N.; Suzuki, Y.; Sakai, H.; Nagaoka, M. On Electrolyte-Dependent Formation of Solid Electrolyte Interphase Film in Lithium-Ion Batteries: Strong Sensitivity to Small Structural Difference of Electrolyte Molecules. *J. Phys. Chem. C* **2014**, *118*, 10874–10882. [CrossRef]
57. Ma, Y.; Feng, L.; Tang, C.-Y.; Ouyang, J.-H.; Dillon, S.J. Effects of Commonly Evolved Solid-Electrolyte-Interphase (SEI) Reaction Product Gases on the Cycle Life of Li-Ion Full Cells. *J. Electrochem. Soc.* **2018**, *165*, A3084. [CrossRef]
58. Xiong, D.J.; Ellis, L.D.; Nelson, K.J.; Hynes, T.; Petibon, R.; Dahn, J.R. Rapid Impedance Growth and Gas Production at the Li-Ion Cell Positive Electrode in the Absence of a Negative Electrode. *J. Electrochem. Soc.* **2016**, *163*, A3069. [CrossRef]
59. Eshetu, G.G.; Diemant, T.; Hekmatfar, M.; Grugeon, S.; Behm, R.J.; Laruelle, S.; Armand, M.; Passerini, S. Impact of the electrolyte salt anion on the solid electrolyte interphase formation in sodium ion batteries. *Nano Energy* **2019**, *55*, 327–340. [CrossRef]
60. Pathan, T.S.; Rashid, M.; Walker, M.; Widanage, W.D.; Kendrick, E. Active formation of Li-ion batteries and its effect on cycle life. *J. Phys. Energy* **2019**, *1*, 044003. [CrossRef]
61. Adenusi, H.; Chass, G.A.; Passerini, S.; Tian, K.V.; Chen, G. Lithium Batteries and the Solid Electrolyte Interphase (SEI)—Progress and Outlook. *Adv. Energy Mater.* **2023**, *13*, 2203307. [CrossRef]
62. Zhuang, G.V.; Xu, K.; Yang, H.; Jow, T.R.; Ross, P.N. Lithium Ethylene Dicarbonate Identified as the Primary Product of Chemical and Electrochemical Reduction of EC in 1.2 M LiPF6/EC:EMC Electrolyte. *J. Phys. Chem. B* **2005**, *109*, 17567–17573. [CrossRef] [PubMed]
63. Aurbach, D.; Markovsky, B.; Weissman, I.; Levi, E.; Ein-Eli, Y. On the correlation between surface chemistry and performance of graphite negative electrodes for Li ion batteries. *Electrochim. Acta* **1999**, *45*, 67–86. [CrossRef]
64. Aurbach, D.; Markovsky, B.; Shechter, A.; Ein-Eli, Y.; Cohen, H. A Comparative Study of Synthetic Graphite and Li Electrodes in Electrolyte Solutions Based on Ethylene Carbonate-Dimethyl Carbonate Mixtures. *J. Electrochem. Soc.* **1996**, *143*, 3809. [CrossRef]
65. Aurbach, D.; Zaban, A.; Schechter, A.; Ein-Eli, Y.; Zinigrad, E.; Markovsky, B. The Study of Electrolyte Solutions Based on Ethylene and Diethyl Carbonates for Rechargeable Li Batteries: I. Li Metal Anodes. *J. Electrochem. Soc.* **1995**, *142*, 2873. [CrossRef]
66. Xu, K. Electrolytes and Interphases in Li-Ion Batteries and Beyond. *Chem. Rev.* **2014**, *114*, 11503–11618. [CrossRef]
67. Xing, L.; Zheng, X.; Schroeder, M.; Alvarado, J.; von Wald Cresce, A.; Xu, K.; Li, Q.; Li, W. Deciphering the Ethylene Carbonate–Propylene Carbonate Mystery in Li-Ion Batteries. *Acc. Chem. Res.* **2018**, *51*, 282–289. [CrossRef]
68. Xu, K.; Lam, Y.; Zhang, S.S.; Jow, T.R.; Curtis, T.B. Solvation Sheath of Li+ in Nonaqueous Electrolytes and Its Implication of Graphite/Electrolyte Interface Chemistry. *J. Phys. Chem. C* **2007**, *111*, 7411–7421. [CrossRef]
69. Tasaki, K.; Goldberg, A.; Winter, M. On the difference in cycling behaviors of lithium-ion battery cell between ethylene carbonate- and propylene carbonate-based electrolytes. *Electrochim. Acta* **2011**, *56*, 10424–10435. [CrossRef]

70. Jeong, S.-K.; Inaba, M.; Iriyama, Y.; Abe, T.; Ogumi, Z. Interfacial reactions between graphite electrodes and propylene carbonate-based solutions: Electrolyte-concentration dependence of electrochemical lithium intercalation reaction. *J. Power Sources* **2008**, *175*, 540–546. [CrossRef]
71. Zhuang, G.V.; Yang, H.; Blizanac, B.; Ross, P.N. A Study of Electrochemical Reduction of Ethylene and Propylene Carbonate Electrolytes on Graphite Using ATR-FTIR Spectroscopy. *Electrochem. Solid-State Lett.* **2005**, *8*, A441. [CrossRef]
72. Wu, J.; Ihsan-Ul-Haq, M.; Chen, Y.; Kim, J.-K. Understanding solid electrolyte interphases: Advanced characterization techniques and theoretical simulations. *Nano Energy* **2021**, *89*, 106489. [CrossRef]
73. Wu, H.; Jia, H.; Wang, C.; Zhang, J.-G.; Xu, W. Recent Progress in Understanding Solid Electrolyte Interphase on Lithium Metal Anodes. *Adv. Energy Mater.* **2021**, *11*, 2003092. [CrossRef]
74. Joho, F.; Rykart, B.; Blome, A.; Novák, P.; Wilhelm, H.; Spahr, M.E. Relation between surface properties, pore structure and first-cycle charge loss of graphite as negative electrode in lithium-ion batteries. *J. Power Sources* **2001**, *97–98*, 78–82. [CrossRef]
75. Winter, M.; Novák, P.; Monnier, A. Graphites for Lithium-Ion Cells: The Correlation of the First-Cycle Charge Loss with the Brunauer-Emmett-Teller Surface Area. *J. Electrochem. Soc.* **1998**, *145*, 428. [CrossRef]
76. Zheng, T.; Gozdz, A.S.; Amatucci, G.G. Reactivity of the Solid Electrolyte Interface on Carbon Electrodes at Elevated Temperatures. *J. Electrochem. Soc.* **1999**, *146*, 4014. [CrossRef]
77. An, S.J.; Li, J.; Daniel, C.; Mohanty, D.; Nagpure, S.; Wood, D.L. The state of understanding of the lithium-ion-battery graphite solid electrolyte interphase (SEI) and its relationship to formation cycling. *Carbon* **2016**, *105*, 52–76. [CrossRef]
78. Verma, P.; Maire, P.; Novák, P. A review of the features and analyses of the solid electrolyte interphase in Li-ion batteries. *Electrochim. Acta* **2010**, *55*, 6332–6341. [CrossRef]
79. Gauthier, M.; Carney, T.J.; Grimaud, A.; Giordano, L.; Pour, N.; Chang, H.-H.; Fenning, D.P.; Lux, S.F.; Paschos, O.; Bauer, C.; et al. Electrode–Electrolyte Interface in Li-Ion Batteries: Current Understanding and New Insights. *J. Phys. Chem. Lett.* **2015**, *6*, 4653–4672. [CrossRef]
80. Xiong, R.; Pan, Y.; Shen, W.; Li, H.; Sun, F. Lithium-ion battery aging mechanisms and diagnosis method for automotive applications: Recent advances and perspectives. *Renew. Sustain. Energy Rev.* **2020**, *131*, 110048. [CrossRef]
81. Ning, G.; Haran, B.; Popov, B.N. Capacity fade study of lithium-ion batteries cycled at high discharge rates. *J. Power Sources* **2003**, *117*, 160–169. [CrossRef]
82. Waldmann, T.; Wilka, M.; Kasper, M.; Fleischhammer, M.; Wohlfahrt-Mehrens, M. Temperature dependent ageing mechanisms in Lithium-ion batteries—A Post-Mortem study. *J. Power Sources* **2014**, *262*, 129–135. [CrossRef]
83. Piao, Z.; Gao, R.; Liu, Y.; Zhou, G.; Cheng, H.-M. A Review on Regulating Li+ Solvation Structures in Carbonate Electrolytes for Lithium Metal Batteries. *Adv. Mater.* **2023**, *35*, 2206009. [CrossRef] [PubMed]
84. Zhang, J.; Li, Q.; Zeng, Y.; Tang, Z.; Sun, D.; Huang, D.; Peng, Z.; Tang, Y.; Wang, H. Non-flammable ultralow concentration mixed ether electrolyte for advanced lithium metal batteries. *Energy Storage Mater.* **2022**, *51*, 660–670. [CrossRef]
85. Zhang, W.; Guo, Y.; Yang, T.; Wang, Y.; Kong, X.; Liao, X.; Zhao, Y. High voltage and robust lithium metal battery enabled by highly-fluorinated interphases. *Energy Storage Mater.* **2022**, *51*, 317–326. [CrossRef]
86. Shi, J.; Xu, C.; Lai, J.; Li, Z.; Zhang, Y.; Liu, Y.; Ding, K.; Cai, Y.-P.; Shang, R.; Zheng, Q. An Amphiphilic Molecule-Regulated Core-Shell-Solvation Electrolyte for Li-Metal Batteries at Ultra-Low Temperature. *Angew. Chem. Int. Ed.* **2023**, *62*, e202218151. [CrossRef]
87. Zhao, Y.; Zhou, T.; Mensi, M.; Choi, J.W.; Coskun, A. Electrolyte engineering via ether solvent fluorination for developing stable non-aqueous lithium metal batteries. *Nat. Commun.* **2023**, *14*, 299. [CrossRef]
88. Fan, X.; Chen, L.; Borodin, O.; Ji, X.; Chen, J.; Hou, S.; Deng, T.; Zheng, J.; Yang, C.; Liou, S.-C.; et al. Non-flammable electrolyte enables Li-metal batteries with aggressive cathode chemistries. *Nat. Nanotechnol.* **2018**, *13*, 715–722. [CrossRef]
89. Zhang, X.-Q.; Cheng, X.-B.; Chen, X.; Yan, C.; Zhang, Q. Fluoroethylene Carbonate Additives to Render Uniform Li Deposits in Lithium Metal Batteries. *Adv. Funct. Mater.* **2017**, *27*, 1605989. [CrossRef]
90. Guo, L.; Huang, F.; Cai, M.; Zhang, J.; Ma, G.; Xu, S. Organic–Inorganic Hybrid SEI Induced by a New Lithium Salt for High-Performance Metallic Lithium Anodes. *ACS Appl. Mater. Interfaces* **2021**, *13*, 32886–32893. [CrossRef]
91. Wang, C.; Fu, X.; Ying, C.; Liu, J.; Zhong, W.-H. Natural protein as novel additive of a commercial electrolyte for Long-Cycling lithium metal batteries. *Chem. Eng. J.* **2022**, *437*, 135283. [CrossRef]
92. Wu, W.; Luo, W.; Huang, Y. Less is more: A perspective on thinning lithium metal towards high-energy-density rechargeable lithium batteries. *Chem. Soc. Rev.* **2023**, *52*, 2553–2572. [CrossRef]
93. Luo, C.; Hu, H.; Zhang, T.; Wen, S.; Wang, R.; An, Y.; Chi, S.-S.; Wang, J.; Wang, C.; Chang, J.; et al. Roll-To-Roll Fabrication of Zero-Volume-Expansion Lithium-Composite Anodes to Realize High-Energy-Density Flexible and Stable Lithium-Metal Batteries. *Adv. Mater.* **2022**, *34*, 2205677. [CrossRef]
94. Zhang, D.; Wang, S.; Li, B.; Gong, Y.; Yang, S. Horizontal Growth of Lithium on Parallelly Aligned MXene Layers towards Dendrite-Free Metallic Lithium Anodes. *Adv. Mater.* **2019**, *31*, 1901820. [CrossRef]
95. Zhang, B.; Ju, Z.; Xie, Q.; Luo, J.; Du, L.; Zhang, C.; Tao, X. Ti3CNTx MXene/rGO scaffolds directing the formation of a robust, layered SEI toward high-rate and long-cycle lithium metal batteries. *Energy Storage Mater.* **2023**, *58*, 322–331. [CrossRef]
96. Chazalviel, J.N. Electrochemical aspects of the generation of ramified metallic electrodeposits. *Phys. Rev. A* **1990**, *42*, 7355–7367. [CrossRef]

97. Monroe, C.; Newman, J. Dendrite Growth in Lithium/Polymer Systems: A Propagation Model for Liquid Electrolytes under Galvanostatic Conditions. *J. Electrochem. Soc.* **2003**, *150*, A1377. [CrossRef]
98. Chen, X.-R.; Yao, Y.-X.; Yan, C.; Zhang, R.; Cheng, X.-B.; Zhang, Q. A Diffusion–Reaction Competition Mechanism to Tailor Lithium Deposition for Lithium-Metal Batteries. *Angew. Chem. Int. Ed.* **2020**, *59*, 7743–7747. [CrossRef]
99. Chen, L.; Zhang, H.W.; Liang, L.Y.; Liu, Z.; Qi, Y.; Lu, P.; Chen, J.; Chen, L.-Q. Modulation of dendritic patterns during electrodeposition: A nonlinear phase-field model. *J. Power Sources* **2015**, *300*, 376–385. [CrossRef]
100. Chen, C.; Liang, Q.; Wang, G.; Liu, D.; Xiong, X. Grain-Boundary-Rich Artificial SEI Layer for High-Rate Lithium Metal Anodes. *Adv. Funct. Mater.* **2022**, *32*, 2107249. [CrossRef]
101. Ramasubramanian, A.; Yurkiv, V.; Foroozan, T.; Ragone, M.; Shahbazian-Yassar, R.; Mashayek, F. Lithium Diffusion Mechanism through Solid–Electrolyte Interphase in Rechargeable Lithium Batteries. *J. Phys. Chem. C* **2019**, *123*, 10237–10245. [CrossRef]
102. Sun, J.; Zhang, S.; Li, J.; Xie, B.; Ma, J.; Dong, S.; Cui, G. Robust Transport: An Artificial Solid Electrolyte Interphase Design for Anode-Free Lithium-Metal Batteries. *Adv. Mater.* **2023**, *35*, 2209404. [CrossRef]
103. Di, J.; Yang, J.-L.; Tian, H.; Ren, P.; Deng, Y.; Tang, W.; Yan, W.; Liu, R.; Ma, J. Dendrites-Free Lithium Metal Anode Enabled by Synergistic Surface Structural Engineering. *Adv. Funct. Mater.* **2022**, *32*, 2200474. [CrossRef]
104. Kang, D.; Sardar, S.; Zhang, R.; Noam, H.; Chen, J.; Ma, L.; Liang, W.; Shi, C.; Lemmon, J.P. In-situ organic SEI layer for dendrite-free lithium metal anode. *Energy Storage Mater.* **2020**, *27*, 69–77. [CrossRef]
105. Zhong, Y.; Chen, Y.; Cheng, Y.; Fan, Q.; Zhao, H.; Shao, H.; Lai, Y.; Shi, Z.; Ke, X.; Guo, Z. Li Alginate-Based Artificial SEI Layer for Stable Lithium Metal Anodes. *ACS Appl. Mater. Interfaces* **2019**, *11*, 37726–37731. [CrossRef]
106. Wu, Q.; Zheng, Y.; Guan, X.; Xu, J.; Cao, F.; Li, C. Dynamical SEI Reinforced by Open-Architecture MOF Film with Stereoscopic Lithiophilic Sites for High-Performance Lithium–Metal Batteries. *Adv. Funct. Mater.* **2021**, *31*, 2101034. [CrossRef]
107. Jiang, G.; Li, K.; Yu, F.; Li, X.; Mao, J.; Jiang, W.; Sun, F.; Dai, B.; Li, Y. Robust Artificial Solid-Electrolyte Interfaces with Biomimetic Ionic Channels for Dendrite-Free Li Metal Anodes. *Adv. Energy Mater.* **2020**, *11*, 2003496. [CrossRef]
108. Zhou, X.; Li, C.; Zhang, B.; Huang, F.; Zhou, P.; Wang, X.; Ma, Z. Difunctional NH2-modified MOF supporting plentiful ion channels and stable LiF-rich SEI construction via organocatalysis for all-solid-state lithium metal batteries. *J. Mater. Sci. Technol.* **2023**, *136*, 140–148. [CrossRef]
109. Gao, Y.; Yan, Z.; Gray, J.L.; He, X.; Wang, D.; Chen, T.; Huang, Q.; Li, Y.C.; Wang, H.; Kim, S.H.; et al. Polymer–inorganic solid–electrolyte interphase for stable lithium metal batteries under lean electrolyte conditions. *Nat. Mater.* **2019**, *18*, 384–389. [CrossRef] [PubMed]
110. Cao, W.; Lu, J.; Zhou, K.; Sun, G.; Zheng, J.; Geng, Z.; Li, H. Organic-inorganic composite SEI for a stable Li metal anode by in-situ polymerization. *Nano Energy* **2022**, *95*, 106983. [CrossRef]
111. Deng, K.; Han, D.; Ren, S.; Wang, S.; Xiao, M.; Meng, Y. Single-ion conducting artificial solid electrolyte interphase layers for dendrite-free and highly stable lithium metal anodes. *J. Mater. Chem. A* **2019**, *7*, 13113–13119. [CrossRef]
112. Xu, R.; Xiao, Y.; Zhang, R.; Cheng, X.-B.; Zhao, C.-Z.; Zhang, X.-Q.; Yan, C.; Zhang, Q.; Huang, J.-Q. Dual-Phase Single-Ion Pathway Interfaces for Robust Lithium Metal in Working Batteries. *Adv. Mater.* **2019**, *31*, 1808392. [CrossRef]
113. Li, Y.; Guo, Q.; Ding, Z.; Jiang, H.; Yang, H.; Du, W.; Zheng, Y.; Huo, K.; Shaw, L.L. MOFs-Based Materials for Solid-State Hydrogen Storage: Strategies and Perspectives. *Chem. Eng. J.* **2024**, *485*, 149665. [CrossRef]
114. Ding, Z.; Li, Y.; Yang, H.; Lu, Y.; Tan, J.; Li, J.; Li, Q.; Chen, Y.A.; Shaw, L.L.; Pan, F. Tailoring MgH2 for hydrogen storage through nanoengineering and catalysis. *J. Magnes. Alloys* **2022**, *10*, 2946–2967. [CrossRef]
115. Lei, X.; Liang, X.; Yang, R.; Zhang, F.; Wang, C.; Lee, C.-S.; Tang, Y. Rational Design Strategy of Novel Energy Storage Systems: Toward High-Performance Rechargeable Magnesium Batteries. *Small* **2022**, *18*, 2200418. [CrossRef]
116. Attias, R.; Salama, M.; Hirsch, B.; Goffer, Y.; Aurbach, D. Anode-Electrolyte Interfaces in Secondary Magnesium Batteries. *Joule* **2019**, *3*, 27–52. [CrossRef]
117. Muldoon, J.; Bucur, C.B.; Oliver, A.G.; Sugimoto, T.; Matsui, M.; Kim, H.S.; Allred, G.D.; Zajicek, J.; Kotani, Y. Electrolyte roadblocks to a magnesium rechargeable battery. *Energy Environ. Sci.* **2012**, *5*, 5941–5950. [CrossRef]
118. Zhao-Karger, Z.; Gil Bardaji, M.E.; Fuhr, O.; Fichtner, M. A new class of non-corrosive, highly efficient electrolytes for rechargeable magnesium batteries. *J. Mater. Chem. A* **2017**, *5*, 10815–10820. [CrossRef]
119. Aurbach, D.; Lu, Z.; Schechter, A.; Gofer, Y.; Gizbar, H.; Turgeman, R.; Cohen, Y.; Moshkovich, M.; Levi, E. Prototype systems for rechargeable magnesium batteries. *Nature* **2000**, *407*, 724–727. [CrossRef] [PubMed]
120. Liu, F.; Wang, T.; Liu, X.; Fan, L.-Z. Challenges and Recent Progress on Key Materials for Rechargeable Magnesium Batteries. *Adv. Energy Mater.* **2021**, *11*, 2000787. [CrossRef]
121. Tang, K.; Du, A.; Du, X.; Dong, S.; Lu, C.; Cui, Z.; Li, L.; Ding, G.; Chen, F.; Zhou, X.; et al. A Novel Regulation Strategy of Solid Electrolyte Interphase Based on Anion-Solvent Coordination for Magnesium Metal Anode. *Small* **2020**, *16*, 2005424. [CrossRef]
122. Tang, K.; Du, A.; Dong, S.; Cui, Z.; Liu, X.; Lu, C.; Zhao, J.; Zhou, X.; Cui, G. A Stable Solid Electrolyte Interphase for Magnesium Metal Anode Evolved from a Bulky Anion Lithium Salt. *Adv. Mater.* **2020**, *32*, 1904987. [CrossRef]
123. Li, Z.; Diemant, T.; Meng, Z.; Xiu, Y.; Reupert, A.; Wang, L.; Fichtner, M.; Zhao-Karger, Z. Establishing a Stable Anode–Electrolyte Interface in Mg Batteries by Electrolyte Additive. *ACS Appl. Mater. Interfaces* **2021**, *13*, 33123–33132. [CrossRef]
124. Sun, Y.; Zou, Q.L.; Wang, W.W.; Lu, Y.C. Non-passivating Anion Adsorption Enables Reversible Magnesium Redox in Simple Non-nucleophilic Electrolytes. *Acs Energy Lett.* **2021**, *6*, 3607–3613. [CrossRef]

125. Sun, Y.; Wang, Y.; Jiang, L.; Dong, D.; Wang, W.; Fan, J.; Lu, Y.-C. Non-nucleophilic electrolyte with non-fluorinated hybrid solvents for long-life magnesium metal batteries. *Energy Environ. Sci.* **2023**, *16*, 265–274. [CrossRef]
126. Yang, H.; Ding, Z.; Li, Y.-T.; Li, S.-Y.; Wu, P.-K.; Hou, Q.-H.; Zheng, Y.; Gao, B.; Huo, K.-F.; Du, W.-J.; et al. Recent advances in kinetic and thermodynamic regulation of magnesium hydride for hydrogen storage. *Rare Met.* **2023**, *42*, 2906–2927. [CrossRef]
127. Zhang, R.; Cui, C.; Xiao, R.; Li, R.; Mu, T.; Huo, H.; Ma, Y.; Yin, G.; Zuo, P. Interface regulation of Mg anode and redox couple conversion in cathode by copper for high-performance Mg-S battery. *Chem. Eng. J.* **2023**, *451*, 138663. [CrossRef]
128. Li, B.; Masse, R.; Liu, C.; Hu, Y.; Li, W.; Zhang, G.; Cao, G. Kinetic surface control for improved magnesium-electrolyte interfaces for magnesium ion batteries. *Energy Storage Mater.* **2019**, *22*, 96–104. [CrossRef]
129. Son, S.-B.; Gao, T.; Harvey, S.P.; Steirer, K.X.; Stokes, A.; Norman, A.; Wang, C.; Cresce, A.; Xu, K.; Ban, C. An artificial interphase enables reversible magnesium chemistry in carbonate electrolytes. *Nat. Chem.* **2018**, *10*, 532–539. [CrossRef] [PubMed]
130. Wan, B.; Dou, H.; Zhao, X.; Wang, J.; Zhao, W.; Guo, M.; Zhang, Y.; Li, J.; Ma, Z.-F.; Yang, X. Three-Dimensional Magnesiophilic Scaffolds for Reduced Passivation toward High-Rate Mg Metal Anodes in a Noncorrosive Electrolyte. *ACS Appl. Mater. Interfaces* **2020**, *12*, 28298–28305. [CrossRef] [PubMed]
131. Tan, Y.-H.; Yao, W.-T.; Zhang, T.; Ma, T.; Lu, L.-L.; Zhou, F.; Yao, H.-B.; Yu, S.-H. High Voltage Magnesium-ion Battery Enabled by Nanocluster Mg3Bi2 Alloy Anode in Noncorrosive Electrolyte. *ACS Nano* **2018**, *12*, 5856–5865. [CrossRef] [PubMed]
132. Chu, H.; Zhang, Z.; Song, Z.; Du, A.; Dong, S.; Li, G.; Cui, G. Facilitated magnesium atom adsorption and surface diffusion kinetics via artificial bismuth-based interphases. *Chem. Commun.* **2021**, *57*, 9430–9433. [CrossRef]
133. Zhao, Y.; Du, A.; Dong, S.; Jiang, F.; Guo, Z.; Ge, X.; Qu, X.; Zhou, X.; Cui, G. A Bismuth-Based Protective Layer for Magnesium Metal Anode in Noncorrosive Electrolytes. *ACS Energy Lett.* **2021**, *6*, 2594–2601. [CrossRef]
134. Yang, B.; Xia, L.; Li, R.; Huang, G.; Tan, S.; Wang, Z.; Qu, B.; Wang, J.; Pan, F. Superior plating/stripping performance through constructing an artificial interphase layer on metallic Mg anode. *J. Mater. Sci. Technol.* **2023**, *157*, 154–162. [CrossRef]
135. Li, Y.; Zuo, P.; Li, R.; Huo, H.; Ma, Y.; Du, C.; Gao, Y.; Yin, G.; Weatherup, R.S. Formation of an Artificial Mg2+-Permeable Interphase on Mg Anodes Compatible with Ether and Carbonate Electrolytes. *ACS Appl. Mater. Interfaces* **2021**, *13*, 24565–24574. [CrossRef] [PubMed]
136. Zhang, R.P.; Cui, C.; Li, R.N.; Li, Y.Q.; Du, C.Y.; Gao, Y.Z.; Huo, H.; Ma, Y.L.; Zuo, P.J.; Yin, G.P. An artificial interphase enables the use of Mg(TFSI)2-based electrolytes in magnesium metal batteries. *Chem. Eng. J.* **2021**, *426*, 130751. [CrossRef]
137. Wen, T.; Qu, B.; Tan, S.; Huang, G.; Song, J.; Wang, Z.; Wang, J.; Tang, A.; Pan, F. Rational design of artificial interphase buffer layer with 3D porous channel for uniform deposition in magnesium metal anodes. *Energy Storage Mater.* **2023**, *55*, 816–825. [CrossRef]
138. Hu, M.; Li, G.; Chen, K.; Zhou, X.; Li, C. A gradient structured SEI enabling record-high areal capacity anode for high-rate Mg metal batteries. *Chem. Eng. J.* **2024**, *480*, 148193. [CrossRef]
139. Li, Y.; Zhou, X.; Hu, J.; Zheng, Y.; Huang, M.; Guo, K.; Li, C. Reversible Mg metal anode in conventional electrolyte enabled by durable heterogeneous SEI with low surface diffusion barrier. *Energy Storage Mater.* **2022**, *46*, 1–9. [CrossRef]
140. Hacker, J.; Rommel, T.; Lange, P.; Zhao-Karger, Z.; Morawietz, T.; Biswas, I.; Wagner, N.; Nojabaee, M.; Friedrich, K.A. Magnesium Anode Protection by an Organic Artificial Solid Electrolyte Interphase for Magnesium-Sulfur Batteries. *ACS Appl. Mater. Interfaces* **2023**, *15*, 33013–33027. [CrossRef]
141. Kong, L.L.; Wang, L.; Ni, Z.C.; Liu, S.; Li, G.R.; Gao, X.P. Lithium–Magnesium Alloy as a Stable Anode for Lithium–Sulfur Battery. *Adv. Funct. Mater.* **2019**, *29*, 1808756. [CrossRef]
142. Li, R.; Liu, Q.; Zhang, R.; Li, Y.; Ma, Y.; Huo, H.; Gao, Y.; Zuo, P.; Wang, J.; Yin, G. Achieving high-energy-density magnesium/sulfur battery via a passivation-free Mg-Li alloy anode. *Energy Storage Mater.* **2022**, *50*, 380–386. [CrossRef]

**Disclaimer/Publisher's Note:** The statements, opinions and data contained in all publications are solely those of the individual author(s) and contributor(s) and not of MDPI and/or the editor(s). MDPI and/or the editor(s) disclaim responsibility for any injury to people or property resulting from any ideas, methods, instructions or products referred to in the content.

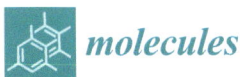 molecules

Article

# Silicon Extraction from a Diamond Wire Saw Silicon Slurry with Flotation and the Flotation Interface Behavior

Lin Zhu [1], Dandan Wu [1,2,*], Shicong Yang [1,2,*], Keqiang Xie [1,2], Kuixian Wei [1,2] and Wenhui Ma [1,2,3,4]

1. Faculty of Metallurgical and Energy Engineering/National Engineering Research Center of Vacuum Metallurgy, Kunming University of Science and Technology, Kunming 650093, China
2. State Key Laboratory of Complex Nonferrous Metal Resources Clean Utilization, Kunming University of Science and Technology, Kunming 650093, China
3. Silicon Industry and Engineering Research Center of Yunnan Province/Silicon Material Industry Research Institution (Innovation Center) of Yunnan Province, Kunming University of Science and Technology, Kunming 650093, China
4. School of Engineering, Yunnan University, Kunming 650500, China
* Correspondence: wdd1006530@sina.com (D.W.); shicongyang@kust.edu.cn (S.Y.)

**Abstract:** Diamond wire saw silicon slurry (DWSSS) is a waste resource produced during the process of solar-grade silicon wafer preparation with diamond wire sawing. The DWSSS contains 6N grade high-purity silicon and offers a promising resource for high-purity silicon recycling. The current process for silicon extraction recovery from DWSSS presents the disadvantages of lower recovery and secondary pollution. This study focuses on the original DWSSS as the target and proposes flotation for efficiently extracting silicon. The experimental results indicate that the maximal recovery of silicon reached 98.2% under the condition of a dodecylamine (DDA) dosage of 0.6 g·L$^{-1}$ and natural pH conditions within 24 min, and the flotation conforms to the first-order rate model. Moreover, the mechanism of the interface behavior between DWSSS and DDA revealed that DDA is adsorbed on the surface of silicon though adsorption, and the floatability of silicon is improved. The DFT calculation indicates that DDA can be spontaneously adsorbed with the silicon. The present study demonstrates that flotation is an efficient method for extracting silicon from DWSSS and provides an available option for silicon recovery.

**Keywords:** diamond wire saw silicon slurry; silicon extraction; flotation kinetics; interface adsorption behavior; DFT calculation

## 1. Introduction

Solar photovoltaic (PV) power generation, as a primary source of energy consumption, is poised to play a crucial strategic role in future energy frameworks [1–3]. Photovoltaic technology, mainly based on crystalline silicon solar cells [4,5], has developed rapidly in recent years with the continuous decrease in the cost of PV power [6,7]. Solar crystalline silicon cells have undoubtedly become a promising new energy material [8–10]. This has led to an increased demand for crystalline silicon and a corresponding waste rise from solar cell production [11,12]. The solar PV waste recovery is an emerging research topic in the new field of energy conversion [13,14]. The production method for solar-grade crystalline silicon wafer is diamond wire cutting, and approximately 30% of the 6N high-purity silicon is transformed into a waste liquid known as diamond wire saw silicon slurry (DWSSS) during the diamond wire cutting process [7,15]. Since the solid silicon contained in DWSSS has a high-purity content, the recycling of DWSSS has become a popular area of research [16–18]. Silicon extraction from DWSSS is vital for resource recycling and the sustainable development of the PV silicon industry [19].

The existing industrial recovery process for silicon extraction from DWSSS involves treating the original DWSSS generated through coagulation, sedimentation, pressure filtration, and flame-retardant treatment to obtain a "silicon sludge" filter cake. Then, the "silicon sludge" filter cake is dried, dehydrated, crushed, and compacted to obtain diamond wire saw silicon powder for further purification treatment, ultimately achieving silicon recovery [13]. However, this lengthy recovery process tends to reintroduce metal impurities [20,21], resulting in reduced silicon recovery [22]. As the particle size of the silicon powder and other contaminants from the diamond wire cutting process is in the micron range, recycling is difficult. To achieve the high-value recycling of DWSSS, this study proposes an efficient approach for silicon extraction from DWSSS through flotation [23].

Flotation is an effective and green method for extracting valuable minerals from different ores based on their physical and chemical surface properties [24]. The target minerals can be separated from raw minerals with the addition of flotation reagents thus achieving the recovery of minerals [25,26]. Based on the characteristics of DWSSS, a process for extracting silicon with low moisture content from DWSSS with flotation by using dodecylamine (DDA) as a collector is proposed in the present study. This process has the advantages of high silicon recovery, easy operation, tight process connection, and easy scalability for sustainable silicon recovery.

## 2. Results and Discussion

### 2.1. Effect of Different Collectors on Feasibility of Flotation

The capturing effect of different reagents on silicon extraction from DWSSS were compared through silicon capture effect experimentation. The experimental phenomena of kerosene, sodium sulfide, and DDA individually as a flotation reagent for the silicon extraction from DWSSS are displayed in Figure 1a–c, respectively. It can be seen that a large amount of mineral-carrying froth appeared when DDA was used as the collector, indicating that DDA had a significant capturing effect on silicon recovery, so the silicon can be effectively recovered from DWSSS with the addition of DDA. However, when kerosene or $Na_2S$ was used alone as a flotation reagent, no mineralized foam was observed, indicating that the collector of kerosene and the oxidized ore vulcanizing agent $Na_2S$ had no significant capture effect on silicon when used alone.

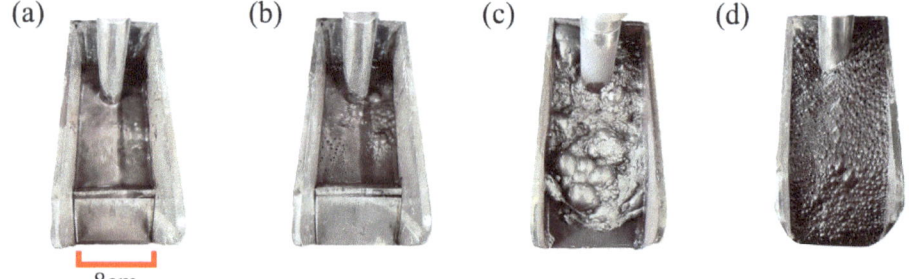

**Figure 1.** Experimental phenomena of different types of collectors: (**a**) kerosene; (**b**) sodium sulfide; (**c**) DDA; and (**d**) DDA and kerosene.

When DDA is used alone as a collector for the flotation silicon from DWSSS, some disadvantages include excessive and sticky mineral-carrying froth, making dehydration challenging and the operation difficult to control. However, a DDA–kerosene mixed collector can alleviate this issue without affecting the silicon recovery [27]. The experimental phenomenon is shown in Figure 1d, where it can be observed that the froth becomes smaller, denser, and thinner with the DDA–kerosene mixed collector [28]. Therefore, the silicon recovery from DWSSS is the highest and the operation is more efficient when DDA and kerosene are used as a combination collector.

## 2.2. Flotation Results of DDA as Collector

To assess the influence of DDA dosage and pH on silicon recovery, the flotation experiments were conducted under DDA concentrations and pH levels, respectively. The effect of different DDA additions on the recovery of silicon was tested at natural pH. The experimental results are shown in Figure 2a, the blue area is the range of 0-1 $g·L^{-1}$ DDA dosage. where it can be observed that the recovery of silicon concentration increased as the DDA dosage increased within the range of 0.1 $g·L^{-1}$ to 0.6 $g·L^{-1}$, and when the DDA dosage reached 0.6 $g·L^{-1}$, the maximal recovery of silicon reached 98.2%. However, the recovery of silicon began to decline when the DDA dosage reached 1.2 $g·L^{-1}$. The optimal DDA dosage was determined to be 0.6 $g·L^{-1}$, at which the recovery of silicon from DWSSS was the maximum of 98.2%.

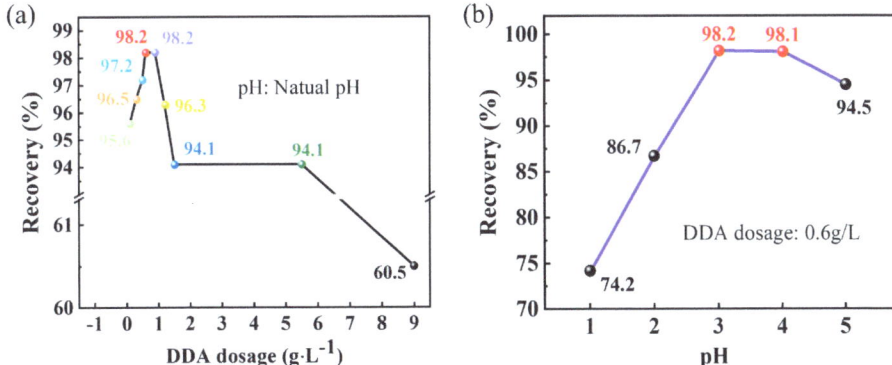

**Figure 2.** Experimental results of DWSSS flotation: (**a**) recovery of silicon under different DDA dosages; and (**b**) recovery of silicon under different pH levels.

To verify the effect of different pH levels on recovery during the flotation experiments, a $H_2SO_4$ or NaOH aqueous solution was used to adjust the pH of the slurry, and the flotation experiments were conducted at different pH values with the DDA dosage of 0.6 $g·L^{-1}$. The experimental results are presented in Figure 2b. The experimental results demonstrate that the prepared slurry is conducive to flotation when the pH level is at the range of 4–5. The original pH of DWSSS is 7–8, and after adding DDA acetate as a collector reagent, the pH of the slurry system is 4–5; this pH is called natural pH. Therefore, the recovery of silicon is the highest with a natural pH of 4–5.

## 2.3. Flotation Kinetics of DWSSS

The first-order classical flotation rate model was used to fit the flotation kinetics for silicon recovery from DWSSS, and the fitting results are shown in Figure 3. The effects of fitting through the first-order classical kinetics model with different DDA dosages are presented in Figure 3(a1–a6). It can be seen that the $R^2$ value reaches 0.98 when the DDA dosage is 0.6 $g·L^{-1}$. The fitting results at different pH values are shown in Figure 3(b1–b6), and it can be seen that the $R^2$ value is closest to 1 at a pH level of 5.

The recovery of silicon from DWSSS can be divided into two stages, as illustrated in Figure 3(a1–a6,b1–b6). In the first stage, the flotation rate is fast, and the cumulative recovery of silicon increases rapidly within approximately 8 min. This is because more silicon particles are floating up within the first 8 min, and the added DDA is kept at a relatively high level. The probability of collision between silicon and DDA is high, resulting in a fast flotation rate and a higher recovery [29]. In the second stage, the cumulative recovery of silicon shows a slow upward trend, and the flotation rate decreases significantly after 8 min. This is because the silicon from DWSSS was selected and adsorbed together with a large amount of DDA as the flotation process continues, and the number of silicon particles that can be floated in the slurry significantly decreases, resulting in the decrease in recovery.

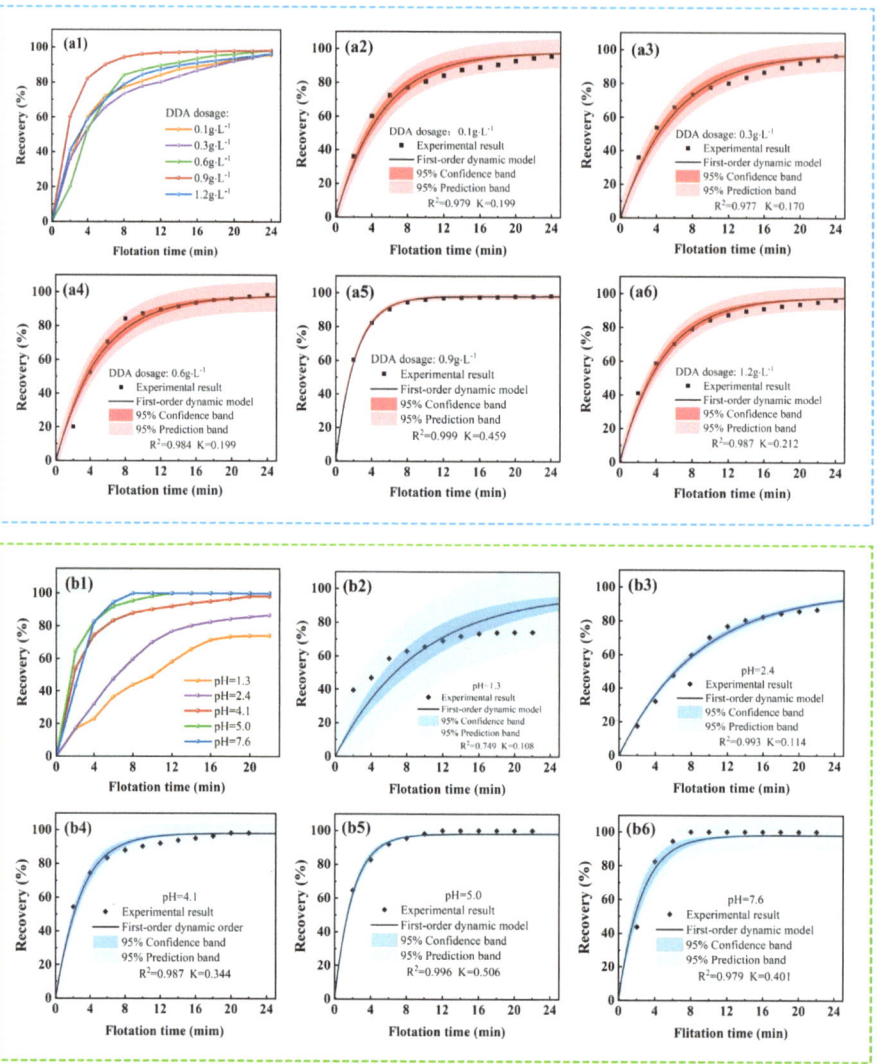

**Figure 3.** The fitting results of the first-order classical flotation rate model for silicon recovery with different conditions: (**a1**) the recovery of silicon under different DDA dosages; (**a2–a6**) the fitting results under different DDA dosages; (**b1**) the recovery of silicon under different pH levels; and (**b2–b6**) the fitting results under different pH levels.

At natural pH, the effects of different DDA amounts on the maximum recovery and flotation rate constant are shown in Figure 4a. It can be seen that both the maximum recovery and flotation rate constant initially increase and then decrease with the increase in DDA dosage. The recovery reaches a maximum of 98.2% when the DDA dosage is 0.6 g·L$^{-1}$, while the flotation ratio constant reaches a maximum of 0.459 when the DDA dosage is 0.9 g·L$^{-1}$. When the DDA dosage is 0.6g·L$^{-1}$, the effects of different pH values of the slurry system on the maximum recovery and flotation rate constant are shown in

Figure 4b. The recovery reaches its maximum of 98.2% at a pH of 4.1; at a pH of 5, the flotation rate constant is 0.506.

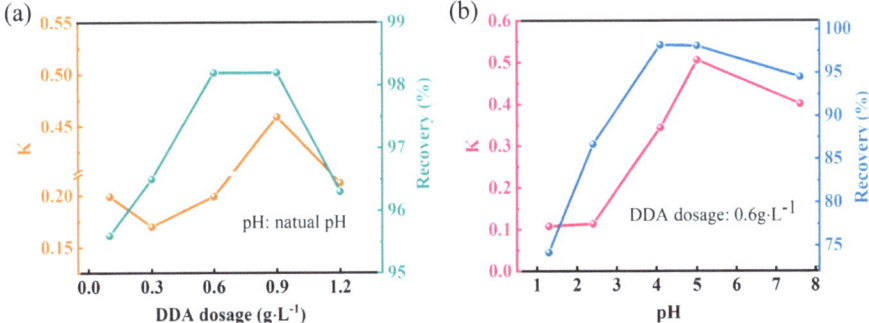

**Figure 4.** (**a**) Effect of DDA dosage on maximum recovery and flotation rate constant at natural pH; (**b**) effect of pH on maximum recovery and flotation rate constant at DDA dosage of $0.6 \text{g} \cdot \text{L}^{-1}$.

### 2.4. Flotation Interface Behavior Analysis

#### 2.4.1. Flotation Interface Behavior Between DDA and Silicon

In the study of the flotation interface behavior of DDA on silicon, the dosage of DDA used for preparing samples for analysis was $6 \text{ g} \cdot \text{L}^{-1}$, and the overall pH range of the slurry was 4–5. The variation in zeta potential at different pH levels before and after the interaction of silicon with DDA is shown in Figure 5a. The zeta potential of silicon decreases with an increasing pH, and the absolute value of the potential increases, indicating that silicon becomes more stable with an increase in pH [30].

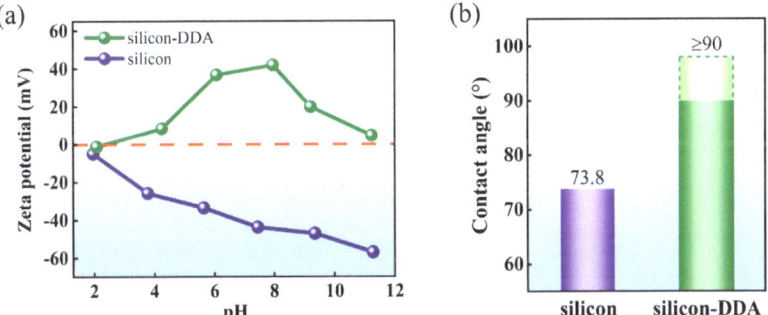

**Figure 5.** (**a**) Effect of DDA on surface zeta potential of silicon; (**b**) contact angle of silicon before and after DDA addition.

The zeta potential of silicon–DDA reached zero at a pH level of approximately 2, indicating a stable flotation system was formed when the pH level was 2. The potential of the silicon–DDA system significantly increases when the pH is 4–8, and the potential change indicates the DDA was adsorbed on the surface of silicon.

The contact angle is a direct indicator of the wetting properties of the mineral surface. The change in the contact angle before and after the interaction of silicon with DDA is presented in Figure 5b. It can be observed that the contact angle of silicon is greater than 90° after the adsorption of DDA. The DDA addition significantly improved the hydrophobicity of the silicon, indicating the increased hydrophobicity of silicon enhances the floatability of silicon in DWSSS. Therefore, the DDA makes the slurry more conducive to the silicon extraction from the DWSSS with flotation.

The infrared spectra of DDA, DWSSS, and DWSSS-DDA are presented in Figure 6. The absorption peak at 3445 cm$^{-1}$, 1632 cm$^{-1}$, and 722 cm$^{-1}$ corresponds to the stretching vibration of N-H, the in-plane bending vibration of N-H, and the out-of-plane bending vibration of N-H [31]. The 2851 cm$^{-1}$ and 2920 cm$^{-1}$ peaks correspond to the symmetric stretching vibration of C-H bonds in the -CH$_3$ and -CH$_2$- groups, respectively [32]. The peaks at 1460 cm$^{-1}$ correspond to the stretching vibration of C-N bonds. After the adsorption of the DDA, the silicon exhibits an absorption band around 1100 cm$^{-1}$, and the peak corresponds to the anti-symmetric stretching vibration of Si-O-Si bonds [33]. The above results indicate that DDA is adsorbed on the surface of silicon after the addition of DDA.

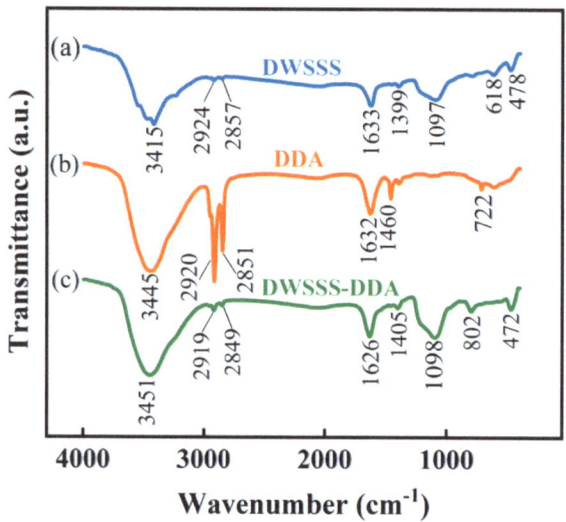

Figure 6. Infrared spectrum results: (a) DWSSS; (b) DDA; (c) DWSSS-DDA.

The three-dimensional height morphology, changes in surface roughness value, two-dimensional geometric morphology, and cross-sectional height of DWSSS before and after DDA addition are presented in Figure 7. According to Figure 7a, it can be understood that the Ra and Rq of DWSSS increased with Rq increasing from 123 nm to 207 nm, whereas Ra increased from 95 nm to 164 nm after the addition of DDA. This indicates an increase in surface roughness after silicon adsorption with DDA [34–36]. Additionally, Figure 7(b1,b2) shows that the maximum cross-sectional height of DWSSP is about 250 nm, and a smooth surface with a minimum value of around −300 nm appeared in the silicon. On the other hand, Figure 7(c1,c2) shows that the surface of the silicon particle becomes rough after the addition of DDA, where the maximum cross-sectional height of the silicon is approximately 500 nm and a minimum value is approximately −400 nm. This is because the surface of silicon particles becomes rough after DDA adsorption thereby increasing the recovery of silicon, which is consistent with the flotation experiment results.

The surface morphology of the DWSSS is shown in Figure 8(a1). It can be seen from Figure 8(a2) that the silicon particles in DWSSS and DWSSS–DDA are light gray and mainly composed of Si, O, and C, where the main elements are silicon and carbon, with a silicon content of 52.8% and a carbon content of 33.5%. The surface morphology of the DWSSS–DDA is shown in Figure 8(b1); the carbon content in DWSSS–DDA is 69.4%, and the silicon content is 14.6%, as shown in Figure 8(b2). The significant increase of carbon content indicates that DDA has adsorbed in the silicon surface of the DWSSS after the addition of DDA.

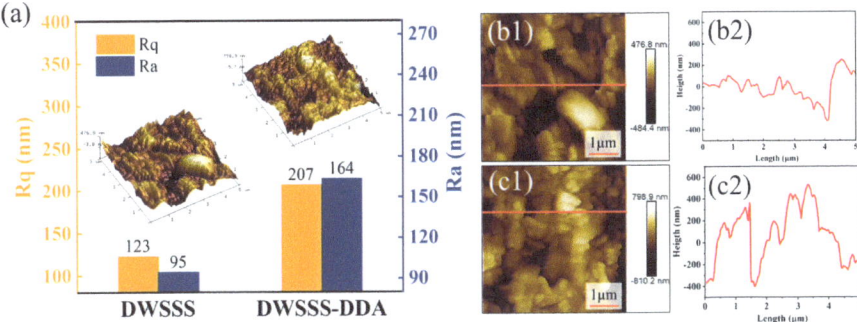

**Figure 7.** (**a**) Three-dimensional height morphology and roughness changes in DWSSS before and after DDA addition; (**b1,b2**) two-dimensional geometric morphology and cross-sectional height of DWSSS; (**c1,c2**) two-dimensional geometric morphology and cross-sectional height of DWSSS-DDA.

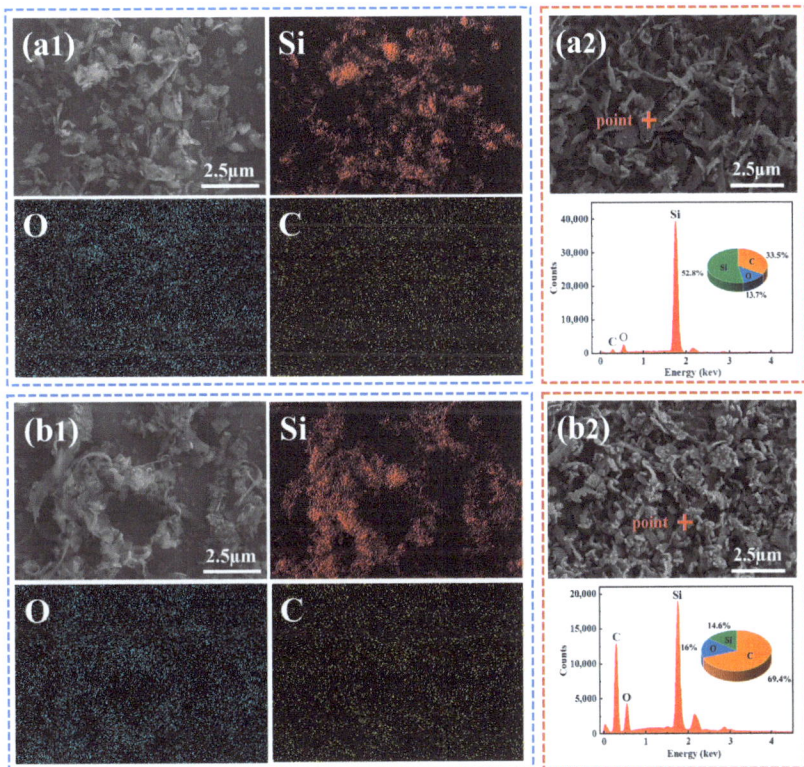

**Figure 8.** (**a1**) SEM image of DWSSS before DDA addition; (**a2**) EDS result of DWSSS before DDA addition; (**b1,b2**) SEM image of DWSSS after DDA addition; (**b2**) EDS result of DWSSS after DDA addition.

### 2.4.2. Interface Adsorption Behavior of DDA

The Adsorption Locator module is used to locate the adsorption position of DDA molecule on the Si surface. To test the adsorption positions of DDA molecules in an aqueous solution system with Si, an adsorption substrate was established with a Si (111) crystal plane cut to a thickness of 6 Å, a supercell of 7 × 7, and a vacuum layer thickness of 40 Å. The adsorbates consisted of 5 DDA molecules and 500 H$_2$O molecules. The calculation results are shown in Figure 9, where Figure 9a presents the optimal adsorption configuration, the green circle is the location of five DDA molecules. It can be seen from the optimal adsorption configuration that DDA, as a macromolecule, has multiple adsorption sites on Si (Top site, Bridge site). The test results indicate that DDA is more inclined to adsorb horizontally on the Si surface. Figure 9b illustrates the most likely adsorption positions of DDA on the Si surface, with the red positions indicating the locations where adsorption is most likely to occur.

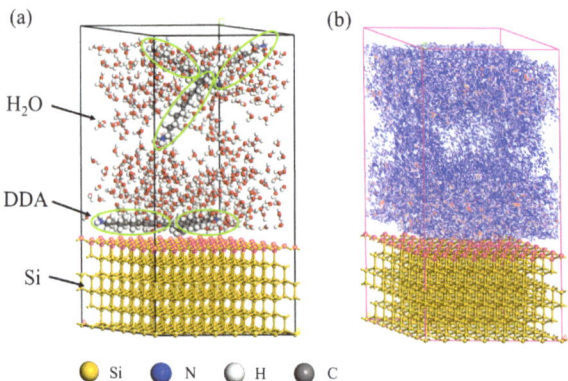

**Figure 9.** (**a**) Best adsorption position of DDA on Si (111) surface in aqueous solution system; (**b**) density map of adsorption region of DDA on Si (111) surface in aqueous solution.

In order to further test the adsorption position of DDA on the Si (111) surface, an adsorption substrate is established, and the Si unit cell is cut to obtain the (111) crystal plane, with a surface layer cutting thickness of 4 Å. A supercell of 5 × 5 is created, and the vacuum layer thickness is set to 15 Å. The adsorbate is a single DDA molecule. The calculation results are shown in Figure 10. The analysis of the adsorption positions of Si (111) and DDA is illustrated in Figure 10a, with the most probable adsorption position marked in red. The stereoscopic and top views of the five positions where Si (111) and DDA are most likely to adsorb are shown in Figure 10b–e, and the DDA molecules adsorbed on Si are macromolecules, and there are many adsorption sites (Top site and Bridge site). The adsorption energy of five different adsorption sites is shown in Table 1. It can be seen that the adsorption reaction between Si (111) and DDA can occur spontaneously, the energy is low, and the adsorption model is stable.

Through DFT calculations, the interfacial adsorption behavior between DDA and silicon in the DWSSS is further revealed from a microscopic perspective. The adsorption site of DDA on Si is the bridge site. A Si-DDA model was established with a Si (111) surface layer thickness of 3 Å, a supercell of 3 × 3, and a vacuum layer thickness of 10 Å to explore the adsorption pathway of Si and DDA. The established adsorption model is shown in Figure 11a. The model underwent geometric structure optimization, and the optimized model is shown in Figure 11b. It can be seen that the positions of the atoms in the adsorption model changed after geometric optimization, and the optimized model was used for DFT calculations involving Si atoms and DDA molecules.

After the adsorption process of the Si-DDA system, the differential charge density map was taken from the plane that intersects the maximum number of atoms, as shown in Figure 12a. The differential charge density maps are illustrated in Figure 12b,c. It can be qualitatively analyzed that after DDA is adsorbed on Si, the charge of the H atoms on DDA increases, while the C atoms, N atoms, and the Si atoms lose charge.

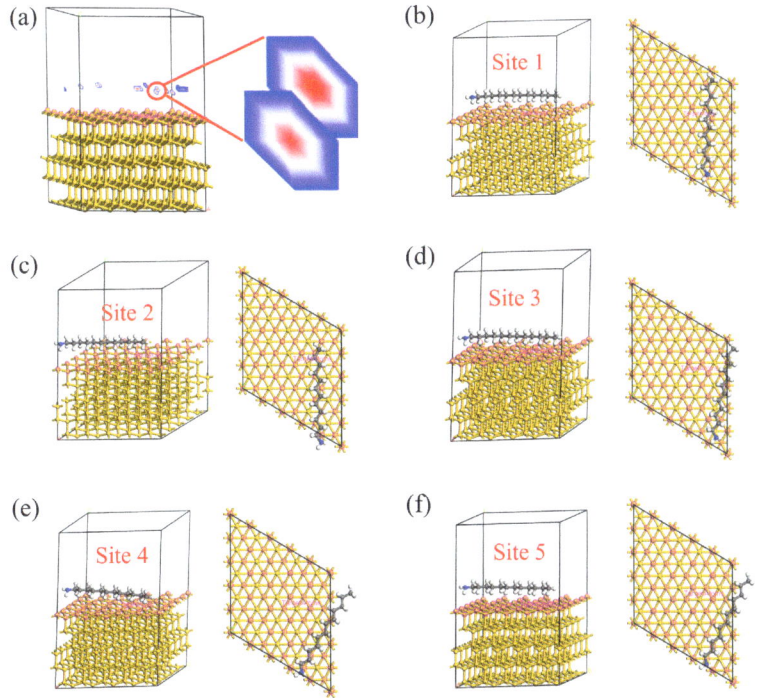

**Figure 10.** (a) Analysis of Si (111) and DDA adsorption sites. Si (111) and DDA possible adsorption position stereogram and top view: (b) Site 1, (c) Site 2, (d) Site 2, (e) Site 2, (f) Site 2.

**Table 1.** Energy results of Si (111) and DDA at different adsorption sites calculated by Adsorption Locator module.

| Model | Site 1 | Site 2 | Site 3 | Site 4 | Site 5 |
| --- | --- | --- | --- | --- | --- |
| Total Energy (kcal/mol) | −59.32 | −59.12 | −58.91 | −58.65 | −58.45 |
| Adsorption Energy (kcal/mol) | −44.09 | −43.89 | −43.69 | −43.43 | −43.22 |
| Adsorption Energy (eV) | −1.90 | −1.89 | −1.88 | −1.87 | −1.86 |

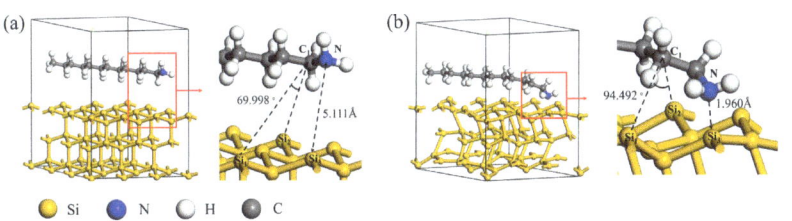

**Figure 11.** DFT calculation model of DDA on Si (111): (a) before geometric optimization; (b) after geometric optimization.

The DFT calculation shows the average Mulliken population distribution of each atom in Si-DDA after adsorption, which is listed in Table 2. It can be observed that C gains electrons from the Si (111) surface, while H, N, and Si lose electrons, indicating a transfer of electrons from H, N, and Si atoms to C atoms after adsorption.

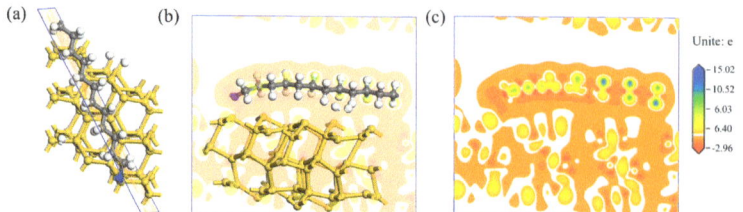

**Figure 12.** (a) Section position of differential charge density diagram of Si-DDA system; (b,c) differential charge density diagram of Si-DDA system.

**Table 2.** Average Mulliken population of atoms in Si (111) surface after DDA molecule adsorption.

| Type of Atom | Atom Orbit | | Total | Charge/e |
|---|---|---|---|---|
| | S | P | | |
| H | 0.37 | 0.00 | 10.09 | 6.81 |
| C | 0.64 | 1.60 | 26.86 | −5.72 |
| N | 0.82 | 2.10 | 2.90 | −0.82 |
| Si | 0.70 | 1.30 | 108.13 | −0.27 |

The Mulliken population distribution of various chemical bonds after Si and DDA adsorption is shown in Figure 13. It can be observed that the population of Si-Si bonds, C-C bonds, H-C bonds, C-N bonds, and N-Si bonds are all greater than 0. However, the population of H-H bonds, H-Si bonds and C-Si bonds are all less than 0, indicating that H-H bonds, H-Si bonds, and C-Si bonds cannot be formed. By comparing the bond lengths, it can be concluded that the H-N bond with a bond length of 1.96 Å is the shortest among the chemical bonds formed, indicating the strongest covalent bond strength for the H-N bond in DDA.

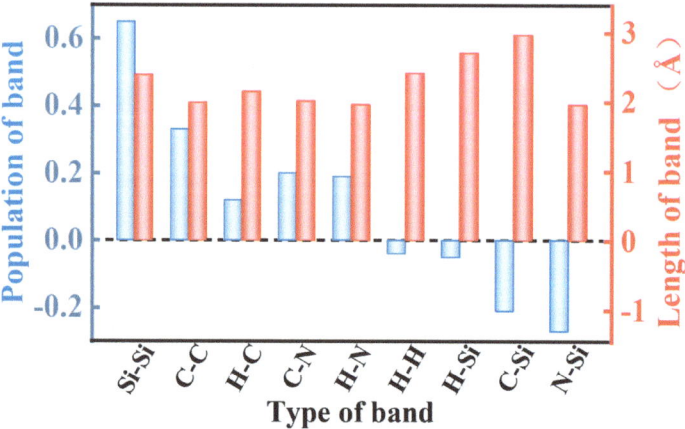

**Figure 13.** Mulliken population of band in Si (111) surface after DDA adsorption.

The band structure and density of states of the DDA and Si (111) surface before and after DDA adsorption were analyzed to reveal the distribution of the electronic states of Si and DDA during the adsorption process. The density of state distribution is shown in Figure 14. The density of states is divided into three valence bands with the upper valence band located at 0.4~17 eV, the middle valence band located at 0.4~−7.5 eV, and the lower valence band located at −7.5~−23 eV before and after DDA adsorption on the Si (111) surface. The upper valence band at 0.4~17 eV and the middle valence band at 0.4~−7.5 eV are mainly contributed by the P orbitals of the silicon atoms. In contrast, the S orbitals of the DDA atoms mainly contribute to the lower valence band at −7.5~−23 eV.

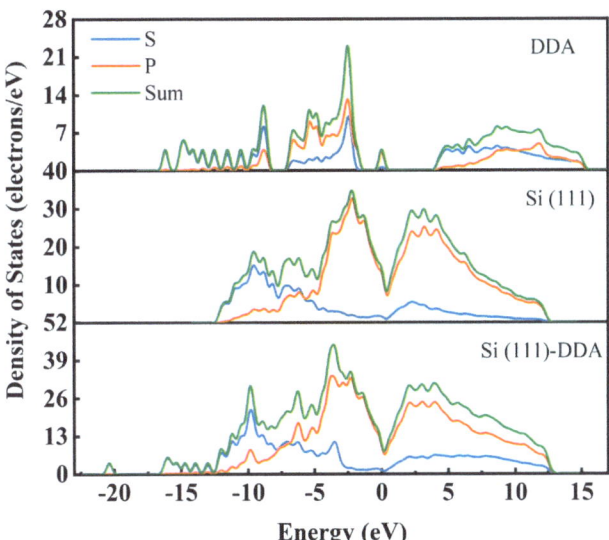

Figure 14. Density of states for DDA, Si (111) surface, and Si-DDA.

According to the DFT calculation results, the adsorption energy of Si before the addition of DDA is −8172.65 eV, and the adsorption energy of DDA is −2604.36 eV. The energy of the Si-DDA system after adsorption is −10,780.29 eV. According to Equation (3), the energy difference $\Delta E$ is −3.28 eV, and the obtained $\Delta E$ indicated that the adsorption process can spontaneously occur. Furthermore, the calculation results demonstrate that, from a microscopic perspective, DDA can be adsorbed with the silicon of the DWSSS thereby allowing the extraction of silicon from the DWSSS by flotation.

According to the research of the flotation interface behavior between DDA and silicon and the interface adsorption behavior of DDA, DDA can spontaneously adsorb onto silicon in the DWSSS. The roughness and hydrophobicity of the silicon surface were changed after DDA was adsorbed to the silicon surface by flotation, making the silicon floatable thereby enabling the separation of silicon in the DWSSS.

## 3. Materials and Methods

### 3.1. Materials and Reagents

The DWSSS used in this study was generated during the diamond wire saw cutting process of a solar-grade crystalline silicon wafer. The image of DWSSS is shown in Figure 15a, where the DWSSS is a gray-black suspension with a solid silicon content of 2.11%. The particle size distribution of the DWSSS is presented in Figure 15b, and the silicon particle in DWSSS has an average particle size of 0.52 μm. The XRD analysis of DWSSS for phase composition is demonstrated in Figure 15c, where it is revealed that the phase component is silicon. Since the metal impurity content in DWSSS is usually less than 1000 ppmw [37], this study does not account for the influence of impurities. The non-polar hydrocarbon kerosene with a dosage of 0.2 mL per 400 mL of DWSSS was used as a common collector. The flotation reagent sodium sulfide ($Na_2S$) with 0.5 g per 400 mL of DWSSS and cationic collector DDA ($CH_3(CH_2)_{11}NH_2$) with a dosage of 0.4 g per 400 mL of DWSSS were used in the flotation experiment, respectively. The DDA acetate was prepared by DDA and glacial acetic acid in a mass ratio of 1:3. A ratio of 2:3 of DDA to kerosene was mixed and shaken, then heated in a water bath at 50 °C for 10min to prepare a homogeneous solution. The DDA, glacial acetic acid, and sodium sulfide reagents were of analytical grade, while the kerosene was of chemical grade. The amount of flotation reagent used in the preparation of the sample for analysis and detection is 10 times that in the flotation experiment.

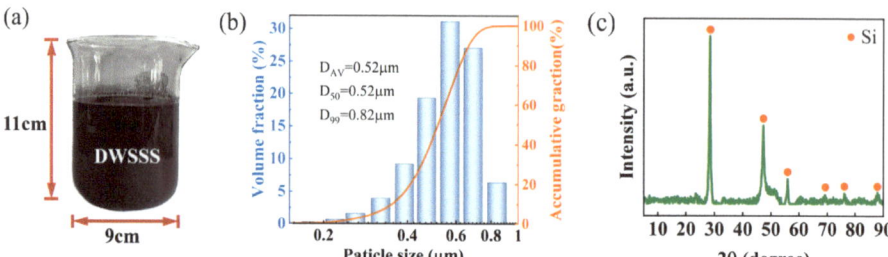

**Figure 15.** (**a**) Image of original DWSSS; (**b**) particle size distribution of DWSSS; (**c**) XRD phase analysis result of DWSSS.

### 3.2. Microflotation Experiment

The flotation experiment was carried out with an XFD$_{IV}$ flotation machine, and the experimental process is shown in Figure 16a,b. The flotation experimental procedure is as follows: (1) 400 mL of DWSSS is placed into a 500 mL flotation cell, then water is added to the flotation cell to maintain the total volume of the slurry at 500 mL; (2) the impeller speed is set at 1920 r·min$^{-1}$ in the flotation process; (3) the DWSSS is stirred in the flotation cell for 2 min to obtain a homogeneous flotation slurry, then the collector is added to the slurry and stirred for 3 min; (4) air is pumped into the flotation cell at 200–300 L/h; (5) once the air is turned on, twelve two-minute concentrates are collected by scraping the froth every five second, a total flotation time of 24 min; and (6) the recovered silicon concentration and tailings are filtered and then dried at 80 °C until a constant weight is maintained. The recovery of the silicon was calculated by weighing, and the samples were then characterized and analyzed.

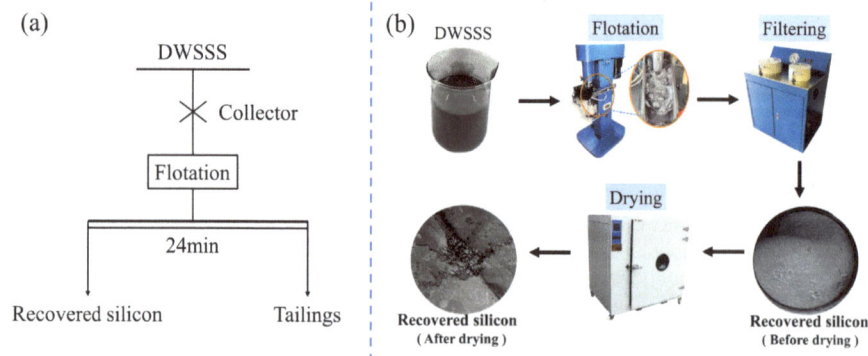

**Figure 16.** Experimental procedure of flotation: (**a**) flow chart of flotation experiment; (**b**) diagram of flotation process.

The recovery of silicon can be calculated through Equation (1) [38].

$$\varepsilon_{silicon} = \frac{Q_k}{Q_k + Q_n} \times 100\% \tag{1}$$

where $Q_k$ (g) is the weight of the silicon concentrate; $Q_n$ (g) is the weight of the tailings; and $\varepsilon_{silicon}$ (%) is the recovery of the silicon in the DWSSS.

*3.3. Flotation Kinetics Analysis*

The experimental results are fitted by using the first-order classical flotation rate model [39], and the equation can be described through Equation (2).

$$\varepsilon = \varepsilon_\infty [1 - \exp(-kt)] \tag{2}$$

where $\varepsilon$ (%) is the recovery of the silicon concentrate; $\varepsilon_\infty$ (%) is the maximum flotation recovery, which is expected to be achieved according to the experimental results, and $\varepsilon_\infty$ is taken as 98%; $k$ is the flotation rate constant; and $t$ (min) is the flotation time.

*3.4. Characterization Methods*

The potential was measured by using a zeta potential analyzer (Zeta, Malvern ZEN-3700, United Kingdom). The contact angle was tested by using a surface tension meter (CA, Krüss K100, Germany), through the dynamic capillary penetration method. The chemical bonds on the surface were analyzed by using a Fourier transform infrared spectrometer (FTIR, Bruker ALPHA, Germany). The change in morphology was determined by using an atomic force microscope (AFM, Bruker Dimension Icon, United States). The changes in the surface morphology were observed by using a scanning electron microscope (SEM-EDS, ZEISS Gemini 300, Germany).

*3.5. DFT Calculation*

The adsorption location of DDA on Si was preliminarily calculated by using the Adsorption Locator module of Materials Studio (2023) software. The force field type in the calculation process is COMPASS II, and the fixed energy window is 100 kcal/mol. Density functional calculations were performed on the adsorption of DDA on Si using the CASTEP module. CASTEP simulates the properties of material interfaces and surfaces based on first-principles density functional theory. Utilizing plane wave pseudopotential theory based on total energy, it predicts properties such as lattice parameters and charge density using the number and type of atoms [40]. This study employs the Broyden–Fletcher–Goldfarb–Shanno (BFGS) optimization algorithm and utilizes the generalized gradient approximation (GGA) for exchange-correlation energy, providing a more comprehensive description of charge systems [41]. The Perdew–Burke–Ernzerhof (PBE) functional is applied to describe the exchange-correlation energy [42]. The Tkatchenko–Scheffler method, based on density functional theory (DFT), enhances the accuracy of electronic structure calculations by considering long-range interactions. To optimize traditional van der Waals corrections and improve computational accuracy while maintaining efficiency, the DFT-D3 dispersion correction uses the Tkatchenko–Scheffler method for calculations [43,44].

The crystal structure of Si has the parameters of $a = b = c = 5.4307$ Å and $\alpha = \beta = \gamma = 90°$. The adsorption energy of DDA on the Si surface could be calculated through Equation (3).

$$\Delta E = E_{Si-DDA} - E_{Si} - E_{DDA} \tag{3}$$

where $\Delta E$ (eV) denotes the adsorption energy; $E_{Si}$ (eV) and $E_{Si-DDA}$ (eV) are the total energy of the Si (111) surface before and after the adsorption, respectively; and $E_{DDA}$ is the energy of the DDA collector.

**4. Conclusions**

Based on the present study, the following three conclusions can be drawn:

(1) The flotation experiments show that silicon could be efficiently extracted from the DWSSS with flotation, and the maximal recovery of silicon can reach 98.2% with a DDA dosage of 0.6 g·L$^{-1}$ and natural pH within 24 min.

(2) The flotation process follows a first-order kinetics model. When the slurry pH is between 4 and 5, the recovery of silicon is highest when the DDA dosage is $0.6 \text{ g·L}^{-1}$, and the flotation rate constant is highest when the DDA dosage is $0.9 \text{ g·L}^{-1}$.

(3) The interface and adsorption behavior between the DDA and DWSSS indicate that DDA adsorbs on the silicon surface during the flotation process, modifying the silicon surface and improving hydrophobicity and floatability.

This study proposes an efficient process for silicon extraction from the DWSSS, which has the advantages of high silicon recovery, a short processing cycle, easy operation, and a low possibility of introducing metal impurity to achieve sustainable silicon waste resource recovery.

**Author Contributions:** Conceptualization, D.W. and S.Y.; Data Curation, L.Z.; Funding Acquisition, K.X. and K.W.; Methodology, L.Z.; Project Administration, K.X.; Resources, W.M.; Writing—Original Draft, L.Z.; Writing—Review and Editing, S.Y. All authors have read and agreed to the published version of the manuscript.

**Funding:** This study was financially supported by the Key Science and Technology Specific Projects of Yunnan Province (No. 202202AG050012), the Yunnan Fundamental Research Projects (No. 202101BE070001-010), and the Yunnan Major Scientific and Technological Projects (No. 202202AB080008).

**Institutional Review Board Statement:** Not applicable.

**Informed Consent Statement:** Not applicable.

**Data Availability Statement:** Dataset available on request from the authors.

**Conflicts of Interest:** The authors declare that they have no known competing financial interests or personal relationships that could have appeared to influence the work reported in this paper.

## References

1. Kwak, J.I.; Nam, S.-H.; Kim, L.; An, Y.-J. Potential environmental risk of solar cells: Current knowledge and future challenges. *J. Hazard. Mater.* **2020**, *392*, 122297. [CrossRef] [PubMed]
2. White, C.M.; Ege, P.; Ydstie, B.E. Size distribution modeling for fluidized bed solar-grade silicon production. *Powder Technol.* **2006**, *163*, 51–58. [CrossRef]
3. Ding, Z.; Li, Y.; Jiang, H.; Zhou, Y.; Wan, H.; Qiu, J.; Jiang, F.; Tan, J.; Du, W.; Chen, Y.; et al. The integral role of high-entropy alloys in advancing solid-state hydrogen storage. *Interdiscip. Mater.* **2024**, 1–34. [CrossRef]
4. Zhang, J.B.; Zhou, X.Y.; Hu, D.L.; Yuan, S.; Cai, E. Phase transformation pre-treatment of diamond wire-sawn multi-crystalline silicon wafers for metal-assisted chemical etching of solar cells. *Surf. Interfaces* **2023**, *36*, 102574. [CrossRef]
5. Yang, F.; Yu, W.; Rao, Z.; Wei, P.; Jiang, W.; Chen, H. A new strategy for de-oxidation of diamond-wire sawing silicon waste via the synergistic effect of magnesium thermal reduction and hydrochloric acid leaching. *J. Environ. Manag.* **2022**, *317*, 115424. [CrossRef]
6. Li, X.F.; Lv, G.Q.; Ma, W.H.; Li, T.; Zhang, R.F.; Zhang, J.H.; Li, S.Y.; Lei, Y. Review of resource and recycling of silicon powder from diamond-wire sawing silicon waste. *J. Hazard. Mater.* **2022**, *424*, 127389. [CrossRef] [PubMed]
7. Wei, K.; Yang, S.; Wan, X.; Ma, W.; Wu, J.; Lei, Y. Review of Silicon Recovery and Purification from Saw Silicon Powder. *JOM* **2020**, *72*, 2633–2647. [CrossRef]
8. Battaglia, C.; Cuevas, A.; De Wolf, S. High-efficiency crystalline silicon solar cells: Status and perspectives. *Energy Environ. Sci.* **2016**, *9*, 1552–1576. [CrossRef]
9. Ding, Z.; Ma, W.; Wei, K.; Wu, J.; Zhou, Y.; Xie, K. Boron removal from metallurgical-grade silicon using lithium containing slag. *J. Non-Cryst. Solids* **2012**, *358*, 2708–2712. [CrossRef]
10. Yang, S.; Wan, X.; Wei, K.; Ma, W.; Wang, Z. Occurrence State and Dissolution Mechanism of Metallic Impurities in Diamond Wire Saw Silicon Powder. *ACS Sustain. Chem. Eng.* **2020**, *8*, 12577–12587. [CrossRef]
11. Nain, P.; Kumar, A. Metal dissolution from end-of-life solar photovoltaics in real landfill leachate versus synthetic solutions: One-year study. *Waste Manag.* **2020**, *114*, 351–361. [CrossRef]
12. Vazquez-Pufleau, M.; Chadha, T.S.; Yablonsky, G.; Biswas, P. Carbon elimination from silicon kerf: Thermogravimetric analysis and mechanistic considerations. *Sci. Rep.* **2017**, *7*, 40535. [CrossRef]
13. Ding, Z.; Li, Y.T.; Yang, H.; Lu, Y.F.; Tan, J.; Li, J.B.; Li, Q.; Chen, Y.A.; Shaw, L.L.; Pan, F.S. Tailoring $MgH_2$ for hydrogen storage through nanoengineering and catalysis. *J. Magnes. Alloys* **2022**, *10*, 2946–2967. [CrossRef]
14. Basu, P.K.; Sreejith, K.P.; Yadav, T.S.; Kottanthariyil, A.; Sharma, A.K. Novel low-cost alkaline texturing process for diamond-wire-sawn industrial monocrystalline silicon wafers. *Sol. Energy Mater. Sol. Cells* **2018**, *185*, 406–414. [CrossRef]

15. Lu, T.; Tan, Y.; Li, J.; Shi, S. Remanufacturing of silicon powder waste cut by a diamond-wire saw through high temperature non-transfer arc assisted vacuum smelting. *J. Hazard. Mater.* **2019**, *379*, 120796. [CrossRef]
16. Zhang, Z.; Guo, X.; Wang, Y.; Wei, D.; Wang, H.; Li, H.; Zhuang, Y.; Xing, P. Leaching kinetic mechanism of iron from the diamond wire saw silicon powder by HCl. *Waste Manag.* **2023**, *169*, 82–90. [CrossRef] [PubMed]
17. Huang, L.; Chen, J.; Fang, M.; Thomas, S.; Danaei, A.; Luo, X.; Barati, M. Clean enhancing elimination of boron from silicon kerf using $Na_2O$-$SiO_2$ slag treatment. *J. Clean. Prod.* **2018**, *186*, 718–725. [CrossRef]
18. Wei, Y.; Lu, F.; Ai, X.; Lei, J.; Bai, Y.; Wei, Z.; Chen, Z. Towards High-Performance Inverted Mesoporous Perovskite Solar Cell by Using Bathocuproine (BCP). *Molecules* **2024**, *29*, 4009. [CrossRef] [PubMed]
19. Li, X.; Wu, J.; Xu, M.; Ma, W. Separation and purification of silicon from cutting kerf-loss slurry waste by electromagnetic and slag treatment technology. *J. Clean. Prod.* **2019**, *211*, 695–703. [CrossRef]
20. Wang, C.D.; Niu, X.X.; Wang, D.H.; Zhang, W.Y.; Shi, H.F.; Yu, L.; Wang, C.; Xiong, Z.H.; Ji, Z.; Yan, X.Q.; et al. Simple preparation of Si/CNTs/C composite derived from photovoltaic waste silicon powder as high-performance anode material for Li-ion batteries. *Powder Technol.* **2022**, *408*, 117744. [CrossRef]
21. Kumar, A.; Kaminski, S.; Melkote, S.N.; Arcona, C. Effect of wear of diamond wire on surface morphology, roughness and subsurface damage of silicon wafers. *Wear* **2016**, *364*, 163–168. [CrossRef]
22. Yang, S.C.; Wan, X.H.; Wei, K.X.; Ma, W.H.; Wang, Z. Silicon recycling and iron, nickel removal from diamond wire saw silicon powder waste: Synergistic chlorination with CaO smelting treatment. *Miner. Eng.* **2021**, *169*, 106966. [CrossRef]
23. Wei, D.; Kong, J.; Gao, S.; Zhou, S.; Zhuang, Y.; Xing, P. Preparation of Al-Si alloys with silicon cutting waste from diamond wire sawing process. *J. Environ. Manag.* **2021**, *290*, 112548. [CrossRef]
24. Zhu, X.D.; He, C.F.; Gu, Z.T. How do local policies and trade barriers reshape the export of Chinese photovoltaic products? *J. Clean. Prod.* **2021**, *278*, 123995. [CrossRef]
25. Cao, J.; Yang, J.; Wu, D.; Wang, Z.; Chen, H. Surface modification of hemimorphite by using ammonium carbamate and its response to flotation. *Appl. Surf. Sci.* **2022**, *605*, 154775. [CrossRef]
26. Mesa, D.; Brito-Parada, P.R. Scale-up in froth flotation: A state-of-the-art review. *Sep. Purif. Technol.* **2019**, *210*, 950–962. [CrossRef]
27. Liu, A.; Fan, M.-q.; Fan, P.-p. Interaction mechanism of miscible DDA-Kerosene and fine quartz and its effect on the reverse flotation of magnetic separation concentrate. *Miner. Eng.* **2014**, *65*, 41–50. [CrossRef]
28. Liu, A.; Fan, M.Q.; Li, Z.H. Synergistic effect of a mixture of dodecylamine and kerosene on separation of magnetite ore. *Physicochem. Probl. Miner. Process.* **2016**, *52*, 647–661.
29. Hu, X.N.; Tong, Z.; Sha, J.; Bilal, M.; Sun, Y.J.; Gu, R.; Ni, C.; Li, C.Q.; Deng, Y.M. Effects of Flotation Reagents on Flotation Kinetics of Aphanitic (Microcrystalline) Graphite. *Separations* **2022**, *9*, 416. [CrossRef]
30. Jada, A.; Akbour, R.A.; Douch, J. Surface charge and adsorption from water onto quartz sand of humic acid. *Chemosphere* **2006**, *64*, 1287–1295. [CrossRef] [PubMed]
31. Nosenko, Y.; Menges, F.; Riehn, C.; Niedner-Schatteburg, G. Investigation by two-color IR dissociation spectroscopy of Hoogsteen-type binding in a metalated nucleobase pair mimic. *Phys. Chem. Chem. Phys.* **2013**, *15*, 8171–8178. [CrossRef] [PubMed]
32. Xia, W.C.; Zhou, C.L.; Peng, Y.L. Enhancing flotation cleaning of intruded coal dry-ground with heavy oil. *J. Clean. Prod.* **2017**, *161*, 591–597. [CrossRef]
33. Ma, C.; Li, X.; Lyu, J.; He, M.; Wang, Z.; Li, L.; You, X. Study on characteristics of coal gasification fine slag-coal water slurry slurrying, combustion, and ash fusion. *Fuel* **2023**, *332*, 126039. [CrossRef]
34. Bai, L.M.; Liu, J.; Han, Y.X.; Jiang, K.; Zhao, W.Q. Effects of Xanthate on Flotation Kinetics of Chalcopyrite and Talc. *Minerals* **2018**, *8*, 369. [CrossRef]
35. Xing, Y.W.; Xu, M.D.; Gui, X.H.; Cao, Y.J.; Babel, B.; Rudolph, M.; Weber, S.; Kappl, M.; Butt, H.J. The application of atomic force microscopy in mineral flotation. *Adv. Colloid Interface Sci.* **2018**, *256*, 373–392. [CrossRef]
36. Li, L.; Zhang, C.; Yuan, Z.; Xu, X.; Song, Z. AFM and DFT study of depression of hematite in oleate-starch-hematite flotation system. *Appl. Surf. Sci.* **2019**, *480*, 749–758. [CrossRef]
37. Yang, H.L.; Liu, I.T.; Liu, C.E.; Hsu, H.P.; Lan, C.W. Recycling and reuse of kerf-loss silicon from diamond wire sawing for photovoltaic industry. *Waste Manag.* **2019**, *84*, 204–210. [CrossRef] [PubMed]
38. Gong, X.L.; Jiang, W.M.; Hu, S.L.; Yang, Z.Y.; Liu, X.W.; Fan, Z.T. Comprehensive utilization of foundry dust: Coal powder and clay minerals separation by ultrasonic-assisted flotation. *J. Hazard. Mater.* **2021**, *402*, 124124. [CrossRef] [PubMed]
39. Cao, S.; Yin, W.; Yang, B.; Zhu, Z.; Sun, H.; Sheng, Q.; Chen, K. Insights into the influence of temperature on the adsorption behavior of sodium oleate and its response to flotation of quartz. *Int. J. Min. Sci. Technol.* **2022**, *32*, 399–409. [CrossRef]
40. Perdew, J.P.; Ruzsinszky, A.; Csonka, G.I.; Vydrov, O.A.; Scuseria, G.E.; Constantin, L.A.; Zhou, X.; Burke, K. Restoring the density-gradient expansion for exchange in solids and surfaces. *Phys. Rev. Lett.* **2008**, *100*, 136406. [CrossRef] [PubMed]
41. Zuo, Q.; Wu, D.D.; Cao, J.; Wang, Z.; Wen, S.M.; Huang, L.Y.; Chen, H.Q. Surface modification of hemimorphite via double-complexion by ammonium fluoride and copper ion to promote sulfidation. *Appl. Surf. Sci.* **2023**, *612*, 155797. [CrossRef]
42. Ciucivara, A.; Sahu, B.R.; Joshi, S.; Banerjee, S.K.; Kleinman, L. Density functional study of Si(001)/Si(110) and Si(100)/Si(110) interfaces. *Phys. Rev. B* **2007**, *75*, 113309. [CrossRef]

43. Ni, C.Q.; Xie, Y.; Liu, C.; Han, Z.W.; Shen, H.R.; Ran, W.; Xie, W.Q.; Liang, Y.T. Exploring the separation mechanism of Gemini surfactant in scheelite froth flotation at low temperatures: Surface characterization, DFT calculations and kinetic simulations. *Sep. Purif. Technol.* **2023**, *305*, 122358. [CrossRef]
44. Li, Y.; Galli, G. Vibrational properties of alkyl monolayers on Si(111) surfaces: Predictions from ab-nitio- calculations. *Appl. Phys. Lett.* **2012**, *100*, 071605. [CrossRef]

**Disclaimer/Publisher's Note:** The statements, opinions and data contained in all publications are solely those of the individual author(s) and contributor(s) and not of MDPI and/or the editor(s). MDPI and/or the editor(s) disclaim responsibility for any injury to people or property resulting from any ideas, methods, instructions or products referred to in the content.

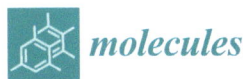 

Article

# An Electrochemical Sensor for Detection of Lead (II) Ions Using Biochar of Spent Coffee Grounds Modified by TiO₂ Nanoparticles

Zaiqiong Liu [1], Yiren Xu [1], Xurundong Kan [1], Mei Chen [1], Jingyang Dai [1], Yanli Zhang [2], Pengfei Pang [2], Wenhui Ma [1,3,*] and Jianqiang Zhang [1,*]

[1] International Union Laboratory of China and Malaysia for Quality Monitoring and Evaluation of Agricultural Products in Yunnan, School of Biology and Chemistry, Pu'er University, Pu'er 665000, China; lzq15025110725@126.com (Z.L.); xuyiren@peu.edu.cn (Y.X.); kanxurundong@163.com (X.K.); mchen1988@126.com (M.C.); 18988150410@163.com (J.D.)

[2] School of Chemistry and Environment, Yunnan Minzu University, Kunming 650500, China; yanli.zhang@yahoo.com (Y.Z.); pfpang@ynni.edu.cn (P.P.)

[3] School of Engineering, Yunnan University, Kunming 650500, China

\* Correspondence: mwhsilicon@126.com (W.M.); drjqzhang@126.com (J.Z.); Tel./Fax: +86-15348798859 (J.Z.)

**Abstract:** Toxic heavy metal ions, such as lead ions, significantly threaten human health and the environment. This work introduces a novel method for the simple and sensitive detection of lead ions based on biochar-loaded titanium dioxide nanoparticles (BC@TiO₂NPs) nanocomposites. Eco-friendly biochar samples were prepared from spent coffee grounds (500 °C, 1 h) that were chemically activated with TiO₂ nanoparticles (150 °C, 24 h) to improve their conductivity. Structural characterizations showed that BC@TiO₂NPs have a porous structure. The BC@TiO₂NPs material was evaluated for lead ion determination by assembling glassy carbon electrodes. Under optimal conditions, the sensor was immersed in a solution containing the analyte (0.1 M NaAc-HAc buffer, pH = 4.5) for the detection of lead ions via differential pulse voltammetry. A linear dynamic range from 1 pM to 10 μM was achieved, with a detection limit of 0.6268 pM. Additionally, the analyte was determined in tap water samples, and a satisfactory recovery rate was achieved.

**Keywords:** coffee grounds-derived biochar; TiO₂ nanoparticles; lead ions electrochemical sensor

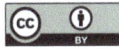

## 1. Introduction

Currently, heavy metal contamination has become much more critical due to the increase in the Industrial Revolution. Lead (Pb) is a relatively abundant heavy metal, present in the Earth's crust with an abundance of 0.0016% [1]. First used by humans as early as 3000 BC, Pb has been considered highly toxic for human health and the environment [2]. Pb is a hazardous non-biodegradable heavy metal. As Pb is smelted from ores and used in gasoline, batteries, pigments, etc., the resulting environmental pollution dramatically impacts ecosystems [3]. The lead ions in mines may cause water pollution when they are slowly released into the water environment through rainwater.

Additionally, it has been reported that lead ions can reach the human body through the gastrointestinal tract, respiratory tract, and skin and damage the nervous system, resulting in kidney, brain, and liver damage [4]. Moreover, lead ions in the human body in concentrations of 30–1000 μg L$^{-1}$ can cause diseases such as atrophy, interstitial nephritis, colic, and anemia, among others [5]. The Drinking Water Quality Act criterion specified the value of 10 μg L$^{-1}$ according to the guidelines established by the World Health Organization; therefore, it is harmful when the concentration of lead ions exceeds this value [6]. Considering the importance of the above, developing rapid and sensitive methods for detecting lead ions is crucial for analytical and environmental disciplines.

A large number of traditional analytical methods have been developed for the determination of lead ions, such as atomic absorption spectrometry [7], colorimetry [8], high-performance liquid chromatography (HPLC) [9], inductively coupled plasma analysis [10,11], mass spectrometry [12], fluorimetry [13,14], and electrochemistry [15], among others. Although these techniques for the detection of trace levels of Pb have their specific applicability and ability to improve the sensitivity, they exhibit typical shortcomings, including requiring expensive instruments, tedious operational procedures, relatively slow detection speeds, the specific design of responsive molecules, etc. Additionally, researchers are still seeking improvements in detection approaches, such as low cost, high sensitivity, simple operation, and ease of use. In comparison, electrochemical methods are more advanced, portable, and sensitive detection technologies, allowing rapid and simultaneous evaluations for lead ions [16].

Several lead ion electrochemical sensors focused on analyzing different surface modifiers have been developed in the past decade. Based on broad prospects for chemically modified electrodes and technological innovations toward advanced materials, developing a novel and effective approach for the electrochemical detection of lead ions has become a research hotspot. At present, studies on lead ion detection mainly focus on using various electrocatalysts, including metal–organic frameworks [17], carbon materials [18], polymers [19], bismuth-based materials [20], and functionalized DNA probes [21]. However, these materials do not meet the global demand for "carbon peaking" and "carbon neutrality" and may cause significant environmental damage. Therefore, it is necessary to develop low-cost and environmentally friendly electronic devices for lead ion detection [22].

Biochar (BC), a carbonaceous product from pyrolysis of biomass resources under a limited oxygen supply, has piqued research interest because of its environmentally friendly precursors [23]. Typically, a wide range of biomass industrial byproducts [24], plants [25], agricultural wastes [26], and forest residues [27] can be used cost-effectively for producing different types of biochar. Furthermore, biomass-derived biochar exhibits several distinctive characteristics, including chemical inertness, a sizable surface area, charged surfaces, and economic favorability. Consequently, it is applied in different fields such as heavy metal ion treatment [28], energy storage conversion devices [29], biomedicine [30], electrochemical sensors [31], photocatalysis [32], and others. Interestingly, these applications are mainly focused on an excellent adsorption capacity for positively charged metal ions because the biomass-derived biochar surface possesses a negative charge [33]. Previous studies indicated that physical and chemical interactions (electrostatic attraction, complexation, etc.) play critical functional roles in the adsorption mechanism [34]. Thus, surface modification has garnered significant attention to enhance raw biochar's catalytic and absorption performances and obtain optimal composites.

Modifying biochar involves various techniques, including physical and chemical methods, to improve specific functionalities or properties. In recent times, acids [35], alkaline agents [36], metal oxides, and salts [37] have been utilized as chemical modifiers for the adsorption of heavy metal ions due to their high potential. Typically, metal oxides ($Co_3O_4$ [38], $Fe_3O_4$ [39], $MoS_2$ [35], $TiO_2$ [40]) have the potential to enhance affinity toward heavy metal contaminants because they can significantly improve the surface sorption, catalytic, and fixation abilities of biochar. Nanobiochar composites modified by metal oxides are an emerging material with exceptional quality. Among them, biochars modified with $TiO_2$ nanomaterials are widely used as photocatalysts and adsorbents for heavy metal ions and organic pollutants [41,42]. In addition, $TiO_2$ nanoparticles with different crystal planes have been applied to improve the catalytic effect of hydrogen absorption [43–45]. However, to the best of our knowledge, an electrochemical sensor based on a biochar–$TiO_2$ nanocomposite has rarely been investigated. On the other hand, designing sustainable BC-based hybrid nanocomposites with appropriate surface functionalization is still challenging [46].

Herein, an electrochemical sensor was fabricated to analyze lead ions by modifying $TiO_2$ nanoparticles on the surface of biochar (BC@$TiO_2$NPs). Porous carbon materials were obtained by using spent coffee grounds. The prepared BC@$TiO_2$NPs exhibited excellent electrical conductivity, which improved the adsorption capacity towards lead ions in aqueous solution. The influence of the experimental conditions on the lead ion detection was investigated. Finally, this work demonstrated that BC@TiO$_2$NPs/GCE possessed good sensitivity for the detection of lead ions.

## 2. Results and Discussion

### 2.1. Detection Principle of the Sensor

This study introduced a rapid and sensitive detection method for Pb$^{2+}$ based on a glass carbon electrode modified with a BC@TiO$_2$NPs nanocomposite. The schematic of the BC@TiO$_2$NPs nanohybrid synthesis and stepwise fabrication of the sensor is shown in Scheme 1. The BC was obtained using coffee grounds as the precursor by the thermal carbonization method (a). Then, TiO$_2$ particles were randomly embedded into the BC network using an easy one-pot hydrothermal method (BC@TiO$_2$NPs) (b). Next, the prepared BC@TiO$_2$NPs composite was used to develop an efficient electrochemical sensing probe. When the probe was exposed to the Pb$^{2+}$ solution, Pb$^{2+}$ was first adsorbed onto the surface of the BC@TiO$_2$NPs nanocomposite and then reduced to a low-valence state. This is because TiO$_2$ nanoparticles can produce electron–hole pairs, and these carriers can redox-react with lead ions under an excitation voltage condition. Additionally, chelate complexes were formed on the surface of the BC@TiO$_2$NPs nanocomposite owing to the empty orbital provided by lead ions and the lone pair electrons produced by the oxygen atoms in TiO$_2$ nanoparticles (c). This greatly facilitated Pb$^{2+}$ adsorption within the micropores and improved the sensitivity of the sensor towards Pb$^{2+}$. Consequently, quantitative detection of Pb$^{2+}$ was achieved by recording the electrochemical signals generated by the lead ion redox process.

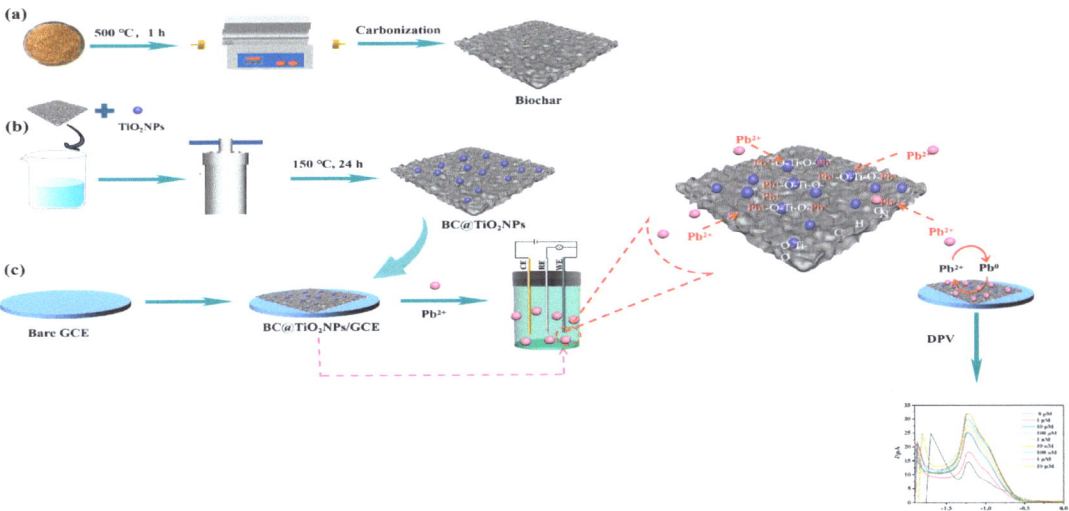

**Scheme 1.** Schematic diagram of the application of BC@TiO$_2$NPs nanomaterial and the detection principle of the electrochemical biosensor for lead ions. The inset in (c) is the photograph of the reaction mechanism of lead ions with the BC@TiO$_2$NPs nanocomposite material.

### 2.2. Characterization of BC and BC@TiO$_2$NPs Nanohybrid

The BC@TiO$_2$NPs were prepared using biochar obtained from coffee grounds as the precursor. A scanning electron microscope (SEM) was employed to inspect the morphology and microstructure of the as-prepared BC and BC@TiO$_2$NPs materials. As illustrated in Figure 1A, the BC showed a blocky porous structure that can facilitate rapid ion transport, and the porosity was roughly calculated as 4.207%, according to the ratio of the porous area to the total area of the SEM image (Table S1). As seen from Figure 1B, small-sized TiO$_2$

nanoparticles (average 0.5218 μm in Figure S1A) were randomly self-assembled on the surface of the BC composite through the interaction between the BC and TiO$_2$. Additionally, we provide real sample images of BC and BC@ TiO$_2$NPs materials in Figure S1B. The results showed a distinct color change between the two materials. Consequently, these results indicated the successful preparation of the BC@TiO$_2$NPs nanohybrid composite, which can be used for the electrochemical sensor construction.

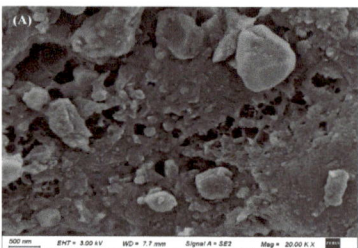 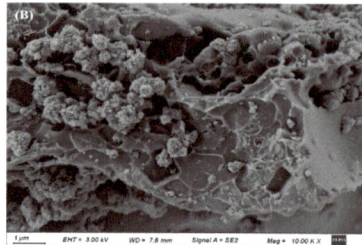

**Figure 1.** SEM images of BC (**A**) and BC@TiO$_2$NPs (**B**).

*2.3. Electrochemical Behavior of Modified Electrodes*

The electrochemical properties of the modified electrode were characterized by cyclic voltammetry (CV) and electrochemical impedance spectroscopy (EIS) using 5.0 mM K$_3$[Fe(CN)$_6$)]$^{3-/4-}$ containing 0.1 M KCl as an electrolyte. The cyclic voltammograms and the Nyquist plots of bare GCE, BC/GCE, and BC@TiO$_2$/GCE are shown in Figure 2. As seen in Figure 2A, the bare GCE produced a pair of well-defined redox peaks (curve a), ascribed to the oxidation and reduction reactions between [Fe(CN)$_6$)]$^{3-/4-}$ ions. However, after BC material modification (BC/GCE), there was a significant reduction in the redox peak (curve b) because of the constraint of the electron transfer toward redox reactions caused by the porous BC with poor electronic conductivity. Notably, after introducing TiO$_2$NPs onto the surface of the BC material to form BC@TiO$_2$/GCE (curve c), the redox peak significantly increased, which could be attributed to parts of TiO$_2$ nanoparticles being electroactive and improving the charge transfer ability. This also confirms the successful decoration of BC and BC@TiO$_2$ onto the surface of GCE. These results were consistent with the corresponding EIS characterizations (Figure 2B), in which the electron transfer resistance varied for the differently assembled electrodes. The semicircular diameter of the impedance equaled the electron transfer resistance (Ret) at the electrode interface, which confirmed the electrode modification process.

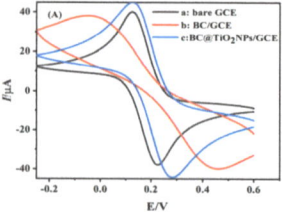 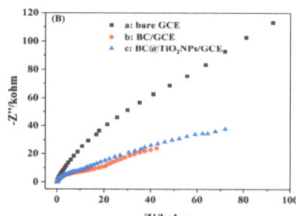

**Figure 2.** Characterization of the Pb$^{2+}$ electrochemical sensor. CV (**A**) and EIS (**B**) of differently assembled electrodes: bare GCE (a), BC/GCE (b), BC@TiO$_2$NPs/GCE (c); EIS and CV were operated in 0.1 M KCl containing 5 mM [Fe (CN)$_6$]$^{3-/4-}$ with the frequency range from 0.1 Hz to 100 kHz, the amplitude of 10 mV, and the scanned potential from −0.2 V to +0.6 V, with a scan rate of 0.05 V/s.

## 2.4. Feasibility Validation of the Electrochemical Sensor

To ensure the success of the subsequent experiment and investigate the electrochemical response of $Pb^{2+}$ by the GCE, BC/GCE, and BC@TiO$_2$NPs/GCE sensors, a differential pulse voltammetry (DPV) experiment was performed in 0.1 M NaAc-HAc buffer (pH = 4.5) containing 10 μM lead ions. As depicted in Figure 3, in the presence of bare GCE, there was almost no peak current at −0.80 V (curve a). In contrast, the modified electrode (BC@TiO$_2$/GCE) exhibited a well-defined oxidation peak current response (curve b), three times higher than that of bare GCE and BC/GCE. The porous structure of BC causes the cationic lead to be adsorbed in the pores. Subsequently, the lead ion is electrochemically reduced to zero valence under the applied voltammetry potential and then oxidized to generate an anodic peak current. These results show that the TiO$_2$NPs decoration on the BC results in a synergy that leads to a notable improvement in the surface area, electronic conductivity, and active functional sites. However, a distinct decrease in the peak current was observed when the BC was immobilized on the bare GCE (curve c). This decrease in the current value indicates that the unmodified biochar can hinder the diffusion of the redox species toward the electrode surface from the electrolyte. These results confirm the efficiency of the designed strategy for detecting lead ions.

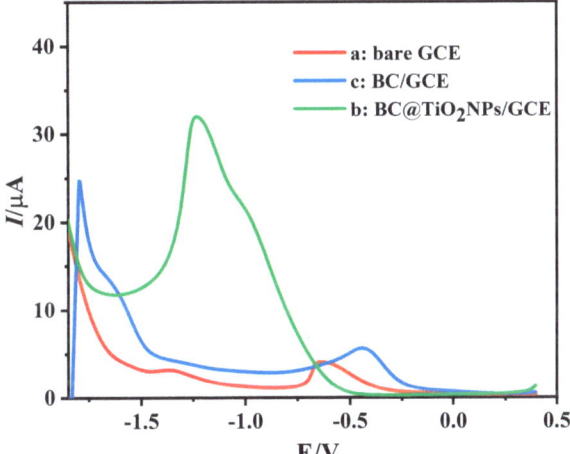

**Figure 3.** DPV responses of the fabricated BC@TiO$_2$NPs sensor in 0.1 M NaAc-HAc solution (pH 4.5) with bare GCE (a), BC/GCE (b), and BC@TiO$_2$NPs/GCE (c). Concentration of lead ions 10 μM. Modulation time of 0.02 s; interval time of 0.5 s; pulse amplitude of 25 mV.

## 2.5. Optimization of Conditions

In order to achieve the best experimental conditions for detecting lead ions, the key factors were optimized, including the type and pH of the electrolyte, concentration of BC@TiO$_2$NPs, and deposition time.

### 2.5.1. Effect of Electrolyte and pH

Supporting electrolytes maintain a homogeneous electric field in electrochemical investigations involving the oxidation and reduction of the analyte molecule. As shown in Figure S2, the current signal and potential peak of the analyte are significantly influenced by various electrolytes, including phosphate acid buffer solution (PBS), acetic acid buffer solution (NaAc-HAc), and ammonium chloride buffer solution (NH$_3$H$_2$O-NH$_4$Cl). The results revealed that the NaAc-HAc buffer displayed the maximum peak current (Ipa). Consequently, the NaAc-HAc buffer was considered the optimal supporting electrolyte for the further detection of lead ions. Next, the effect of pH on the lead ion response in

NaAc-HAc buffer was evaluated. The DPV response of BC@TiO$_2$NPs/GCE sensor was recorded in various pH values (4.0–6.5) of NaAc-HAc buffer. The current response reached the highest value when the solution pH was 4.5 (Figure S3), probably because overly acidic or basic solutions affect the target's molecular structure. Therefore, the following sensing process was carried out under pH = 4.5.

2.5.2. Effect of Concentration of BC@TiO$_2$NPs Composite

The concentration of the BC@TiO$_2$NPs composites during the electrocatalytic process directly affected the electrochemical performance for determining lead ions. As seen in Figure S4, when the BC@TiO$_2$NPs concentration increased from 2 mg/mL to 12 mg/mL, the oxidation current intensity increased and reached its maximum value at 10 mg/mL. The porous structure of BC@TiO$_2$NPs composite offers electroactive sites at the electrolyte–electrode interface. However, overloading can affect the thickness of this composite, hindering lead ion diffusion and increasing electron transport resistance. Thus, 10 mg/mL BC@TiO$_2$NPs was utilized for the following detection experiments.

2.5.3. Effect of Deposition Time

The effect of the deposition time of lead ions on BC@TiO$_2$NPs/GCE was studied within the range of 1 to 12 s (Figure S5). It was observed that the current value exhibited a gradual increase with the extension of the deposition time up to 3 s. Hence, an adsorption time of 3 s was selected for practical purposes in the subsequent experiment.

*2.6. Analytical Performance of the Proposed Method*

Under the optimized experimental conditions (pH = 4.5, NaAc-HAc buffer, 10 mg/mL BC@TiO$_2$NPs, 3 s deposition time), DPV was employed to detect Pb$^{2+}$ adsorption behavior on BC@TiO$_2$NPs/GCE. As depicted in Figure 4 A, the oxidation peak current ($I_{pa}$) increased with the increase in Pb$^{2+}$ concentration. $I_{pa}$ presented a well-defined linear relationship with the logarithm of Pb$^{2+}$ concentration in the 1 pM-10 μM range. The corresponding linear regression equation was expressed as $I$ (μA) = 2.23541log$C_{Pb2+}$ + 31.8198 ($R^2$ = 0.9667), and the detection limit was determined to be 0.6268 pM according to the calibration curve method. The calculation formula of LOD is LOD = 3σ/S, where σ is the standard deviation of the detection value of blank samples, and S is the slope of the calibration curve. This result indicated that more lead ions were adsorbed onto the cavities of the porous biochar owing to abundant binding sites at the BC@TiO$_2$NPs nanocomposite. Compared with previously reported electrochemical sensors for lead ions (Table 1), the proposed BC@TiO$_2$NPs-modified electrode presented better analytical performance. Therefore, the fabricated sensor significantly improved the detection sensitivity toward lead ions.

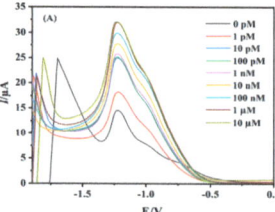
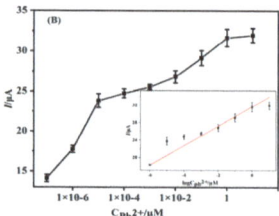

**Figure 4.** (**A**) Electrochemical responses of the BC@TiO$_2$NPs/GCE sensor to different concentrations of Pb$^{2+}$ from 0 pM to 10 μM recorded in 0.1 M NaAc-HAc solution (pH 4.5). (**B**) Calibration plots between the current and the log$C_{Pb2+}$. Error bars, SD, $n$ = 3.

Table 1. Comparisons of the proposed electrochemical sensor with the reported methods.

| Strategy | Technique | Linear Range/μM | LOD/μM | Reference |
| --- | --- | --- | --- | --- |
| G-C-4/SPE | SWASV | 0.05–1 | 0.0089 | [1] |
| PA-PPy@SPCE | DPASV | 0.01–6 | $0.43 \times 10^{-3}$ | [47] |
| CHO/CS-GO/Pb(II)/Aptmer/MCH/AuNPs/GCE | DPV | $0.483 \times 10^{-6}$–$0.965 \times 10^{-5}$ | $0.384 \times 10^{-6}$ | [48] |
| BC@TiO$_2$NPs/GCE | DPV | $1 \times 10^{-6}$–10 | $0.6268 \times 10^{-6}$ | This method |

### 2.7. Selectivity, Reproducibility, and Stability Investigation

To assess the selection accuracy of the prepared BC@TiO$_2$NPs sensor, the selectivity was estimated using 100 μM solutions of different cations ($Cd^{2+}$, $Ca^{2+}$, $Cu^{2+}$, $Mg^{2+}$, $Ba^{2+}$, $Al^{3+}$, $Zn^{2+}$). The results revealed that the current signal of $Pb^{2+}$ ions exhibited a maximum value (Figure 5A). However, the sensor's response to different ions ($Cd^{2+}$, $Ca^{2+}$, $Cu^{2+}$, $Mg^{2+}$, $Ba^{2+}$, $Al^{3+}$, $Zn^{2+}$) was almost equivalent, which may mean that changes in the ionic strength can affect the electrode response. In addition, the interfering ions may react chemically with the electrode membrane, resulting in a change in the properties of the electrode membrane, which then produces a potential response. In general, the proposed method based on the BC@TiO$_2$NPs composites possessed good specificity for $Pb^{2+}$ detection.

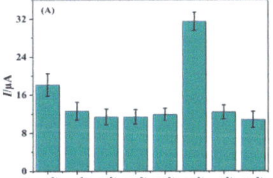
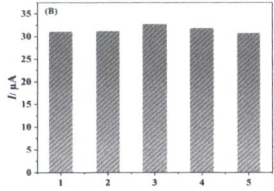
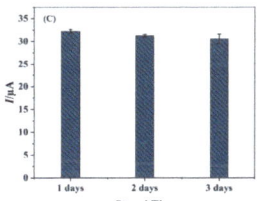

**Figure 5.** (**A**) High selectivity of the designed sensor for $Pb^{2+}$ detection. One μM of $Pb^{2+}$ and various ions, including $Cd^{2+}$, $Ca^{2+}$, $Cu^{2+}$, $Mg^{2+}$, $Ba^{2+}$, $Al^{3+}$, and $Zn^{2+}$ (100 μM), were used in the experiments. (**B**) Reproducibility of the $Pb^{2+}$ electrochemical sensor was evaluated by measuring 10 μM of lead ions with different electrodes. (**C**) Stability evaluated by the BC@TiO$_2$NPs/GCE sensor in the presence of lead ions.

To evaluate the reproducibility of the sensor, further investigations were conducted by preparing five BC@TiO$_2$NPs/GCE sensors using the same modification process and testing them with 10 μM lead ions in NaAc-HAc buffer solution (pH = 4.5). It was observed that the peak current of lead ions was roughly the same (Figure 5B), and the relative standard deviation (RSD) value was found to be 2.50% ($n = 5$), indicating good repeatability of the developed sensor. In addition, one independent BC@TiO$_2$NPs/GCE electrode was also used to test the reproducibility experiment under same conditions. The results are shown in Figure S6A, and the RSD was calculated as 14.8%, which indicated that the BC@TiO$_2$NPs/GCE can operate under different lead ion concentrations.

Stability is also crucial in assessing the sensor's performance and service life. Here, 10 mg/mL of BC@TiO$_2$NPs-altered GCE was stored for 1 day, 2 days, and 3 days at room temperature, respectively. Furthermore, the DPV signals are shown in Figure 5C, and there were fewer changes in the observed current signals for each measurement, demonstrating commendable storage stability with an RSD of 2.70%. To estimate the lifetime of BC@TiO$_2$NPs/GCE electrode, cyclic experiments were carried out via cyclic voltammetry (CV) technology (Figure S6B). The results shown that as the number of cycles increased, the oxidation peak current of lead ions gradually enhanced, possibly due to the electro-adsorption and desorption reactions of lead ions on the BC@TiO$_2$NPs/GCE electrode surface. The capacity retention rate of the sensor was about 116.0% even after

50 cycles according to the formula: Capacity Retention Ratio = $I_n/I_0$, where $I_n$ is the peak current value after 50 cycles, and $I_0$ is the initial peak current value, indicating that the sensor had excellent storage capacity.

*2.8. Analysis of Water Samples*

To evaluate the practical performance of the fabricated BC@TiO$_2$NPs/GCE sensor, it was applied to analyze the content of lead ions in a natural water sample. Initially, the quantification of lead ions was conducted through the standard addition method, and different concentrations of lead ions (1, 10, and 100 nM) were spiked into tap water samples, respectively. Next, the current response was determined using the DPV technique under the same conditions. As presented in Table 2, the recovery rates of lead ions from the water samples ranged between 100.09 and 103.0% with RSD values from 0.8792 to 1.0910%, suggesting the high potential of the BC@TiO$_2$NPs/GCE sensor for the reliable determination of lead ions in the actual water samples.

**Table 2.** Detection of Pb$^{2+}$ in an actual water sample ($n$ = 3).

| Sample (Tap Water) | Added (nM) | Found (nM) | Recovery (%) | RSD (%) |
|---|---|---|---|---|
| 1 | 0 | 0 | 0 | 0 |
| 2 | 1 | 1.030 | 103.00 | 0.9324 |
| 3 | 10 | 10.046 | 100.46 | 0.8792 |
| 4 | 100 | 100.088 | 100.088 | 1.0910 |

## 3. Materials and Methods

*3.1. Reagent and Apparatus*

Waste coffee grounds were purchased from Arabica-Cardim Coffee in Nandu River, Pu'er, Yunnan province. Titanium dioxide (TiO$_2$), ammonia water (NH$_3$ H$_2$O), ethyl alcohol (CH$_3$CH$_2$OH, 95%), glacial acetic acid (CH$_3$COOH), and sodium anhydrous acetate (CH$_3$COONa) were provided by Shanghai Titan Scientific Co., Ltd. (Shanghai, China). Sodium dihydrogen phosphate dihydrate (NaH$_2$PO4 2H$_2$O), disodium hydrogen phosphate dodecahydrate (Na$_2$HPO$_4$ 12H$_2$O), potassium hexacyanoferrate (III) (K$_3$Fe(CN)$_6$), and potassium hexacyanoferrate (II) (K$_4$Fe(CN)$_6$ 3H$_2$O) were purchased from Tianjin Damao Chemicals Reagent Factory (China). Anhydrous sodium sulfate (Na$_2$SO$_4$) was supplied by Tianjin Zhiyuan Chemicals Reagent Co., Ltd. (Tianjin, China). Lead chloride (PbCl$_2$) was obtained from Shanghai Reagent Factory No.1 Co., Ltd. (Shanghai, China), and solid potassium chloride (KCl) was purchased from Sichuan Xilong Science Co., Ltd. (Sichuan, China). For evaluation of the sensor performance, calcium (Ca$^{2+}$), cadmium (Cd$^{2+}$), copper (Cu$^{2+}$), and magnesium (Mg$^{2+}$) standard solutions were acquired from The National Center for Analysis and Testing of Nonferrous Metals and Electronic Materials. All solutions were prepared using ultrapure water.

Field emission scanning electron microscopy (SEM) images of the BC@TiO$_2$NPs nanohybrid were obtained using a German Zeiss Sigma 300 microscope. Cyclic voltammetry (CV), differential pulse voltammetry (DPV), and electrochemical impedance spectroscopy (EIS) measurements were performed using a CHI660C electrochemical workstation (ChenHua Instrument Co., Shanghai, China) at room temperature. A typical three-electrode system, composed of a bare or modified glass–carbon electrode (GCE) as the working electrode, a saturated calomel electrode (SCE) as the reference electrode, and a platinum wire as the auxiliary electrode, was used for electrochemical measurements.

*3.2. Preparation of BC@TiO$_2$NPs Nanocomposite*

The BC@TiO$_2$NPs nanocomposite was prepared using the following two steps. First, the coffee grounds were boiled five times in ultrapure water and then dried at 80 °C for three days. To obtain biochar (BC), the dried coffee grounds were carbonized at 500 °C for 1 h in a tube furnace under a nitrogen atmosphere (10 °C/min). After screening with a

0.125 mm sieve, the pyrolyzed coffee BC material was stored in sealed bottles for further use. Afterwards, 2.1 g of pyrolyzed BC material and 0.9 g of TiO$_2$ nanoparticles were mixed in a Teflon-lined stainless-steel autoclave with 30 mL of ultrapure water. The mixture was then heated to 150 °C for 24 h. Finally, the resulting product was centrifuged and rinsed with Milli-Q water and ethyl alcohol repeatedly. After that, the obtained sample was dried at 60 °C for 24 h and named BC@TiO$_2$NPs.

### 3.3. Fabrication of Electrochemical Sensor for Lead Ions

Before preparing the modified electrode, a GCE was initially polished with 0.3 and 0.05 μm Al$_2$O$_3$ powder to improve its surface kinetics. Then, it was ultrasonically cleaned with ethanol and ultrapure water for 1 min, respectively. Next, 10 mg of BC@TiO$_2$NPs nanocomposite was dispersed in 1 mL of ultrapure water (10 mg/mL) and treated in a sonicator for 2 h; then, 10 μL of the uniform solution was withdrawn and dripped onto the surface of the smooth and polished GCE, followed by drying naturally in air at 25 °C for 1 h. The modified electrode served as a working electrode for electrochemical detection.

### 3.4. Electrochemical Measurement

The electrochemical performance of the fabricated GCE was determined by cyclic voltammetry (CV) and electrochemical impedance spectra (EIS) measurements. The CV and EIS experiments were conducted using 5 mM [Fe(CN)$_6$]$^{3-}$/$^{4-}$ electrolyte containing 0.1 M KCl over the voltage range of −0.2–0.6 V, at a scan rate of 0.05 V/s, a frequency range of 0.1 Hz to 100 kHz, and a potential amplitude of 10 mV. Differential pulse voltammetry (DPV) curves were constructed using 0.1 M NaAc-HAc buffer (pH = 4.5) as the electrolyte with the potential between −2.0 and 0.6 V, at a pulse time of 0.02 s, pulse period of 0.5 s, and amplitude of 25 mV.

### 3.5. Optimization of Experimental Conditions

In order to achieve the best experimental conditions for detecting lead ions, this experiment further studied the influence of possible factors, including the type of buffer solution, pH, modification concentration of BC@TiO$_2$NPs nanocomposite, and deposition time. The selection of these experimental conditions was achieved using DPV technology, with specific details described in Section 2.5.

### 3.6. Determination of Lead Ions

Lead ions were detected using DPV technology under the optimal experimental conditions presented in Section 3.5. First, 40 mL of 0.1 M NaAc-HAc buffer solution with a pH of 4.5 was taken in beaker, and an appropriate amount of lead standard solution was added to prepare eight standard solutions with different concentrations of 1 pM, 10 pM, 100 pM, 1 nM, 10 nM, 100 nM, 1 μM, and 10 μM. Then, the pretreated three-electrode system was inserted into the electrolysis tank and connected to the electrochemical workstation. Referring to Section 3.4, the parameters of the DPV were set, and a scan was performed in the potential range of −2 V to 0.6 V. The peak current values corresponding to lead ions in the DPV curves were recorded, and a standard curve was plotted with the lead ion concentration as the horizontal coordinate and the peak current value as the vertical coordinate. The experimental result in Section 2.6 is based on this step.

### 3.7. Real Sample Tests

To investigate the practical application of the proposed sensor in routine analysis, BC@TiO$_2$/GCE was employed to detect Pb$^{2+}$ in Pu'er water samples. First, local water samples from Pu'er City were treated using a membrane filter with a pore size of 0.45 μm, and the pH of the water samples was adjusted to 4.5 using a 0.1 M NaAc-HAc buffer solution. A precise volume of 40 mL of the pretreated actual water sample was then placed in a beaker, and known concentrations of lead ions within the linear range of the standard curve, such as 1, 10, and 100 nM, were added as standard solutions. According to the electrochemical detection conditions in Section 3.6, the spiked water samples were tested to obtain the desorption peak current. Based on the linear regression equation of the standard curve, the concentration of spiked lead ions was calculated, and the recovery rate was determined.

## 4. Conclusions

A simple, green, and sensitive BC@TiO$_2$NPs-modified working electrode was successfully fabricated and applied to detect lead ions. First, a BC@TiO$_2$NPs nanocomposite derived from coffee residue was synthesized and characterized using SEM, CV, and EIS techniques. Then, TiO$_2$ nanoparticles were successfully dispersed throughout the surface of the mesoporous BC, which enormously improved the peak currents for lead ion determination. The resulting electrode demonstrated outstanding sensitivity, a low limit of detection (0.6268 pM), a wide linear range (1 pM–10 μM), good interference, good repeatability, and practical stability. Additionally, this sensor was employed to monitor lead ions in real samples and displayed remarkable recovery values (100.09–103.0%). Therefore, the results indicate that carbon materials derived from waste coffee residues can be utilized to manufacture high-value devices. Additionally, the BC@TiO$_2$NPs/GCE sensor has an expectation for serving as a reliable electrochemical platform in the field of environmental monitoring, demonstrating significant potential for reducing carbon footprints.

**Supplementary Materials:** The following supporting information can be downloaded at: https://www.mdpi.com/article/10.3390/molecules29235704/s1, Figure S1: (A) The particle size distribution histogram of TiO$_2$ nanoparticles. (B) The real samples of BC and BC@TiO$_2$NPs; Figure S2: (A) Effects of various electrolytes including PBS, NaAc-HAc, NH$_3$H$_2$O-NH$_4$Cl. (B) The error bars represent the standard deviation of three independent experiments, $n$ = 3; Figure S3: Effects of the pH on the sensor in the NaAc-HAc buffer. The error bars represent the standard deviation of three independent experiments, $n$ = 3; Figure S4: Effects of the BC@TiO$_2$NPs concentration. The error bars represent the standard deviation of three independent experiments, $n$ = 3; Figure S5: Effects of the deposition time on the Pb$^{2+}$ detection. The error bars represent the standard deviation of three independent experiments, $n$ = 3; Figure S6 (A) DPV responses of one BC@TiO$_2$NPs/GCE electrode for detecting lead ions at different concentrations including 1 pM, 10 pM, 100 pM, 1 nM, 10 nM in 0.1 M NaAc-HAc buffer (pH 4.5). (B) Cyclic voltammograms of 10 μM of lead ions recorded at the BC@TiO$_2$NPs/GCE sensor in 0.1 M NaAc-HAc of pH 7.0 at a scan rate of 0.05 V/s, 50 cycles, and a potential range of -1.80 to 0.4 V; Table S1: Porosity data of BC material.

**Author Contributions:** Z.L.: Conceptualization, Formal analysis, Investigation, Writing-original draft. Y.X.: Data curation, Formal analysis, Investigation. X.K.: Investigation, Resources, Formal analysis. M.C.: Resources, Supervision, Validation. J.D.: Conceptualization, Methodology. Y.Z.: Investigation, Resources, Formal analysis. P.P.: Resources, Supervision, Validation. W.M.: Conceptualization, Methodology, Supervision, Project administration, Funding acquisition. J.Z.: Resources, Supervision, Validation, Writing-review & editing. All authors have read and agreed to the published version of the manuscript.

**Funding:** The authors gratefully acknowledge the financial support from the Science and Technology Plan project of Yunnan Provincial Science and Technology Department (Grant No. 202403AP140027); the Scientific Research project of Yunnan Pu'er University (Grant No. PEXYXJYB202314); Pu'er City Science and Technology Bureau's first batch of municipal-level science and technology plan projects for 2024 (self-funded) (Grant No. ZCXM20240132); the Basic Research in Local Undergraduate Universities Fund of Yunnan Provincial Science and Technology Department (Nos. 202101BA070001-025; 202301BA070001-126); the Research on Coffee Quality Control and Utilization of Residues Based on Nanomultifunctional Materials and Endophytic Fungi (Project No.: FWCY-ZNT2024030); the Yunnan China–Laos International Joint Research and Development Center for Energy and Mineral Analysis and Technology Innovation (Project No.: 202203AP140148); the International Union Laboratory of China and Malaysia for Quality Monitoring and Evaluation of Agricultural Products in Yunnan (Project No.: 202403AP140027); and the financial support for this work from the Major Science and Technology Projects in Yunnan Province (No. 202402AF080005).

**Institutional Review Board Statement:** Not applicable.

**Informed Consent Statement:** Not applicable.

**Data Availability Statement:** The data presented in this study are available in the article and can be shared upon request.

**Acknowledgments:** The authors wish to express their gratitude for the financial support from the Science and Technology Plan project of Yunnan Provincial Science and Technology Department; the Basic Research in Local Undergraduate Universities Fund of Yunnan Provincial Science and Technology Department; the Young Talents Special Fund of Yunnan Provincial "Promoting Yunnan Talents"; the Research on Coffee Quality Control and Utilization of Residues Based on Nanomultifunctional Materials and Endophytic Fungi; the Yunnan China–Laos International Joint Research and Development Center for Energy and Mineral Analysis and Technology Innovation; the International Union Laboratory of China and Malaysia for Quality Monitoring and Evaluation of Agricultural Products in Yunnan; and the financial support for this work from the Major Science and Technology Projects in Yunnan Province.

**Conflicts of Interest:** There are no conflicts of interest to declare.

# References

1. Fan, G.J.; Luo, X.Y. Disposable electrochemical sensor for the detection of lead(II) ions in the natural water. *Int. J. Electrochem. Sci.* **2021**, *16*, 210924. [CrossRef]
2. Baghayeria, M.; Amiria, A.; Malekia, B.; Alizadeha, Z.; Reiser, O. A simple approach for simultaneous detection of cadmium(II) and lead(II) based on glutathione coated magnetic nanoparticles as a highly selective electrochemical probe. *Sens. Actuators B Chem.* **2018**, *273*, 1442–1450. [CrossRef]
3. Kamran, U.; Lee, S.Y.; Rhee, K.Y.; Park, S.J. Rice husk valorization into sustainable Ni@TiO$_2$/biochar nanocomposite for highly selective Pb (II) ions removal from an aqueous media. *Chemosphere* **2023**, *323*, 138210. [CrossRef]
4. Zaynab, M.; Al-Yahyai, R.; Ameen, A.; Sharif, Y.; Ali, L.; Fatima, M.; Khan, K.A.; Li, S.F. Health and environmental effects of heavy metals. *J. King Saud Univ. Sci.* **2022**, *34*, 101653. [CrossRef]
5. Flora, J.S.; Flora, G.; Saxena, G. Environmental occurrence, health effects and management of lead poisoning. In *Lead*; Elsevier: Amsterdam, The Netherlands, 2006; pp. 158–228.
6. WHO. *Guidelines for Drinking-Water Quality*, 4th ed.; World Health Organization: Geneva, Switzerland, 2011; p. 383.
7. Huang, Y.F.; Peng, J.H.; Huang, X.J. Allylthiourea functionalized magnetic adsorbent for the extraction of cadmium, copper and lead ions prior to their determination by atomic absorption spectrometry. *Microchim. Acta* **2019**, *186*, 51. [CrossRef]
8. Singh, H.; Bamrah, A.; Bhardwaj, S.K.; Deep, A.; Khatri, M.; Brown, R.J.C.; Bhardwaj, N.; Kim, K.H. Recent advances in the application of noble metal nanoparticles in colorimetric sensors for lead ions. *Environ. Sci. Nano* **2021**, *8*, 863–889. [CrossRef]
9. Chen, L.; Wang, Z.Z.; Pei, J.X.; Huang, X.J. Highly Permeable Monolith-based Multichannel In-Tip Microextraction Apparatus for Simultaneous Field Sample Preparation of Pesticides and Heavy Metal Ions in Environmental Waters. *Anal. Chem.* **2020**, *92*, 2251–2257. [CrossRef]
10. Zhao, N.; Biana, Y.W.; Donga, X.Y.; Gao, X.; Zhao, L.S. Magnetic solid-phase extraction based on multi-walled carbon nanotubes combined ferroferric oxide nanoparticles for the determination of five heavy metal ions in water samples by inductively coupled plasma mass spectrometry. *Water Sci. Technol.* **2021**, *84*, 1417–1427. [CrossRef]
11. Huang, J.; Cui, W.R.; Liang, R.P.; Zhang, L.; Qiu, J.D. Porous BMTTPA-CS-GO nanocomposite for the efficient removal of heavy metal ions from aqueous solutions. *RSC Adv.* **2021**, *11*, 3725–3731. [CrossRef] [PubMed]
12. Wua, H.Y.; Unnikrishnana, B.; Huang, C.C. Membrane-based detection of lead ions in seawater, urine and drinking straws through laser desorption/ionization. *Sens. Actuators B Chem.* **2014**, *203*, 880–886. [CrossRef]
13. Liu, X.M.; Luo, Y.J.; Lin, T.F.; Xie, Z.Q.; Qi, X.H. Gold nanoclusters-based fluorescence resonance energy transfer for rapid and sensitive detection of Pb$^{2+}$. *Spectrochim. Acta Part A Mol. Biomol. Spectrosc.* **2024**, *315*, 124302. [CrossRef] [PubMed]
14. Teng, W.Q.; Li, Q.; Zhao, J.; Shi, P.F.; Zhang, J.; Yan, M.; Zhang, S.S. A novel dual-mode aptasensor based on a multiple amplification system for ultrasensitive detection of lead ions using fluorescence and surface-enhanced Raman spectroscopy. *Analyst* **2024**, *149*, 1817–1824. [CrossRef]
15. Dhaffouli, A.; Salazar-Carballo, P.A.; Carinelli, S.; Holzinger, M.; Barhoumi, H. Improved electrochemical sensor using functionalized silica nanoparticles (SiO$_2$-APTES) for high selectivity detection of lead ions. *Mater. Chem. Phys.* **2024**, *318*, 129253. [CrossRef]
16. Li, Y.; Huang, H.; Cui, R.L.; Wang, D.M.; Yin, Z.; Wang, D.; Zheng, L.R.; Zhang, J.; Zhao, Y.D.; Yuan, H.; et al. Electrochemical sensor based on graphdiyne is effectively used to determine Cd$^{2+}$ and Pb$^{2+}$ in water. *Sens. Actuators. B. Chem.* **2021**, *332*, 129519. [CrossRef]
17. Qi, T.Y.; Yuan, Z.Y.; Meng, F.L. Highly sensitive and highly selective lead ion electrochemical sensor based on zn/cu-btc-nh$_2$ bimetallic MOFs with nano-reticulated reinforcing microstructure. *Anal. Chim. Acta* **2024**, *1318*, 342896. [CrossRef] [PubMed]
18. Boselli, E.; Wu, Z.Z.; Haynes, E.N.; Papautsky, I. Screen-Printed Sensors Modified with Nafion and Mesoporous Carbon for Electrochemical Detection of Lead in Blood. *J. Electrochem. Soc.* **2024**, *171*, 027513. [CrossRef]

19. Chabbah, T.; Chatti, S.; Jaffrezic-Renault, N.; Weidner, S.; Marestin, C.; Mercier, R. Impedimetric sensors based on diethylphosphonate-containing poly(arylene ether nitrile)s films for the detection of lead ions. *Polym. Adv. Technol.* **2023**, *34*, 2471–2481. [CrossRef]
20. Ren, X.; Wang, M.; Chen, J.G.; Zhao, J.X.; Wang, H.; Wu, D.; Xu, R.; Zhang, Y.; Ju, H.X.; Wei, Q. Sulfur defect-engineered $Bi_2S_{3-x}/In_2S_{3-y}$ mediated signal enhancement of photoelectrochemical sensor for lead ions detection. *Talanta* **2024**, *273*, 125871. [CrossRef]
21. Sun, X.Y.; Dong, S.L.; Zhao, W.Y. Catalytic hairpin assembly assisted target-dependent DNAzyme nanosystem coupled with AgPt@Thi for the detection of lead ion. *Anal. Chim. Acta* **2022**, *1205*, 339735. [CrossRef]
22. Qu, K.; Hu, X.; Li, Q.L. Electrochemical environmental pollutant detection enabled by waste tangerine peel-derived biochar. *Diam. Relat. Mater.* **2023**, *131*, 109617. [CrossRef]
23. Zhang, C.X.; Meng, L.B.; Fang, Z.H.; Xu, Y.X.; Zhou, Y.; Guo, H.S.; Wang, J.Y.; Zhao, X.T.; Zang, S.Y.; Shen, H.L. Experimental and Theoretical Studies on the Adsorption of Bromocresol Green from Aqueous Solution Using Cucumber Straw Biochar. *Molecules* **2024**, *29*, 4517. [CrossRef] [PubMed]
24. Cardozo, R.E.; Clauser, N.M.; Felissia, F.E.; Areaa, M.S.; Vallejosa, M.E. Design of an integrated biorefinery for bioethylene production from industrial forest byproducts. *Green Chem.* **2024**, *26*, 4092–4102. [CrossRef]
25. Liu, Q.H.; Sun, H.Y.; Yang, Z.M. Role of KOH-activated biochar on promoting anaerobic digestion of biomass from *Pennisetum gianteum*. *J. Environ. Manag.* **2024**, *353*, 120165. [CrossRef]
26. Nie, W.; Che, Q.Q.; Chen, D.; Cao, H.Y.; Deng, Y.H. Comparative Study for Propranolol Adsorption on the Biochars from Different Agricultural Solid Wastes. *Materials* **2024**, *17*, 2793. [CrossRef] [PubMed]
27. Desjardins, S.M.; Ter, M.T.; Chen, J.X. Cradle-to-gate life cycle analysis of slow pyrolysis biochar from forest harvest residues in Ontario, Canada. *Biochar* **2024**, *6*, 58. [CrossRef]
28. Djebbi, M.A.; Allagui, L.; Ayachi, M.S.E.; Boubakri, S.; Jaffrezic-Renault, N.; Namour, P.; Amara, A.B.H. Zero-Valent Iron Nanoparticles Supported on Biomass-Derived Porous Carbon for Simultaneous Detection of $Cd^{2+}$ and $Pb^{2+}$. *ACS Appl. Nano Mater.* **2022**, *5*, 546–558. [CrossRef]
29. Kouchachvili, L.; Gagnon-Caya, G.; Djebbar, R. Wood-derived biochar as a matrix for cost-effective and high performing composite thermal energy storage materials. *J. Porous Mater.* **2024**, *31*, 1–12. [CrossRef]
30. Joshi, M.; Bhatt, D.; Srivastava, A. Enhanced Adsorption Efficiency through Biochar Modification: A Comprehensive Review. *Ind. Eng. Chem. Res.* **2023**, *62*, 13748–13761. [CrossRef]
31. Zou, J.; Liu, J.W.; Peng, G.W.; Huang, H.Y.; Wang, L.Y.; Lu, L.M.; Gao, Y.S.; Hu, D.N.; Chen, S.X. An Electrochemical Sensor Based on a Porous Biochar/Cuprous Oxide ($BC/Cu_2O$) Composite for the Determination of Hg(II). *Molecules* **2023**, *28*, 5352. [CrossRef]
32. Liu, M.; Guan, L.Q.; Wen, Y.J.; Su, L.Z.; Hu, Z.; Peng, Z.J.; Li, S.K.; Tang, Q.Y.; Zhou, Z.; Zhou, N. Rice husk biochar mediated red phosphorus for photocatalysis and photothermal removal of *E. coli*. *Food Chem.* **2023**, *410*, 135455. [CrossRef]
33. Zhu, Z.Y.; Duan, W.Y.; Chang, Z.F.; Du, W.; Chen, F.Y.; Li, F.F.; Oleszczuk, P. Stability of Functionally Modified Biochar: The Role of Surface Charges and Surface Homogeneity. *Sustainability* **2023**, *15*, 7745. [CrossRef]
34. Premalatha, R.P.; Bindu, J.P.; Nivetha, E.; Malarvizhi, P.; Manorama, K.; Parameswari, E.; Davamani, V. A review on biochar's effect on soil properties and crop growth. *Front. Energy Res.* **2023**, *11*, 1092637. [CrossRef]
35. Zhu, H.S.; Tan, X.L.; Tan, L.Q.; Chen, C.L.; Alharbi, N.S.; Hayat, T.; Fang, M.; Wang, X.K. Biochar Derived from Sawdust Embedded with Molybdenum Disulfide for Highly Selective Removal of $Pb^{2+}$. *ACS Appl. Nano Mater.* **2018**, *1*, 2689–2698. [CrossRef]
36. Choudhary, V.; Philip, L. Sustainability assessment of acid-modified biochar as adsorbent for the removal of pharmaceuticals and personal care products from secondary treated wastewater. *J. Environ. Chem. Eng.* **2022**, *10*, 107592. [CrossRef]
37. Liu, C.; Wang, W.D.; Wu, R.; Liu, Y.; Lin, X.; Kan, H.; Zheng, Y.W. Preparation of Acid-and Alkali-Modified Biochar for Removal of Methylene Blue Pigment. *ACS Omega* **2020**, *5*, 30906–30922. [CrossRef]
38. Bhattacharya, S.; Hossain, A.; Bhowal, P.D. Integral approach of adsorption and photo-degradation of Bisphenol A using pyrolyzed rice straw biochar coated with metal oxide: Batch, mechanism and optimization. *Sadhana Acad. Proc. Eng. Sci.* **2024**, *49*, 38. [CrossRef]
39. Peng, J.; Zhang, Z.Y.; Wang, Z.W.; Zhou, F.; Yu, J.X.; Chi, R.; Xiao, C.Q. Adsorption of $Pb^{2+}$ in solution by phosphate-solubilizing microbially modified biochar loaded with $Fe_3O_4$. *J. Taiwan Inst. Chem. Eng.* **2024**, *156*, 105363. [CrossRef]
40. Zhang, Y.Y.; Chen, K.D.; Zhang, J.C.; Huang, K.Z.; Liang, Y.H.; Hu, H.W.; Xu, X.J.; Chen, D.C.; Chang, M.L.; Wang, Y.Z. Dense and uniform growth of $TiO_2$ nanoparticles on the pomelo-peel-derived biochar surface for efficient photocatalytic antibiotic degradation. *J. Environ. Chem. Eng.* **2023**, *11*, 109358. [CrossRef]
41. Wang, J.W.; Wang, G.Q.; Yu, T.; Ding, N.J.; Wang, M.C.; Chen, Y. Photocatalytic performance of biochar-modified $TiO_2$ ($C/TiO_2$) for ammonia–nitrogen removal. *RSC Adv.* **2023**, *13*, 24237–24249. [CrossRef]
42. Manpetch, P.; Singhapong, W.; Jaroenworaluck, A. Synthesis and characterization of a novel composite of ricehusk-derived graphene oxide with titania microspheres ($GO-RH/TiO_2$)for effective treatment of cationic dye methylene blue in aqueous solutions. *Environ. Sci. Pollut. Res.* **2022**, *29*, 63917–63935. [CrossRef]
43. Ding, Z.; Li, H.; Shaw, L. New Insights into the Solid-State Hydrogen Storage of Nanostructured $LiBH_4$-$MgH_2$ System. *Chem. Eng. J.* **2020**, *385*, 123856. [CrossRef]

44. Ding, Z.; Li, Y.T.; Yang, H.; Lu, Y.F.; Tan, J.; Li, J.B.; Chen, Q.L.Y.A.; Shaw, L.L.; Pan, F.S. Tailoring MgH$_2$ for hydrogen storage through nanoengineering and catalysis. *J. Magnes. Alloys* **2022**, *10*, 2946–2967. [CrossRef]
45. Yang, H.; Ding, Z.; Li, S.Y.; Wu, P.K.; Hou, Q.H.; Zheng, Y.; Gao, B.; Huo, K.F.; Du, W.J.; Shaw, L.L. Recent advances in kinetic and thermodynamic regulation of magnesium hydride for hydrogen storage. *Rare Met.* **2023**, *42*, 2906–2927. [CrossRef]
46. Yameen, M.Z.; Naqvi, S.R.; Juchelková, D.; Aslam Khan, M.N. Harnessing the power of functionalized biochar: Progress, challenges, and future perspectives in energy, water treatment, and environmental sustainability. *Biochar* **2024**, *6*, 25. [CrossRef]
47. Zhang, H.C.; Li, Y.R.; Zhang, Y.P.; Wu, J.F.; Li, S.X.; Li, L.L. A Disposable Electrochemical Sensor for Lead Ion Detection Based on In Situ Polymerization of Conductive Polypyrrole Coating. *J. Electron. Mater.* **2023**, *52*, 1819–1828. [CrossRef]
48. Zhu, N.X.; Liu, X.N.; Peng, K.M.; Cao, H.; Yuan, M.; Ye, T.; Wu, X.X.; Yin, F.Q.; Yu, J.S.; Hao, L.L.; et al. A Novel Aptamer-Imprinted Polymer-Based Electrochemical Biosensor for the Detection of Lead in Aquatic Products. *Molecules* **2022**, *28*, 196. [CrossRef]

**Disclaimer/Publisher's Note:** The statements, opinions and data contained in all publications are solely those of the individual author(s) and contributor(s) and not of MDPI and/or the editor(s). MDPI and/or the editor(s) disclaim responsibility for any injury to people or property resulting from any ideas, methods, instructions or products referred to in the content.

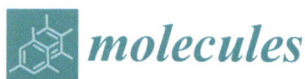 

Article

# Natural Silkworm Cocoon-Derived Separator with Na-Ion De-Solvated Function for Sodium Metal Batteries

Zhaoyang Wang [1], Zihan Zhou [1], Xing Gao [1], Qian Liu [1], Jianzong Man [1], Fanghui Du [1] and Fangyu Xiong [2,3,*]

[1] Shandong Provincial Key Laboratory of Chemical Energy Storage and Novel Cell Technology, College of Chemistry Engineering, Liaocheng University, Liaocheng 252059, China; wzy9218@126.com (Z.W.); 13884971808@163.com (Z.Z.); 18764792075@163.com (X.G.); 13562862100@163.com (Q.L.); manjianzong@lcu.edu.cn (J.M.); dufanghui@lcu.edu.cn (F.D.)
[2] College of Materials Science and Engineering, Chongqing University, Chongqing 400044, China
[3] Chongqing Institute of New Energy Storage Materials and Equipment, Chongqing 401135, China
* Correspondence: xfy@cqu.edu.cn

**Abstract:** The commercialization of sodium batteries faces many challenges, one of which is the lack of suitable high-quality separators. Herein, we presented a novel natural silkworm cocoon-derived separator (SCS) obtained from the cocoon inner membrane after a simple degumming process. A Na||Na symmetric cell assembled with this separator can be stably cycled for over 400 h under test conditions of 0.5 mA cm$^{-2}$–0.5 mAh cm$^{-2}$. Moreover, the Na||SCS||Na$_3$V$_2$(PO$_4$)$_3$ full cell exhibits an initial capacity of 79.3 mAh g$^{-1}$ at 10 C and a capacity retention of 93.6% after 1000 cycles, which far exceeded the 57.5 mAh g$^{-1}$ and 42.1% of the full cell using a commercial glass fiber separator (GFS). The structural origin of this excellent electrochemical performance lies in the fact that cationic functional groups (such as amino groups) on silkworm proteins can de-solvate Na-ions by anchoring the ClO$_4^-$ solvent sheath, thereby enhancing the transference number, transport kinetics and deposition/dissolution properties of Na-ions. In addition, the SCS has significantly better mechanical properties and thinness indexes than the commercial GFS, and, coupled with the advantages of being natural, cheap, non-polluting and degradable, it is expected to be used as a commercialized sodium battery separator material.

**Keywords:** sodium metal battery; separator materials; natural silkworm cocoon; Na-ion de-solvated function; mechanistic analysis

Citation: Wang, Z.; Zhou, Z.; Gao, X.; Liu, Q.; Man, J.; Du, F.; Xiong, F. Natural Silkworm Cocoon-Derived Separator with Na-Ion De-Solvated Function for Sodium Metal Batteries. *Molecules* **2024**, *29*, 4813. https://doi.org/10.3390/molecules29204813

Academic Editor: Chaoji Chen

Received: 26 August 2024
Revised: 3 October 2024
Accepted: 9 October 2024
Published: 11 October 2024

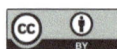

**Copyright:** © 2024 by the authors. Licensee MDPI, Basel, Switzerland. This article is an open access article distributed under the terms and conditions of the Creative Commons Attribution (CC BY) license (https:// creativecommons.org/licenses/by/ 4.0/).

## 1. Introduction

The growing energy demand has greatly prompted researchers to explore electrochemical energy storage systems (EESs) with low-cost, high energy density and environmental friendliness characteristics [1,2]. Among all available EESs, sodium metal batteries (SMBs) are considered to be the most promising substitutes to Li-ion batteries (LIBs) owing to the following unique advantages [3]: (i) SMBs work similarly to LIBs, so the research experience with LIBs can be utilized to develop SMBs [4]. (ii) Sodium resources are abundant and evenly distributed worldwide, which leads to a potential low cost of sodium metal anodes (SMAs) [5]. (iii) Sodium metal anodes possess low redox potential ($-2.71$ V vs. the standard hydrogen potential), light weight (23 g mol$^{-1}$) and high theoretical specific capacity (1166 mAh g$^{-1}$), endowing SMBs with high working voltage and high energy density [6]. Despite the attractive advantages, the development of SMBs has encountered various bottlenecks, one of which is the lack of high-quality separators [7].

As an important component of battery, the separator, on the one hand, bears the task of isolating the flow of electrons between the cathode and anode within the battery; on the other hand, it is also responsible for allowing ions to pass through smoothly [8]. There is no doubt that the quality of the separator determines the final performance of the battery. Compared to Na-ion batteries, SMBs place a higher demand on the electrolyte wettability and uptake capability, thermal stability, mechanical strength and ion distribution regulation ability of the separator [9]. Currently, the commercial Na-ion battery utilizes an LIB separator, i.e., a polypropylene (PP) or polyethylene (PE) separator. However, due to the drawbacks such as inferior electrolyte wettability, poor thermal stability and low electrolyte uptake capability, PP/PE separators are unsuitable for SMBs [10]. Although glass fiber separators (GFSs) can solve the above problems and are therefore widely used in laboratory research, their excessive thickness and poor mechanical properties make them difficult to apply in industrial production [11,12].

Scientists have made tremendous efforts to develop high-quality separators for SMBs [13]. Among them, biomass-derived separators have gained increasing attention due to their environmental friendliness, renewability and resource abundance [14]. Casas et al. cross-linked carboxymethyl cellulose (CMC) and hydroxyethyl cellulose (HEC) to prepare membranes with large specific surface area [15]. The Na | | Na$_3$V$_2$(PO$_4$)$_3$(NVP) battery assembled with this biomass membrane as a separator delivered a residual capacity of 74 mAh g$^{-1}$ after 10 cycles at 0.1 C with a nearly 100% Coulombic efficiency, which were both higher than that of the battery using a commercial Whatman GFS (61 mAh g$^{-1}$, 96%). Wang's group used electrospinning technology to construct cellulose nanocrystals into flexible bifunctional separators and applied them to SMBs [16]. This kind of separator can not only promote the uniform deposition of Na-ions on the anode by regulating the ion flow and nucleation behavior, but can also take advantage of the mechanical strength to block the continuous vertical growth of sodium dendrites, thus avoiding the occurrence of short circuits. These studies confirm the potential of biomass-derived separators for SMB applications and inspire subsequent researchers to continue to delve deeper into the natural treasure trove.

The silkworm cocoon is an amazing biological material that is naturally porous and layered, and therefore has morphological similarities to battery separators. Based on this similarity, silkworm cocoons have been initially developed as separators for LIBs [17–22]. Pereira et al. tested the suitability of silkworm cocoons as LIBs separators in carbonate-based and trifluoromethylsulfonyl-based electrolytes, and the results prove that the former electrolyte is more suitable for LIBs using cocoon separators [17]. In view of the multilayer structure of cocoons, Guo et al. examined the electrochemical performance of sublayers at different positions in cocoons and after stacking, and the results show that the inner layer is more suitable as a separator for LIBs, and the multilayer structure is more beneficial to the electrochemical performance [18]. It is well known that micro-morphology is an important factor affecting the electrochemical performance of the separator, and in order to regulate the pore structure in cocoon-based separators, Reizabal et al. treated cocoons by a salting method [19]. The battery using a cocoon separator with a pore size range of 106–250 μm showed the best electrochemical performance, i.e., a discharge capacity of 66.9 mAh g$^{-1}$ at 2 C and a residual capacity of 56.9 mAh g$^{-1}$ after 55 cycles. In addition to this, the lyophilization [20] and plasma treatment [21] of silk have been used to optimize the morphology of cocoon-based separators with exciting progress.

In this paper, we reported a novel natural silkworm cocoon separator (SCS) for SMBs. The unique advantage of SCSs over commercially available GFSs is that they can anchor ClO$_4^-$ in the electrolyte by virtue of the abundant amino functional groups in the protein molecular chain, thus enabling Na-ions to exhibit superior transport kinetics. Benefiting from this, the Na | | SCS | | Na symmetric cell is able to cycle stably for more than 400 h at a current density of 0.5 mA cm$^{-2}$ with an areal capacity of 0.5 mAh cm$^{-2}$, which far exceeds the effective cycling time (~20 h) of the Na | | GFS | | Na symmetric cell under the same test conditions. In addition, the Na | | SCSs | | NVP full cell exhibits a discharge capacity of 79.3 mAh g$^{-1}$ at 10 C with a capacity retention rate of 93.6% after 1000 cycles. In order to facilitate the reader to compare the differences in electrochemical performance between the present work and previous cocoon separator studies, we summarize these findings in Table S1.

## 2. Results

### 2.1. Electrochemical Performance

In order to optimize the pore structure of silkworm cocoons and to expose the functional groups on their protein molecules, natural silkworm cocoons were boiled in a weak alkaline solution to remove the sericin [22]. The SCS sample has four broadened crystal diffraction peaks located at 9.1°, 20.5°, 23.0° and 29.4° (Figure 1a). These diffraction peaks should be attributed to the (100), (210), (002) and (300) crystal planes of β-sheet silkworm protein, respectively [23–25]. Table S2 summarizes the structural parameters of each grain surface calculated using Jade 6 software and the Debye–Scherrer formula, where a small grain size (<4 nm) implies the poor crystallinity of the SCS sample [26,27]. In contrast, no crystal diffraction peaks are observed in the XRD patterns of the GFS sample due to the disordered characteristics of glass fiber [28]. Scanning electron microscopy (SEM) was employed to observe the morphology features of the samples at the micron scale [29–31]. As shown in Figure 1b,c, the morphology of the inner and outer layers of the cocoon varies greatly: the silkworm in the outer layer of cocoon is fluffy and stacked with large pores; the silkworm in the inner layer of the cocoon is flat and stacked with small pores, and an obvious bonding phenomenon can be observed. This bonding phenomenon is significantly reduced after boiling (Figure 1d). In view of the advantages in regularity and pore structure, the inner layer of the cocoon was selected as the separator for SMBs. The GFS also exhibits a large pore structure and has no bonding points between its fibers (Figure 1e). The bonding between fibers is likely to be the structural root cause of the superior mechanical properties of the SCS over the GFS [32].

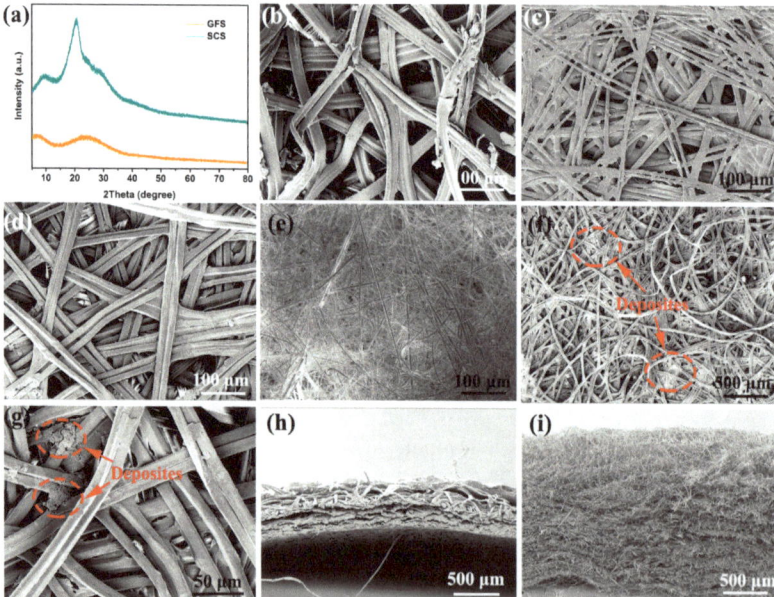

**Figure 1.** (a) XRD of the SCS and GFS. SEM top view images of the outer layer (b), pristine (c)/boiled (d) inner layers of the cocoon and the glass fiber separator (e). (f,g) SEM images of SCS samples after cyclic testing. SEM cross-section view images of the cocoon (h) and GFS (i).

SEM images of the SCS samples after 100 cycles at 5 C show no significant changes in the SCS except that some deposits can be observed (as shown in Figure 1f,g). Based on previous studies, it is known that these sediments are metallic sodium crystals and sodium salt crystals, of which the former is predominant [33]. In order to evaluate the pore structure of the separators more comprehensively, SEM tests were performed on the cross-sections of the cocoons and GFS, respectively. As shown in Figure 1h, the cocoons were clearly stratified, with the inner layer being more regular and tightly packed compared to the outer layer, which is consistent with the results observed in Figure 1b,c. The SCS, taken from the inner layer of the cocoon, is much lower than the GFS (Figure 1i) in both porosity and tortuosity.

The Na∥Cu asymmetric and Na∥Na symmetric cells using SCSs and GFSs as separators were assembled for testing. As shown in Figure S1, the assembled Na∥SCS∥Cu battery shows a lower nucleation over-potential of 0.065 V than that of the Na∥GFS∥Cu battery (0.113 V), indicating that the SCS could decrease the nucleation resistance and local current density during Na deposition [34]. Figure 2 presents the voltage–time profiles of Na∥Na symmetric cells with the SCS and the GFS. Notably, the Na∥SCS∥Na symmetric cell can stably cycle for ~480 h and the polarization voltage is stabilized at only 0.04 V throughout under 0.2 mA cm$^{-2}$–0.2 mAh cm$^{-2}$ test conditions (Figure 2a). As for the Na∥GFS∥Na battery, the polarization voltage under the same test conditions is close to 0.075 V and short circuit occurs when the battery run for about 100 h. At the test conditions of 0.5 mA cm$^{-2}$–0.5 mAh cm$^{-2}$, the Na∥SCS∥Na symmetric cell exhibits a polarization voltage of ~0.05 V (Figure 2b). After 400 h of steady operation, the polarization voltage of this battery rises slightly to ~0.09 V and eventually fails completely after 427 h of operation. As a comparison, the Na∥GFS∥Na cell displays an initial polarization voltage as high as 0.125 V and only stably cycles for about 20 h. The above results indicate that SCS is more beneficial as a battery separator for Na-ion transport and deposition/dissolution [35].

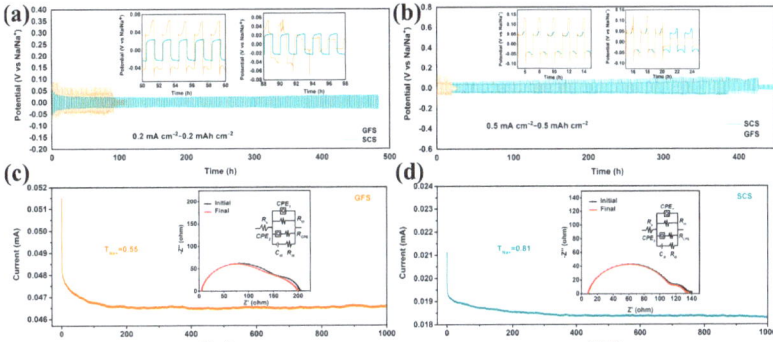

**Figure 2.** Characterization of sodium plating/stripping behavior in symmetric batteries. Voltage profiles of the symmetrical Na∥GFS∥Na and Na∥SCS∥Na cells under current areal capacities of (**a**) 0.2 mAh cm$^{-2}$ and (**b**) 0.5 mAh cm$^{-2}$. The *i–t* curves of Na∥GFS∥Na (**c**) and Na∥SCS∥Na (**d**) cells; the insets are the corresponding EIS curves before and after chronoamperometry test.

To clarify the effect of the SCS on Na-ion transport in batteries, chronoamperometry (CA) and corresponding electrochemical impedance spectroscopy (EIS) tests were performed on the Na∥GFS∥Na and Na∥SCS∥Na cells. After careful comparison, all the EIS curves in Figure 2c,d are well matched to the "$R_s(QR_{ct}(QR_{CPE})(C_{dl}R_{dl}))$" equivalent circuit with errors of less than 4.1%. Here, $Q$ represents the constant phase element (CPE); $C_{dl}$ represents double layer capacitance; and $R_s$, $R_{ct}$, $R_{CPE}$ and $R_{dl}$ represent solution impedance, charge transfer impedance, CPE impedance and double capacitance impedance, respectively [36,37]. As reported by the ZSimpwin 3.60 software fitting parameter (Table S3), the initial $R_{ct}$ of the Na∥SCS∥Na cell (134.6 Ω) is much smaller than that of the Na∥GFS∥Na cell (205.7 Ω), indicating that the interfacial impedance between the SCS and the sodium metal anode is smaller. The Na$^+$ transference number ($T_{Na+}$) of the above symmetric cell can be calculated using the following equation [38,39]:

$$T_{Na+} = (I_s \times (\Delta V - I_0 \times R_0))/(I_0 \times (\Delta V - I_s \times R_s))$$

where $\Delta V$, $I_0$, $I_s$, $R_0$ and $R_s$ are the constant applied voltage (10 mV), initial and steady-state currents, and the $R_{ct}$ before and after the CA test. The calculated $T_{Na^+}$ of the Na||SCS||Na cell is 0.81, which is higher than the 0.55 of Na||GFS||Na cell.

To further demonstrate the application potential of SCSs, the electrochemical performances of Na||NVP full batteries using the SCS and the GFS were tested. As shown in Figure 3a,b, the Na||GFS||NVP and Na||SCS||NVP cells exhibit similar electrochemical reaction potentials (~3.4 V) and discharge capacities (~100 mAh g$^{-1}$) at 0.1 C. When the charge/discharge rate is increased to 10 C, the Na||SCS||NVP cell still displays a discharge capacity of 79.3 mAh g$^{-1}$, which is much higher than that of the Na||GFS||NVP cell (60 mAh g$^{-1}$). It should be noted that the potential hysteresis in the charge–discharge curves of the Na||SCS||NVP cell is only about 1/2 of that of the Na||GFS||NVP cell at 10 C (Figure S2a,b). This phenomenon suggests that Na-ions are able to pass through SCSs more easily and are not over−enriched on the surface of SCSs even at high current densities [40,41]. The rate performance test reveals that the Na||SCS||NVP cell consistently outperforms the Na||GFS||NVP cell in terms of discharge capacity at 0.5–10 C, and the higher the rate, the more pronounced this advantage becomes (Figure 3c). Furthermore, the Na||SCS||NVP cell also exhibits better cycling performance than the Na||GFS||NVP cell at 10 C (Figure 3d). The discharge capacity of the Na||SCS||NVP cell remains 74.2 mAh g$^{-1}$ after 1000 cycles, corresponding to a capacity retention rate of 93.6%. In contrast, the discharge capacity and capacity retention rate of the Na||GFS||NVP cell are only 24.2 and 42.1%, respectively. Moreover, the discharge medium voltage of the full cell using the SCS gradually increases with cycling until it stabilizes near 3.2 V, while that of the full cell using the GFS keeps decreasing (Figure S2c).

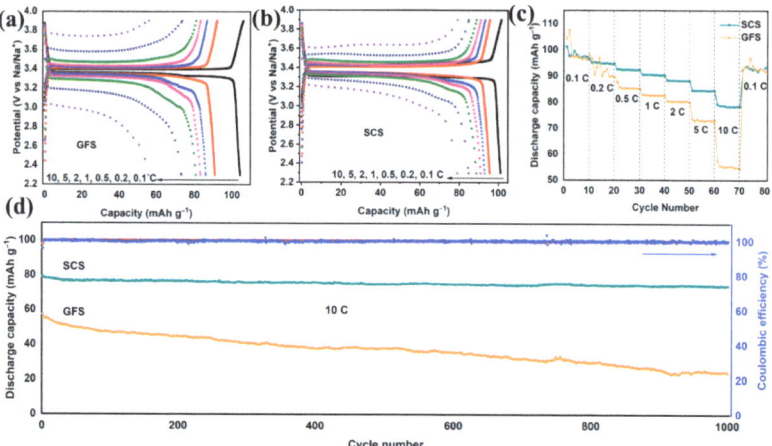

**Figure 3.** Comparison of electrochemical performances of Na||NVP full cells assembled with SCSs and GFSs. Galvanostatic charging–discharging profile curves of the Na||SCS||NVP (**a**) and Na||GFS||NVP full cells (**b**) from 0.1 C to 10 C. Rate capabilities (**c**) and long-term cycling performances (**d**) of the Na||SCS||NVP and Na||GFS||NVP full cells.

In order to understand the chemical stability of SCSs during electrochemical reactions, cyclic voltammetry (CV) tests of both the Na||SCS||NVP and Na||GFS||NVP full cells were executed. Compared with the Na||GFS||NVP cell, the Na||SCS||NVP cell also exhibits only a pair of $V^{3+}/V^{4+}$ redox peaks attributed to NVP cathode materials (Figure S3a), which implies that the SCS is in a chemically stable state during electrochemical processes. Electrochemical impedance spectroscopy (EIS) is an efficient testing technique to analyze the internal resistance distribution of a battery. The Na||SCS||NVP and the Na||GFS||NVP share the same EIS graphic characteristics (Figure S3b), i.e., both consist of a semicircle in the high-frequency region and a diagonal line in the low−frequency region. The semicircle is mainly associated with the $R_{ct}$ [42]. The Na||SCS||NVP cell displays a smaller semicircle diameter than the Na||GFS||NVP cell, indicating that the former has smaller values of $R_{ct}$ than the latter, which implies superior transport kinetics of Na-ions in the former [43]. In addition to this, the diffusion coefficient of Na-ions can be quantitatively calculated using the following equation:

$$D_{Na+} = \frac{R^2 T^2}{2A^2 n^4 F^4 C^2 \sigma^2}$$

Since the parameters $R$ (gas constant, 8.314 J mol$^{-1}$ K$^{-1}$), $T$ (room temperature, 298.15 K), $A$ (area of the electrode, 1.13 cm$^2$), $n$ (the number of electrons involved in electrochemical reactions, 2), $F$ (Faraday constant, 96485.4 C mol$^{-1}$) and $C$ (the concentration of Na-ions in the unit cell volume, $6.92 \times 10^{-23}$ mol cm$^{-3}$) in the above equations are the same for both the GFS and SCS cells, the Na-ion transport efficiency of these two cells should be inversely related to the $\sigma$ value. By fitting $-Z'-\omega^{-1/2}$ plots to the straight lines in the low-frequency region of the EIS curves (Figure S3c), it is found that the $\sigma$-values for cells using SCSs and GFSs are 684.2 and 740.1 $\Omega$ s$^{-0.5}$ (see Table S4 for details), respectively, which implies a higher $D_{Na+}$ in the cell using SCSs.

## 2.2. Mechanical Properties and Functional Group Characterization

The mechanical properties of the separator are not only related to the safety of the battery, but also to whether it can match the winding process for industrial production of the battery. As shown in Figure 4b, the maximum tensile strength of the GFS is only 0.16 MPa which is much lower than the minimum tensile strength value (6.9 MPa) in the winding process, and therefore, the GFS cannot be applied to commercialized column batteries [44]. By comparison, the SCS exhibits a much higher tensile strength (17.72 MPa, Figure 4a) and Young's modulus (64.12 MPa, Figure 4c). In terms of mechanical properties, the SCS has met the basic requirements for commercialized separators.

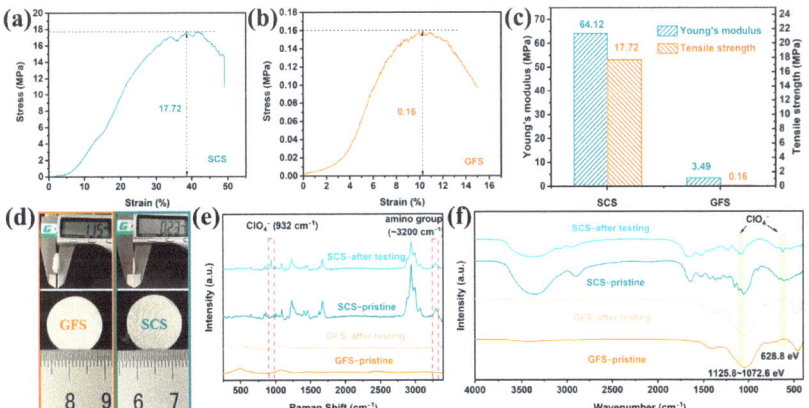

**Figure 4.** Characterization of mechanical properties and functional groups of the SCS and GFS. Stress–strain curves of the GFS (**a**) and the SCS (**b**). (**c**) Tensile mechanical properties (Young's modulus, strength). (**d**) Comparison of the appearance and thickness of the SCS and the GFS. (**e**) Raman and (**f**) FT-IR spectra of the SCS and the GFS before and after electrochemical reaction.

The appearance characteristics of the GFS and SCS are shown in Figure 4d, and the flatness of the SCS is slightly worse than that of the GFS, which is due to the slight shrinkage of the sample during the drying process of the SCS. The thicknesses of the SCS and GFS are 0.23 ± 0.01 mm and 1.15 ± 0.02 mm, respectively, and the SCS is clearly more advantageous in the demand for a thinner and lighter separator. Raman and FT−IR spectroscopy were performed on the SCS before and after charging and discharging, respectively. As shown in Figure 4e, a characteristic peak is present at around 3200 cm$^{-1}$ for both SCS samples, which could be attributed to the amino group upon careful comparison with the literature [45]. In addition, the SCS sample after electrochemical testing also exhibits a characteristic peak belonging to $ClO_4^-$ at 932 cm$^{-1}$ that is not found in any other samples [46], suggesting that the SCS sample may anchor the $ClO_4^-$ anion in the electrolyte during the electrochemical reaction. Two sets of characteristic peaks belonging to $ClO_4^-$ at 628.8 and 1125–1072 cm$^{-1}$ are also observed in the FT-IR spectrum of the SCS after the electrochemical test, reconfirming the inference of a possible interaction between silkworm and $ClO_4^-$ (Figure 4f) [47,48].

It is noteworthy that the XPS spectra also reveal not only the ability of the SCS sample to interact with $ClO_4^-$ but also the presence of amino groups in the silkworm. As shown in Figure 5a, the SCS and GFS exhibit completely different O1s spectra. Specifically, the O1s spectra of the GFS samples before and after the electrochemical reaction did not change significantly, and only one characteristic peak of bridging oxygen was found at 531.5 eV [49]. Meanwhile, the SCS sample has the characteristic peak representing O=C−NH$_2$ at 530.6 eV [50], and the characteristic peaks representing the Cl−O (532.1 eV) bond and Na−auger (536.5 eV) are added to the electrochemically reacted SCS sample [51,52]. Combined with the Cl 2p spectrum (Figure 5c), the presence of a $ClO_4^-$ group in the electrochemically reacted SCS sample can be determined [53]. For the C 1s spectra (Figure 5b), three characteristic peaks are observed for the SCS whether it undergoes electrochemical reaction or not, which correspond to a C−C bond at 283.9 eV, a C−COO bond at 285.4 eV and a C−N bond at 287.4 eV [54–56]. In addition, although all samples responded to N 1s spectral detection, the low signal-to-noise ratio of the N 1s spectra of the two GFS samples implies that these samples contain less elemental nitrogen. The high signal-to-noise ratio and good symmetry of the characteristic peaks of the N 1s spectra of the SCS samples indicate that these samples have a high content of nitrogen. The high similarity in the shape and position of the N 1s peaks suggests that the electrochemical reaction does not significantly change the valence state of elemental N.

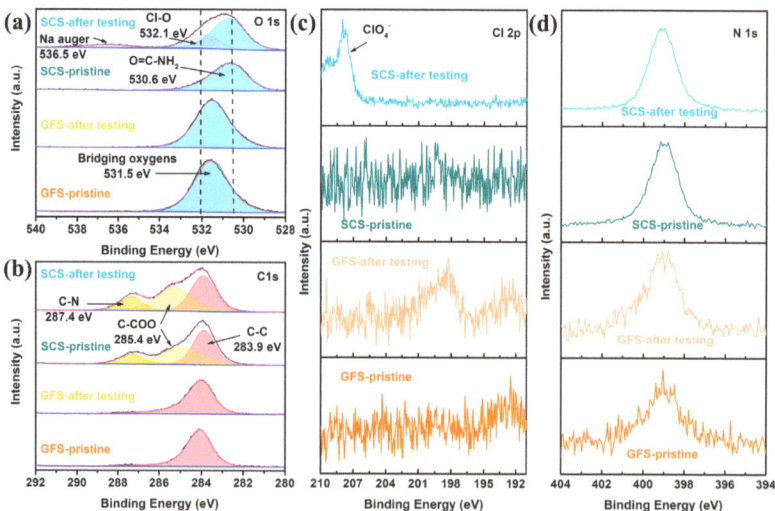

Figure 5. (a) O 1s, (b) C 1s, (c) Cl 2p and (d) N 1s XPS spectra of the GFS and SCS samples.

## 3. Discussion

The low nucleation over-potential of 0.065 V (Figure S1) and the stable cycling of 427 h under test conditions of 0.5 mA cm$^{-2}$–0.5 mAh cm$^{-2}$ (Figure 2b) demonstrate that the Na-ion deposition/dissolution in SCS-assembled cells is not only easier but also has excellent reversibility [57]. In addition to this, the small charge transfer resistance (Figure S3b) implies excellent transport kinetics of Na-ions in the cell using the SCS [58]. Under the synergistic effect of excellent Na-ion transport and deposition/dissolution kinetics, the batteries using SCSs exhibit superior high-rate cycling performance. Therefore, the Na‖SCS‖NVP full battery displays an initial capacity of 79.3 mAh g$^{-1}$ at 10 C and a capacity retention of 93.6% after 1000 cycles (Figure 3d), which far exceeds the 57.5 mAh g$^{-1}$ and 42.1% of the Na‖GFS‖NVP full battery. There is a significant effect of separator thickness on the electrochemical performance and that the thickness of the SCS in this work is much lower than that of the GFS (Figure 4d). In order to clarify the specific effect of separator thickness on electrochemical performance, the commercial GFA separator (only 0.34 ± 0.01 mm in thickness), which is thinner than the GFS, was used for a comparison experiment. As shown in Figure S4, the Na‖GFA‖NVP cell experiences a rapid capacity decline in the multifold test, with the capacity decaying from 115 mAh g$^{-1}$ at 0.1 C to 44 mAh g$^{-1}$ at 5 C until the cell fails at 10 C. The results of this test show that the thinner the separator, the harder it is to obtain excellent electrochemical performance.

Characteristic peaks belonging to $ClO_4^-$ are observed in the Raman (Figure 4e), FT-IR (Figure 4f) and XPS patterns (Figure 5a,c) of the SCS samples after electrochemical testing, which are not observed in the pristine SCS or the GFS before and after electrochemical testing, suggesting that $ClO_4^-$ could be firmly attached to the SCS fibers. Combined with the previous literature, it can be reasonable to assume that this phenomenon is most likely caused by cationic functional groups (such as amino groups) on the protein molecule [59,60]. From the conclusions of previous studies, it is known that Na-ions undergo solvation reactions with anions and solvents during transport in the electrolyte [61,62]. The solvated Na-ions increase in both mass and volume, which undoubtedly reduces the transport kinetics of the Na-ions [63]. As shown in Figure 6, when solvated Na-ions pass through the SCS, the amino functional groups on silkworm proteins disrupt the solvent sheath by anchoring $ClO_4^-$, thereby releasing free Na-ions. As a result, the transference number ($T_{Na+}$ = 0.81), transport kinetics and deposition/solvent properties of Na-ions are improved. On this basis, the advantages in mechanical strength and thinness make SCSs more promising than GFSs for commercialized sodium batteries.

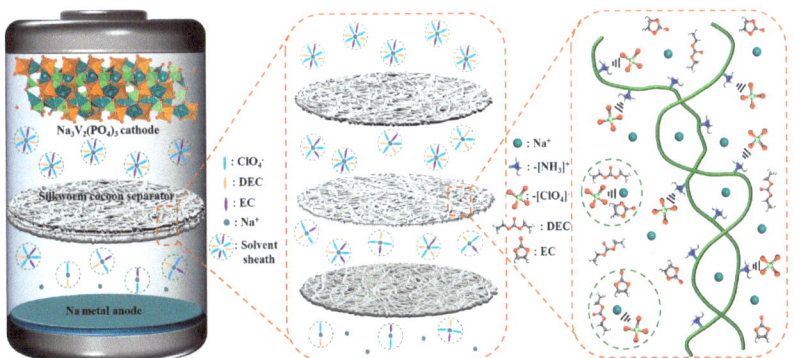

**Figure 6.** Schematic diagram of the cell structure and the SCS' action mechanism.

## 4. Materials and Methods

### 4.1. Fabricating SCS

The SCS fabrication process is shown in Figure 7. First, 0.04 mol $Na_2CO_3$ (99.8%, Shanghai Macklin Biochemical Technology Co., Ltd., Shanghai, China) was dissolved in 2 L deionized water to prepare the washing solution and heated to boiling. The mulberry silkworm cocoons (Beijing Tong Ren Tang group Co., Ltd., Beijing, China) were then poured into the boiling liquid and treated for 20 min to remove the sericin. Next, the cocoons were fished out, washed three times with deionized water and exfoliated of their inner layers. Subsequently, the inner layer of the cocoon was flattened, sandwiched between two glass plates to fix the shape, and transferred to a vacuum oven at 80 °C until dry. The dried cocoons' inner layer was cut into 16 mm discs to be used as separators, which were named SCS. Thick (Whatman GF/D) and thin (Whatman GF/A) glass fiber separators were used as comparison samples, named GFS and GFA, respectively.

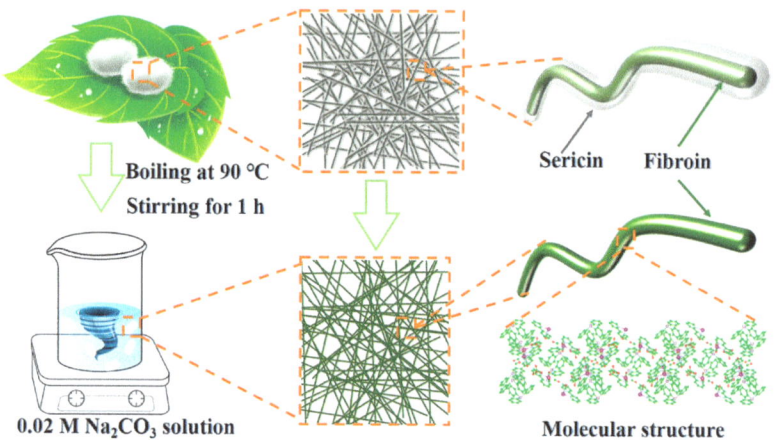

**Figure 7.** Schematic diagram of the preparation process of silkworm cocoon separator.

*4.2. Material Characterization*

The microscopic morphology of the SCS, GFS and sodium metal anode was observed by field-emission scanning electron microscopy (FESEM, Thermo Fisher Scientific FIB-SEM GX4, Waltham, MA, USA). The XRD data were measured by a Bruker D8 diffractometer at a sweep speed of $0.3° \ s^{-1}$ over a range of 5–80° with Cu Kα (λ = 1.5418 Å). FT-IR absorption spectroscopy (Thermo Scientific Nicolet iS50, Waltham, MA, USA) was used to test the functional groups of different separators in the range of $600 \ cm^{-1} \sim 4000 \ cm^{-1}$; all samples were washed three times in water under sonication for 10 min before testing. An electronic universal testing machine was employed to test the mechanical properties of different separators. An X-ray photoelectron spectrometer (ThermoFischer, ESCALAB 250Xi, Waltham, MA, USA) was used in this experiment for XPS tests. In this case, the vacuum of the analysis chamber was $2 \times 10^{-8}$ Pa, the excitation source was an Al Kα ray (hυ = 1486.6 eV) and the operating voltage was 12.5 kV. Raman spectroscopy tests were performed on a ThermoFischer Dxr3xi Raman microscopy (Waltham, MA, USA) instrument equipped with an $Ar^+$ laser (λ = 532 nm).

*4.3. Electrochemical Measurements*

All the electrochemical performance tests were performed based on CR2025-type coin batteries, and the battery assembly was completed in an argon-filled glovebox ($H_2O$ < 0.1 ppm, $O_2$ < 0.1 ppm, Mikrouna, Shanghai, China). For the preparation of the NVP cathode, NVP (Guangdong Canrd New Energy Technology Co., Ltd., Dongguan, China), polyvinylidene fluoride (PVDF) and acetylene black with a mass ratio of 8:1:1 were dispersed in N-methyl-2-pyrrolidine (NMP) to form a uniform slurry and then coated on aluminum foils. After they were dried in a vacuum oven at 110 °C for 10 h, these aluminum foils were cut into discs with a diameter of 14 mm to be the NVP cathode. An amount of 50 μL of electrolytes (1 M $NaClO_4$ dissolved in EC:DEC=1:1 (*v/v*) with 5% FEC) was used for each battery. All batteries used Na foil (~100 μm) as the anode, and the difference was that the working electrodes were NVP, Cu foil or Na foil, with the GFS or SCS as the separator. The galvanostatic charging–discharging, over-potential and cycling performance of the batteries were measured on a Land BT 2000 battery test systems at 25 °C. The potentiostatic modal EIS (frequency range from $10^{-2}$ to $10^5$ Hz with an amplitude value of 10 mV), CV (voltage range from 2.3 to 3.9 V with a scanning rate of 0.1 mV s$^{-1}$) and CA (open-circuit voltage used as initial voltage, executed for 1000 s at 10 mV bias) curves were tested on a CHI660e electrochemical workstation.

## 5. Conclusions

In summary, we developed a novel natural SCS for sodium metal batteries. Systematic structural characterization reveals that the cationic functional groups (such as amino groups) enriched in the SCS samples can anchor the $ClO_4^-$ solvent sheath around the Na-ions, realizing a high Na$^+$ transference number ($T_{Na+}$ = 0.81) and substantially enhancing the transport kinetics. Benefiting from this, the Na||SCS||Na symmetric cell can be stably cycled for over 400 h at 0.5 mA cm$^{-2}$–0.5 mAh cm$^{-2}$. Moreover, the Na||SCS||NVP full battery displays a reversible discharge specific capacity of 79.3 mAh g$^{-1}$ at 10 C and a remaining capacity of up to 74.2 mAh g$^{-1}$ after 1000 cycles. In addition, the mechanical properties and thickness of the SCS are also completely superior to those of the GFS, which means that the SCS has more potential for commercial application than the GFS.

**Supplementary Materials:** The following supporting information can be downloaded at https://www.mdpi.com/article/10.3390/molecules29204813/s1: Figure S1: Voltage-capacity curves of Cu||SCS||Na and Cu||GFS||Na asymmetric cell at a current density of 0.5 mA cm$^{-2}$; Figure S2: Charge-discharge voltage profiles for Na||NVP full batteries using GFS (a) and SCS (b) separator. The discharge medium voltage at different cycles of Na||GFS||NVP and Na||SCS||NVP full batteries; Figure S3: (a) CV curves at a scan rate of 0.1 mV s$^{-1}$, (b) EIS curves (inset: equivalent circuit diagram) and (c) relationship plots of the impedance as a function of the inverse square root of angular frequency in a low-frequency region of Na||SCS||NVP and Na||GFS||NVP full cells; Figure S4: Galvanostatic charging-discharging profile curves of Na||GFA||NVP; Table S1: Comparative table of electrochemical properties of cocoon based separators; Table S2: Summary table of structural parameters of SCS sample; Table S3: Parameters reported for EIS curves in Figure 2c,d fitted by equivalent circuits. Table S4: Parameters reported of the EIS curves in Figure S3 after equivalent circuits and linear fitting.

**Author Contributions:** Conceptualization, Z.W. and F.X.; methodology, Z.Z.; validation, X.G. and Q.L.; investigation, X.G.; data curation, Z.Z. and Q.L.; writing—original draft preparation, Z.Z., X.G. and Q.L.; writing—review and editing, Z.W., J.M., F.D. and F.X.; funding acquisition, Z.W. All authors have read and agreed to the published version of the manuscript.

**Funding:** This research was funded by the PhD Initiation Program of Liaocheng University, grant number 318052012, and the Open Project Program of Shandong Provincial Key Laboratory of Chemical Energy Storage and Novel Cell Technology, Liaocheng University, China.

**Institutional Review Board Statement:** Not applicable.

**Informed Consent Statement:** Not applicable.

**Data Availability Statement:** The data that support the findings of this study are available from the corresponding author upon reasonable request.

**Acknowledgments:** The authors acknowledge Liaocheng University for the financial support.

**Conflicts of Interest:** The authors declare no conflicts of interest.

## References

1. Huang, X.Z.; He, R.; Li, M.; Chee, M.O.L.; Dong, P.; Lu, J. Functionalized separator for next-generation batteries. *Mater. Today* **2020**, *41*, 143–155. [CrossRef]
2. Lizundia, E.; Kundu, D. Advances in natural biopolymer-based electrolytes and separators for battery applications. *Adv. Funct. Mater.* **2021**, *31*, 2005646. [CrossRef]
3. Sullivan, M.; Tang, P.; Meng, X.B. Atomic and molecular layer deposition as surface engineering techniques for emerging alkali metal rechargeable batteries. *Molecules* **2022**, *27*, 6170. [CrossRef]
4. Lie, C. Sustainable battery materials from biomass. *ChemSusChem* **2020**, *13*, 2110–2141.

5. Vaalma, C.; Buchholz, D.; Weil, M.; Passerini, S. A cost and resource analysis of sodium-ion batteries. *Nat. Rev. Mater.* **2018**, *3*, 18013. [CrossRef]
6. Lee, B.; Paek, E.; Mitlin, D.; Lee, S.W. Sodium metal anodes: Emerging solutions to dendrite growth. *Chem. Rev.* **2019**, *119*, 5416–5460. [CrossRef]
7. Li, Y.C.; Fu, X.W.; Wang, Y.; Zhong, W.H.; Li, R.F. "See" the invisibles: Inspecting battery separator defects via pressure drop. *Energy Storage Mater.* **2019**, *16*, 589–596. [CrossRef]
8. Lagadec, M.F.; Zahn, R.; Wood, V. Characterization and performance evaluation of lithium-ion battery separators. *Nat. Energy* **2018**, *4*, 16–25. [CrossRef]
9. Wang, J.M.; Gao, Y.; Liu, D.; Zou, G.D.; Li, L.J.; Fernandez, C.; Zhang, Q.R.; Peng, Q.M. A sodiophilic amyloid fibril modified separator for dendrite-free sodium-metal batteries. *Adv. Mater.* **2024**, *36*, 2304942. [CrossRef]
10. Zhang, L.P.; Li, X.L.; Yang, M.R.; Chen, W.H. High-safety separators for lithium-ion batteries and sodium-ion batteries: Advances and perspective. *Energy Storage Mater.* **2021**, *41*, 522–545. [CrossRef]
11. Zhu, J.D.; Yanilmaz, M.; Fu, K.; Chen, C.; Lu, Y.; Ge, Y.Q.; Kim, D.; Zhang, X.W. Understanding glass fiber membrane used as a novel separator for lithium–sulfur batteries. *J. Membr. Sci.* **2016**, *504*, 89–96. [CrossRef]
12. Zhang, X.Y.; Cheng, S.A.; Huang, X.; Logan, B.E. The use of nylon and glass fiber filter separators with different pore sizes in air-cathode single-chamber microbial fuel cells. *Energy Environ. Sci.* **2010**, *3*, 659–664. [CrossRef]
13. Liu, Z.F.; Jiang, Y.J.; Hu, Q.M.; Guo, S.T.; Yu, L.; Li, Q.; Liu, Q.; Hu, X.L. Safer lithium-ion batteries from the separator aspect: Development and future perspectives. *Energy Environ. Mater.* **2021**, *4*, 336–362. [CrossRef]
14. Jin, C.B.; Nai, J.W.; Sheng, O.W.; Yuan, H.D.; Zhang, W.K.; Tao, X.Y.; Lou, X.W. Biomass-based materials for green lithium secondary batteries. *Energy Environ. Sci.* **2021**, *14*, 1326. [CrossRef]
15. Casas, X.; Niederberger, M.; Lizundia, E. A sodium-ion battery separator with reversible voltage response based on water-soluble cellulose derivatives. *ACS Appl. Mater. Interfaces* **2020**, *12*, 29264–29274. [CrossRef]
16. Wang, J.; Xu, Z.; Zhang, Q.C.; Song, X.; Lu, X.K.; Zhang, Z.Y.; Onyianta, A.J.; Wang, M.N.; Titirici, M.M.; Eichhorn, S.J. Stable sodium-metal batteries in carbonate electrolytes achieved by bifunctional, sustainable separators with tailored alignment. *Adv. Mater.* **2022**, *34*, 2206367. [CrossRef]
17. Reizabal, A.; Fidalgo-Marijuan, A.; Gonçalves, R.; Gutiérrez-Pardo, A.; Aguesse, F.; Pérez-Álvarez, L.; Vilas-Vilela, J.L.; Costa, C.M.; Lanceros-Mendez, S. Silk-fibroin and sericin polymer blends for sustainable battery separators. *J. Colloid Interface Sci.* **2022**, *611*, 366–376. [CrossRef]
18. Guo, X.S.; Li, J.Y.; Xing, J.X.; Zhang, K.; Zhou, Y.G.; Pan, C.; Wei, Z.Z.; Zhao, Y. Silkworm cocoon layer with gradient structure as separator for lithium-ion battery. *Energy Technol.* **2022**, *10*, 2100996. [CrossRef]
19. Reizabal, A.; Gonçalves, R.; Fidalgo-Marijuan, A.; Costa, C.M.; Pérez, L.; Vilas, J.-L.; Lanceros-Mendez, S. Tailoring silk fibroin separator membranes pore size for improving performance of lithium ion batteries. *J. Membr. Sci.* **2020**, *598*, 117678. [CrossRef]
20. Pereira, R.F.P.; Brito-Pereira, R.; Gonçalves, R.; Silva, M.P.; Costa, C.M.; Silva, M.M.; Bermudez, V.D.Z.; Lanceros-Méndez, S. Silk fibroin separators: A step towards lithium ion batteries with enhanced sustainability. *ACS Appl. Mater. Interfaces* **2018**, *10*, 5385–5394. [CrossRef]
21. Pereira, R.F.P.; Gonçalves, R.; Gonçalves, H.M.R.; Correia, D.M.; Costa, C.M.; Silva, M.M.; Lanceros-Méndez, S.; Bermudez, V.D.Z. Plasma-treated Bombyx mori cocoon separators for high-performance and sustainable lithium-ion batteries. *Mater. Today Sustain.* **2020**, *9*, 100041. [CrossRef]
22. Biswal, B.; Dan, A.K.; Sengupta, A.; Das, M.; Bindhani, B.K.; Das, D.; Parhi, P.K. Extraction of silk fibroin with several sericin removal processes and its importance in tissue engineering: A review. *J. Polym. Environ.* **2022**, *30*, 2222–2253. [CrossRef]
23. Chen, X.D.; Wang, Y.F.; Wang, Y.J.; Li, Q.Y.; Liang, X.Y.; Wang, G.; Li, J.L.; Peng, R.J.; Sima, Y.H.; Xu, S.Q. Ectopic expression of sericin enables efficient production of ancient silk with structural changes in silkworm. *Nat. Commun.* **2023**, *13*, 6295. [CrossRef]
24. Drummy, L.F.; Farmer, B.L.; Naik, R.R. Correlation of the β-sheet crystal size in silk fibers with the protein amino acid sequence. *Soft Matter* **2007**, *3*, 877–882. [CrossRef]
25. Cho, S.Y.; Yun, Y.S.; Lee, S.; Jang, D.; Park, K.Y.; Kim, J.K.; Kim, B.H.; Kang, K.; Kaplan, D.L.; Jin, H.J. Carbonization of a stable β-sheet-rich silk protein into a pseudographitic pyroprotein. *Nat. Commun.* **2015**, *6*, 7145. [CrossRef] [PubMed]
26. Dash, P.; Yang, J.M.; Lin, H.; Lin, A.S. Preparation and characterization of zinc gallate phosphor for electrochemical luminescence. *J. Lumin.* **2020**, *228*, 117593. [CrossRef]
27. Ding, Z.; Li, H.; Shaw, L. New insights into the solid-state hydrogen storage of nanostructured $LiBH_4$-$MgH_2$ system. *Chem. Eng. J.* **2020**, *385*, 123856. [CrossRef]
28. Liu, Y.J.; Tai, Z.X.; Rozen, I.; Yu, Z.P.; Lu, Z.Y.; LaGrow, A.P.; Bondarchuk, O.; Chen, Q.Q.; Goobes, G.; Li, Y.; et al. Ion flux regulation through PTFE nanospheres impregnated in glass fiber separators for long-lived lithium and sodium metal batteries. *Adv. Energy Mater.* **2023**, *13*, 2204420. [CrossRef]
29. Ding, Z.; Li, Y.T.; Yang, H.; Lu, Y.F.; Tan, J.; Li, J.B.; Li, Q.; Chen, Y.A.; Shaw, L.L.; Pan, F.S. Tailoring $MgH_2$ for hydrogen storage through nanoengineering and catalysis. *J. Magnes. Alloys* **2022**, *10*, 2946–2967. [CrossRef]
30. Li, Y.T.; Guo, Q.F.; Ding, Z.; Jiang, H.; Yang, H.; Du, W.J.; Zheng, Y.; Huo, K.F.; Shaw, L.L. MOFs-based materials for solid-state hydrogen storage: Strategies and perspectives. *Chem. Eng. J.* **2024**, *485*, 149665. [CrossRef]
31. Yang, H.; Ding, Z.; Li, Y.-T.; Li, S.-Y.; Wu, P.-K.; Hou, Q.-H.; Zheng, Y.; Gao, B.; Huo, K.-F.; Du, W.-J.; et al. Recent advances in kinetic and thermodynamic regulation of magnesium hydride for hydrogen storage. *Rare Met.* **2023**, *42*, 2906–2927. [CrossRef]

32. Nurazzi, N.M.; Asyraf, M.R.M.; Fatimah Athiyah, S.; Shazleen, S.S.; Rafiqah, S.A.; Harussani, M.M.; Kamarudin, S.H.; Razman, M.R.; Rahmah, M.; Zainudin, E.S.; et al. A review on mechanical performance of hybrid natural fiber polymer composites for structural applications. *Polymers* **2021**, *13*, 2170. [CrossRef] [PubMed]
33. Ma, X.H.; Cheng, Z.Y.; Zhang, T.W.; Zhang, X.Q.; Ma, Y.; Guo, Y.Q.; Wang, X.Y.; Zheng, Z.H.; Hou, Z.G.; Zi, Z.F. High efficient recycling of glass fiber separator for sodium-ion batteries. *Ceram. Int.* **2023**, *49*, 23598–23604. [CrossRef]
34. Li, M.H.; Lu, G.J.; Zheng, W.K.; Zhao, Q.N.; Li, Z.P.; Jiang, X.P.; Yang, Z.G.; Li, Z.Y.; Qu, B.H.; Xu, C.H. Multifunctionalized safe separator toward practical sodium-metal batteries with high-performance under high mass loading. *Adv. Funct. Mater.* **2023**, *33*, 2214759. [CrossRef]
35. Hou, J.R.; Xu, T.T.; Wang, B.Y.; Yang, H.Y.; Wang, H.; Kong, D.Z.; Lyu, L.L.; Li, X.J.; Wang, Y.; Xu, Z.L. Self-confinement of Na metal deposition in hollow carbon tube arrays for ultrastable and high-power sodium metal batteries. *Adv. Funct. Mater.* **2024**, *34*, 2312750. [CrossRef]
36. Gannon, W.J.F.; Dunnil, C.W. Apparent disagreement between cyclic voltammetry and electrochemical impedance spectroscopy explained by time-domain simulation of constant phase elements. *Int. J. Hydrogen Energy* **2020**, *45*, 22383–22393. [CrossRef]
37. Xiong, F.Y.; Li, J.T.; Zuo, C.L.; Zhang, X.L.; Tan, S.S.; Jiang, Y.L.; An, Q.Y.; Chu, P.K.; Mai, L.Q. Mg-doped $Na_4Fe_3(PO_4)_2(P_2O_7)/C$ composite with enhanced intercalation pseudocapacitance for ultra-stable and high-rate sodium-ion storage. *Adv. Funct. Mater.* **2023**, *33*, 2211257. [CrossRef]
38. Bruce, P.G.; Vincent, C.A. Steady state current flow in solid binary electrolyte cells. *J. Electroanal. Chem.* **1987**, *225*, 1–17. [CrossRef]
39. Evans, J.; Vincent, C.A.; Bruce, P.G. Electrochemical measurement of transference numbers in polymer electrolytes. *Polymer* **1987**, *28*, 2324–2328. [CrossRef]
40. Wei, Q.L.; Chang, X.Q.; Wang, J.; Huang, T.Y.; Huang, X.J.; Yu, J.Y.; Zheng, H.F.; Chen, J.H.; Peng, D.L. An ultrahigh-power mesocarbon microbeads | $Na^+$-diglyme | $Na_3V_2(PO_4)_3$ sodium-ion battery. *Adv. Mater.* **2022**, *34*, 2108304. [CrossRef]
41. Cao, J.L.; Wang, Y.; Wang, L.; Yu, F.; Ma, J. $Na_3V_2(PO_4)_3$@C as faradaic electrodes in capacitive deionization for high performance desalination. *Nano Lett.* **2019**, *19*, 823–828. [CrossRef] [PubMed]
42. Panda, P.K.; Cho, T.S.; Hsieh, C.T.; Yang, P.C. Cobalt- and copper-doped NASICON-type LATP polymer composite electrolytes enabling lithium titania electrode for solid-state lithium batteries with high-rate capability and excellent cyclic performance. *J. Energy Storage* **2024**, *95*, 112559. [CrossRef]
43. Huang, R.; Yan, D.; Zhang, Q.Y.; Zhang, G.W.; Chen, B.B.; Yang, H.Y.; Yu, C.Y.; Bai, Y. Unlocking charge transfer limitation in NASICON structured $Na_3V_2(PO_4)_3$ cathode via trace carbon incorporation. *Adv. Energy Mater.* **2024**, *14*, 2400595. [CrossRef]
44. Huang, X.S. A lithium-ion battery separator prepared using a phase inversion process. *J. Power Sources* **2012**, *216*, 216–221. [CrossRef]
45. Berger, E.; Niemelä, J.; Lampela, O.; Juffer, A.H.; Komsa, H.P. Raman spectra of amino acids and peptides from machine learning polarizabilities. *J. Chem. Inf. Model.* **2024**, *64*, 4601–4612. [CrossRef] [PubMed]
46. Sun, Y.L.; Ji, X.; Wang, X.; He, Q.F.; Dong, J.C.; Le, J.B.; Li, J.F. Visualization of electrooxidation on palladium single crystal surfaces via in situ Raman spectroscopy. *Angew. Chem. Int. Ed.* **2024**, e202408736. [CrossRef]
47. Yu, J.M.; Guo, T.L.; Wang, C.; Shen, Z.H.; Dong, X.Y.; Li, S.H.; Zhang, H.G.; Lu, Z.D. Engineering two-dimensional metal–organic framework on molecular basis for fast $Li^+$ conduction. *Nano Lett.* **2021**, *21*, 5805–5812. [CrossRef] [PubMed]
48. Shen, L.; Bin Wu, H.; Liu, F.; Brosmer, J.L.; Shen, G.; Wang, X.; Zink, J.I.; Xiao, Q.; Cai, M.; Wang, G.; et al. Creating lithium-ion electrolytes with biomimetic ionic channels in metal–organic frameworks. *Adv. Mater.* **2018**, *30*, 1707476. [CrossRef]
49. Harizanova, R.; Tashava, T.; Gaydarov, V.; Avramova, I.; Lilova, V.; Nedev, S.; Zamfirova, G.; Nedkova-Shtipska, M.; Rüssel, C. Structure and physicochemical characteristics of the glasses in the system $Na_2O/BaO/ZrO_2/TiO_2/SiO_2/B_2O_3/Al_2O_3$-Influence of the $ZrO_2$ addition on the physico-chemical and mechanical properties. *Solid State Sci.* **2024**, *151*, 107515. [CrossRef]
50. Hurisso, B.B.; Lovelock, K.R.J.; Licence, P. Amino acid-based ionic liquids: Using XPS to probe the electronic environment via binding energies. *Phys. Chem. Chem. Phys.* **2011**, *13*, 17737–17748. [CrossRef]
51. Martin-Vosshage, D.; Chowdari, B.V.R. XPS studies on $(PEO)_nLiClO_4$ and $(PEO)_nCu(ClO_4)_2$ polymer electrolytes. *J. Electrochem. Soc.* **1995**, *142*, 1442. [CrossRef]
52. Zhou, X.Z.; Chen, X.M.; Yang, Z.; Liu, X.H.; Hao, Z.Q.; Jin, S.; Zhang, L.H.; Wang, R.; Zhang, C.F.; Li, L.; et al. Anion receptor weakens $ClO_4^-$ solvation for high-temperature sodium-ion batteries. *Adv. Funct. Mater.* **2024**, *34*, 2302281. [CrossRef]
53. Amin, M.A. Metastable and stable pitting events on Al induced by chlorate and perchlorate anions-Polarization, XPS and SEM studies. *Electrochim. Acta* **2009**, *54*, 1857–1863. [CrossRef]
54. Sreedhar, B.; Sairam, M.; Chattopadhyay, D.K.; Mitra, P.P.; Rao, D.V.M. Thermal and XPS studies on polyaniline salts prepared by inverted emulsion polymerization. *J. Appl. Polym. Sci.* **2006**, *101*, 499–508. [CrossRef]
55. Stevens, J.S.; Luca, A.C.D.; Pelendritis, M.; Terenghi, G.; Downes, S.; Schroeder, S.L.M. Quantitative analysis of complex amino acids and RGD peptides by X-ray photoelectron spectroscopy (XPS). *Surf. Interface Anal.* **2013**, *45*, 1238–1246. [CrossRef]
56. Tan, S.S.; Jiang, Y.L.; Ni, S.Y.; Wang, H.; Xiong, F.Y.; Cui, L.M.; Pan, X.L.; Tang, C.; Rong, Y.G.; An, Q.Y.; et al. Serrated lithium fluoride nanofibers-woven interlayer enables uniform lithium deposition for lithium-metal batteries. *Natl. Sci. Rev.* **2022**, *9*, nwac183. [CrossRef]
57. Sun, B.; Li, P.; Zhang, J.Q.; Wang, D.; Munroe, P.; Wang, C.Y.; Notten, P.H.L.; Wang, G.X. Dendrite-free sodium-metal anodes for high-energy sodium-metal batteries. *Adv. Mater.* **2018**, *30*, 1801334. [CrossRef]

58. Wang, Z.Y.; Du, Z.J.; Li, Z.; Zhang, X.H.; Liu, J.T.; Dai, Y.H.; Zhang, W.; Wang, D.; Wang, Y.Y.; Li, H.X.; et al. Super-lattices enabled performances of vanadate-phosphate glass-ceramic composite cathode in lithium-ion batteries. *Ceram. Int.* **2024**, *50*, 15407–15416. [CrossRef]
59. Fu, X.W.; Hurlock, M.J.; Ding, C.F.; Li, X.Y.; Zhang, Q.; Zhong, W.H. MOF-enabled ion-regulating gel electrolyte for long-cycling lithium metal batteries under high voltage. *Small* **2022**, *18*, 2106225. [CrossRef]
60. Zhu, F.L.; Bao, H.F.; Wu, X.S.; Tao, Y.L.; Qin, C.; Su, Z.M.; Kang, Z.H. High-performance metal–organic framework-based single ion conducting solid-state electrolytes for low-temperature lithium metal batteries. *ACS Appl. Mater. Interfaces* **2019**, *11*, 43206–43213. [CrossRef]
61. Sheng, L.; Wang, Q.Q.; Liu, X.; Cui, H.; Wang, X.L.; Xu, Y.L.; Li, Z.L.; Wang, L.; Chen, Z.H.; Xu, G.L.; et al. Suppressing electrolyte-lithium metal reactivity via $Li^+$-desolvation in uniform nano-porous separator. *Nat. Commun.* **2022**, *13*, 172. [CrossRef] [PubMed]
62. Chang, Z.; Qiao, Y.; Deng, H.; Yang, H.J.; He, P.; Zhou, H.S. A liquid electrolyte with de-solvated lithium ions for lithium-metal battery. *Joule* **2020**, *4*, 1776–1789. [CrossRef]
63. Ma, W.H.; Wang, S.; Wu, X.W.; Liu, W.W.; Yang, F.; Liu, S.D.; Jun, S.C.; Dai, L.; He, Z.X.; Zhang, Q.B. Tailoring desolvation strategies for aqueous zinc-ion batteries. *Energy Environ. Sci.* **2024**, *17*, 4819–4846. [CrossRef]

**Disclaimer/Publisher's Note:** The statements, opinions and data contained in all publications are solely those of the individual author(s) and contributor(s) and not of MDPI and/or the editor(s). MDPI and/or the editor(s) disclaim responsibility for any injury to people or property resulting from any ideas, methods, instructions or products referred to in the content.

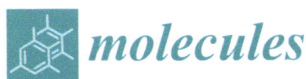

*Article*

# The Impact of Biowaste Composition and Activated Carbon Structure on the Electrochemical Performance of Supercapacitors

Alisher Abdisattar [1,2,3], Meir Yerdauletov [4,5,*], Mukhtar Yeleuov [1,3,4], Filipp Napolskiy [5,6], Aleksey Merkulov [6], Anna Rudnykh [6], Kuanysh Nazarov [4,5], Murat Kenessarin [4,5], Ayazhan Zhomartova [4,5] and Victor Krivchenko [6]

1. Bes Saiman Group, 050057 Almaty, Kazakhstan
2. Satbayev University, 050000 Almaty, Kazakhstan
3. Engineering and Science Hub, 050004 Almaty, Kazakhstan
4. Institute of Nuclear Physics, 050032 Almaty, Kazakhstan; k.nazarov@inp.kz (K.N.)
5. Joint Institute for Nuclear Research, 141980 Dubna, Russia
6. Dubna State University, 141980 Dubna, Russia
* Correspondence: meyir2008@mail.ru

**Abstract:** The increasing demand for sustainable and efficient energy storage materials has led to significant research into utilizing waste biomass for producing activated carbons. This study investigates the impact of the structural properties of activated carbons derived from various lignocellulosic biomasses—barley straw, wheat straw, and wheat bran—on the electrochemical performance of supercapacitors. The Fourier Transform Infrared (FTIR) spectroscopy analysis reveals the presence of key functional groups and their transformations during carbonization and activation processes. The Raman spectra provide detailed insights into the structural features and defects in the carbon materials. The electrochemical tests indicate that the activated carbon's specific capacitance and energy density are influenced by the biomass source. It is shown that the wheat-bran-based electrodes exhibit the highest performance. This research demonstrates the potential of waste-biomass-derived activated carbons as high-performance materials for energy storage applications, contributing to sustainable and efficient supercapacitor development.

**Keywords:** biomass composition; wheat bran; wheat straw; barley straw; activated carbon; FTIR spectra; supercapacitor

**Citation:** Abdisattar, A.; Yerdauletov, M.; Yeleuov, M.; Napolskiy, F.; Merkulov, A.; Rudnykh, A.; Nazarov, K.; Kenessarin, M.; Zhomartova, A.; Krivchenko, V.. The Impact of Biowaste Composition and Activated Carbon Structure on the Electrochemical Performance of Supercapacitors. *Molecules* **2024**, *29*, 5029. https://doi.org/10.3390/molecules29215029

Academic Editors: Zhao Ding, Liangjuan Gao and Shicong Yang

Received: 7 September 2024
Revised: 14 October 2024
Accepted: 15 October 2024
Published: 24 October 2024

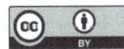

**Copyright:** © 2024 by the authors. Licensee MDPI, Basel, Switzerland. This article is an open access article distributed under the terms and conditions of the Creative Commons Attribution (CC BY) license (https://creativecommons.org/licenses/by/4.0/).

## 1. Introduction

The increasing demand for sustainable and efficient materials has driven significant research into the utilization of waste biomass as a renewable source for producing activated carbons for high-power energy storage systems such as supercapacitors and Li-ion capacitors [1,2]. Waste biomass, a byproduct of various agricultural and industrial processes, offers an abundant and low-cost precursor for activated carbon production. This approach not only addresses waste management challenges but also provides a sustainable pathway for creating high-value materials with diverse applications [3,4].

Activated carbons are renowned for their high surface area, porosity, and adsorption capacitance, making them ideal candidates for environmental and energy storage applications, particularly in the development of electric double-layer capacitors (i.e., supercapacitors) [2,5]. These energy storage devices require materials with high electrical conductivity, electrochemical stability, and a large surface area to achieve high energy and power density [6,7]. The activated carbons derived from waste biomass possess these characteristics, making them promising materials for supercapacitor electrodes.

The composition of lignocellulosic biomass significantly influences the development of pores in activated carbon [8]. Cellulose primarily contributes to the formation of micropores, while lignin helps maintain structural integrity as well as contributes to specific surface area development [9]. The activation process, whether physical or chemical, further refines the pore structure, enhancing the overall adsorption capacitance and effectiveness of the activated carbon.

Traditional wet chemical methods using two-step sulfuric acid hydrolysis for biomass composition analysis are time-consuming and labor-intensive and do not provide structural information, limiting their suitability for industrial applications or large-scale energy storage systems. In contrast, infrared techniques offer rapid, cost-effective analysis that is non-destructive and have shown promising results [10].

FTIR spectroscopy, a robust analytical technique, provides detailed information on the chemical structure and functional groups present in materials [11,12]. It has been successfully utilized to analyze the composition of lignocellulosic biomass. By analyzing the FTIR spectra of waste biomasses as well as carbonized and activated carbons, we can identify the key functional groups and compositional changes that occur during the activation process. This spectral analysis is essential for understanding how the initial composition of the biomass influences the properties of activated carbons and, ultimately, their performance as supercapacitor electrodes.

In this research, we systematically investigated the FTIR spectra of various waste biomasses and their corresponding carbonized and activated carbons. We aimed to correlate the spectral data with the electrochemical properties of the activated carbons to provide a comprehensive understanding of the relationship between the initial biomass composition, the activation-induced changes, and the electrode performance.

In this work, we investigated the structural and electrochemical characteristics of activated carbons synthesized from barley straw (BS), wheat straw (WhS), and wheat bran (WhB). The resulting activated carbons had a specific surface area of 1866 to 2036 $m^2/g$.

The study of electrochemical characteristics revealed that the activated carbon synthesized from wheat bran had the highest specific capacitance, reaching 143 F/g at 0.1 A/g.

At the same time, all samples demonstrated high cyclability, which was expressed by a retention of approximately 94% of the initial capacitance after 6000 cycles at a current density of 1 A/g.

This study not only enhances the fundamental knowledge of biomass-derived activated carbons but also offers practical insights for developing high-performance supercapacitor electrodes from sustainable resources.

## 2. Results and Discussion

### 2.1. Characterization

The Fourier Transform Infrared (FTIR) spectroscopy analysis of the biomass samples revealed characteristic peaks, indicating the presence of various functional groups (Figure 1). The b broad peak at 3330 $cm^{-1}$ indicates O-H stretching vibration (Figure 1a). This peak is characteristic of hydroxyl groups, which are prevalent in the cellulose, hemicellulose, and lignin components of biomass [13]. The presence of this peak suggests a significant amount of hydrogen bonding, which is typical in polysaccharides and water molecules within biomass.

The absorption bands observed in the range of 3000–2780 $cm^{-1}$ correspond to the C-H stretching vibrations of aliphatic hydrocarbons. These bands indicate the presence of methylene (CH2) and methyl (CH3) groups, which are common in lignocellulosic materials [14]. The distinct peak at 1727 $cm^{-1}$ is associated with the C=O stretching vibration of carbonyl groups [15]. This peak is typically attributed to esters, aldehydes, and ketones, suggesting the presence of hemicellulose and lignin derivatives in biomass.

The peak at 1640 $cm^{-1}$ is attributed to H-O-H deformation vibration. This peak is often associated with absorbed water and indicates the presence of moisture in the biomass sample [15]. The peaks in the range of 1500–1280 $cm^{-1}$ are assigned to the bending vibrations of $CH_3$ groups. These peaks suggest the presence of methyl groups, which are part of the lignin and hemicellulose structures in biomass.

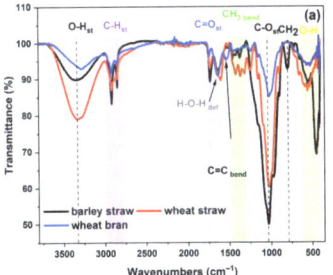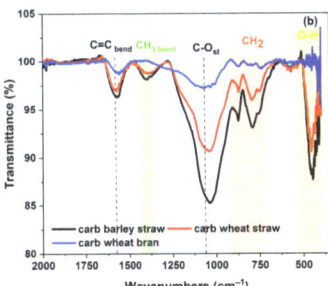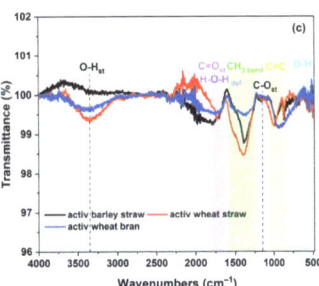

**Figure 1.** FTIR spectra and composition of functional groups of (**a**) original biomass; (**b**) carbonized biomass; (**c**) activated biomass.

The peak at 1030 cm$^{-1}$ indicates C-O stretching vibration. This peak is commonly associated with the C-O-C linkages in cellulose and hemicellulose, confirming the polysaccharide nature of the biomass [9].

As illustrated in Figure 1a, there were no qualitative differences among the various lignocellulosic biomasses; the distinctions were solely in the quantitative ratios of their components. Following carbonization (heat treatment up to 550 °C), the functional groups in the range of 1600–3500 cm$^{-1}$ and the H-O-H deformation vibration at 1640 cm$^{-1}$, associated with absorbed water, completely disappeared due to the volatilization of these substances. Additionally, the intensity of the remaining peaks significantly decreased, indicating the decomposition of the hemicellulose and its associated functional groups, as well as the partial decomposition of the cellulose and lignin.

Notably, a C=C peak representing aromatic rings emerged after carbonization (Figure 1b) at 1540 cm$^{-1}$, likely formed due to the loss of functional groups. It was interesting to observe that the intensity of this peak was higher for barley and wheat straw, which initially exhibited more intense functional groups that volatilized during heat treatment (1600–3500 cm$^{-1}$) compared to wheat bran. This suggests that the more functional groups are lost, the more aromatic rings are formed. Consequently, the remaining functional groups play a crucial role in influencing the structure and properties of activated carbon during further activation of the carbonized mass. The yield of the carbonaceous products after the carbonization process for all the biomass samples was 29–30%.

Of particular interest was the peak at 1500–1280 cm$^{-1}$, corresponding to the CH$_3$ group, the intensity of which did not significantly decrease after both carbonization and activation (Figure 1). Methyl groups are exceptionally stable, comprising a central carbon atom connected to three hydrogen atoms, and generally remain unreactive even when exposed to strong acids or bases [16]. The intensity of this group remained higher for barley and wheat straw after carbonization and activation, suggesting that these biomasses exhibited the smallest total pore volume in the activated state (Table 1). It appeared that these stable groups blocked the pores during the activation process, as they did not evaporate or decompose at high temperatures or in the presence of KOH.

**Table 1.** Specific surface area and total pore volume of the activated carbons.

| Activated Carbon | SSA (BET Method), m$^2$/g | Total Pore Volume, cm$^3$/g |
|---|---|---|
| WhB | 1866.24 | 1.42 |
| BS | 1970 | 1.39 |
| WhS | 2036 | 1.23 |

The FTIR spectra of the activated carbons (Figure 1c) show significantly fewer bands, indicating that most functional groups decomposed during carbonization and activation. This decomposition process is crucial for understanding the structural transformations and the resultant properties of the activated carbons. The yield of the activated carbons after the activation process was 44.7% for wheat bran, 41.75% for barley straw, and 49.5% for wheat straw.

The nitrogen adsorption/desorption isotherm of the samples exhibited a Type Ib isotherm with an H4 hysteresis loop (Figure 2a), indicating the presence of wider micropores and narrow mesopores with high surface area and slit shape [17,18]. The BET surface area and the total pore volume for activated carbons are represented in Table 1.

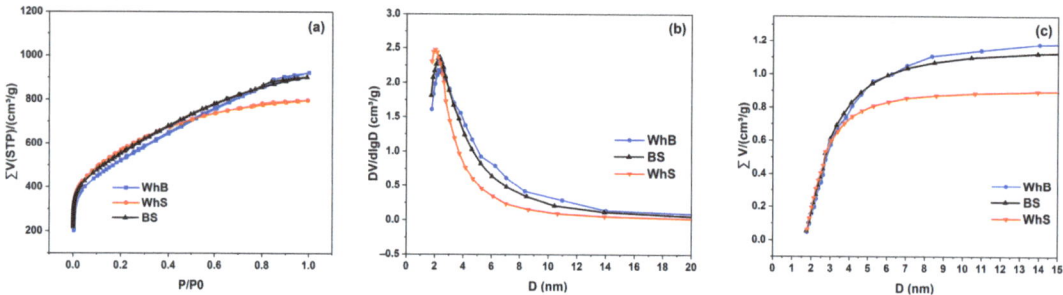

Figure 2. (a) Nitrogen adsorption/desorption isotherms, (b) differential PSDs, and (c) cumulative PSDs for the activated biomasses.

The differential pore size distribution showed a peak at 2–2.4 nm, confirming the dominance of mesopores in this range (Figure 2b). The cumulative pore size distribution demonstrated a steady increase in pore volume with increasing pore diameter, with a significant rise between 1.7 nm and 3 nm, aligning with the micro- and mesoporous nature of the material (Figure 2c). The cumulative pore volume reached a plateau at around 5 nm, signifying that most of the pore volume was due to mesopores. The consistent pore size distribution across all samples indicated that the activation process effectively generated micropores in the 2.2 nm range, which is beneficial for various adsorption and filtration applications.

Comparing the specific surface area of the activated carbons (Table 1) and the intensity of the peaks at 1030 cm$^{-1}$ corresponding to C-O stretching vibrations (Figure 1b), it was evident that a higher presence of this functional group correlated with a greater specific surface area. This is consistent with findings by Catalina et al. [9], who demonstrated that cellulose possesses the largest specific surface area.

The wheat bran activated carbon exhibited a layered structure with both micro- and macropores (Figure 3a). The SEM images showed a mix of sheet-like formations and irregularly shaped particles. The particle size varied in a range of few hundred micrometers. The SEM images of wheat straw (Figure 3b) activated carbon revealed a heterogeneous porosity with a mix of micropores and macropores. The surface texture was rough, and remnants of the straw's cellular structure were evident. The activated carbon derived from barley straw (Figure 3c) displayed a porous network with visible vascular bundles. The surface was rough with notable cracks and fissures, indicative of the breakdown of the straw's cellular structure. The particles were predominantly elongated and ranged in size in a range of a few hundred micrometers.

The Raman spectra of the RH, BS, WhS, and WhB samples, recorded in the spectral range of 1000–2000 cm$^{-1}$, are presented in Figure 4. The spectra were deconvoluted using Lorentzian functions to accurately isolate the first-order modes: the D*, D, D″, G, and D′ bands. This deconvolution method allowed for a more precise analysis of the structural features and defects in the carbon materials, addressing the limitations of the traditional I(D)/I(G) ratio, which can be skewed by band overlap.

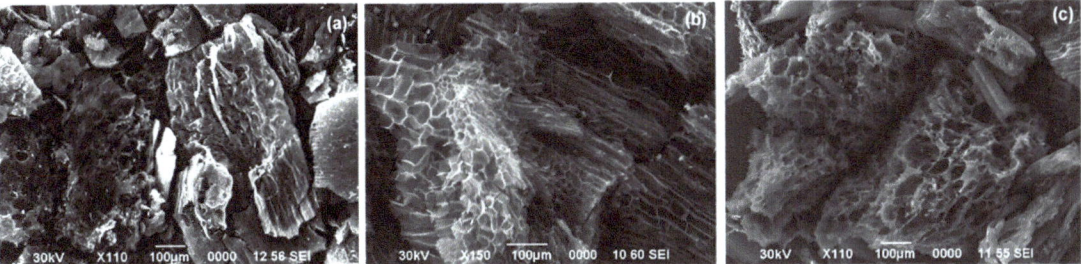

**Figure 3.** SEM images of activated carbon derived from (**a**) wheat bran; (**b**) wheat straw; (**c**) barley straw.

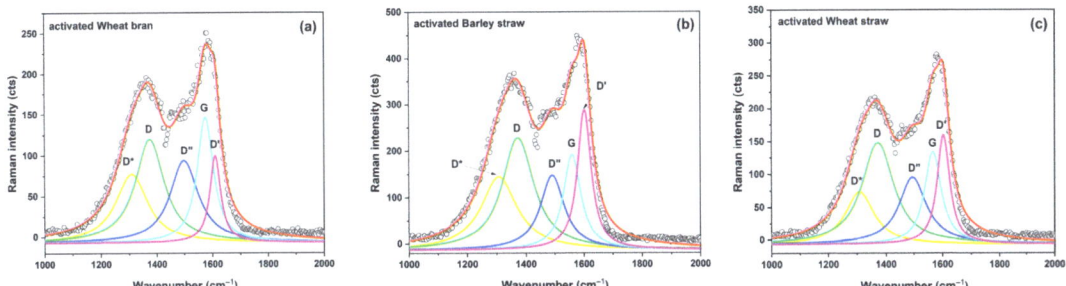

**Figure 4.** Raman spectra of activated wheat bran (**a**), barley straw (**b**), and wheat straw (**c**).

The G band, observed at 1583 cm$^{-1}$, corresponds to the E2g optical phonon mode, characteristic of sp2-hybridized carbon atoms in graphite-like materials [19]. This band is a key indicator of the degree of crystallinity of and structural changes in carbon materials. The D band, located between 1330 and 1350 cm$^{-1}$, is attributed to defects and disorders in the carbon lattice, as well as double-resonance processes near the K point of the Brillouin zone [19]. The D″ band, appearing in the 1500–1550 cm$^{-1}$ range, is associated with the amorphous phase, with its intensity inversely proportional to crystallinity [20]. The D′ band at 1620 cm$^{-1}$ corresponds to the disorder-induced phonon mode associated with crystal defects. The D* band, found between 1050 and 1200 cm$^{-1}$, depends on the remaining oxygen-containing groups [21].

The degree of graphitization for each sample was calculated using the ratio of the area under the G peak (A(G)) to the total area of all peaks (A$_{total}$), as defined by the following equation [22]:

$$Gf = \frac{A(G)}{A_{total}} \quad (1)$$

The WhB sample exhibited the highest degree of graphitization at 12.3%, indicating superior crystallinity and fewer defects relative to the other samples. The WhS sample displayed a graphitization degree of 10.0% but with lower-intensity the D and G bands, suggesting a different structural organization. The BS sample showed the lowest graphitization degree of 6.8%, correlating with the low intensity of the D and G bands, indicative of a more amorphous structure.

*2.2. Electrochemical Test*

The electrochemical performance of activated-carbon-based supercapacitor electrodes can vary significantly depending on the biomass source used for their derivation. This variation is primarily due to the differences in the pore structure and specific surface area that arise during the carbonization and activation processes.

These factors influence the double-layer capacitance of the electrodes during constant current charge/discharge cycles. Figure 5a illustrates the galvanostatic charge/discharge curves at a current density of 1 A/g for the electrodes derived from different biomass sources.

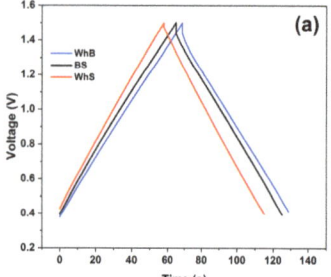
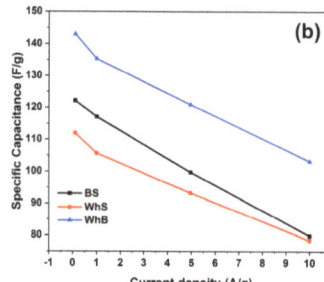
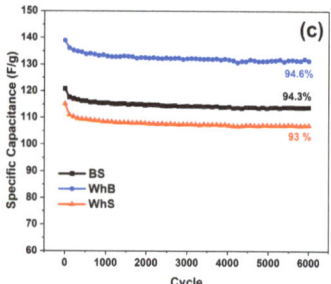

**Figure 5.** Electrochemical characteristics of supercapacitor electrodes obtained from barley straw, wheat straw, and wheat bran: (**a**) galvanostatic charge/discharge curves from 0.4 to 1.5 V at 1 A/g; (**b**) specific capacitances of the electrodes in a current range of 0.1–10 A/g; (**c**) cyclic stability test at 1 A/g from 0.4 to 1.5 V.

The curves exhibit a typical behavior of electrical double-layer capacitor electrodes. No significant redox processes on the surface of the carbon electrodes in the given voltage ranges were observed.

Figure 5b presents the specific capacitances of the electrodes based on barley (BS), wheat straw (WhS), and wheat bran (WhB) as a function of charge/discharge current density. Among the tested materials, the electrodes based on wheat bran exhibited the highest specific capacitance, reaching up to 143 F/g at 0.1 A/g. This was followed by the electrodes based on barley and wheat straw, with specific capacitances of 122 F/g and 112 F/g, respectively.

As the charge/discharge current density increased to 10 A/g, the specific capacitance of the wheat-bran-based electrodes decreased to 103.2 F/g, maintaining 72.1% of its maximum value. In comparison, the wheat-straw-based electrodes showed a capacitance retention of 70%, while the performance of the barley-straw-based sample dropped to 65.3%.

Table 1 shows that the activated carbon from the wheat straw possessed the largest specific surface area, followed by barley and wheat bran. However, this order did not correlate with the specific capacitances, where the electrodes based on wheat bran exhibited the highest specific capacitance, followed by those based on barley and wheat straw. This discrepancy was likely due to the significant proportion of microscopic pores in these activated carbons, rendering the BET calculation method inaccurate.

Moreover, the higher graphitization degree of the active material (Figure 4) correlated with a greater retention of the specific capacitance as the charge/discharge current density increased. A high ratio of the intensities of the D and G peaks indicates a higher degree of crystalline structure destruction, leading to deteriorated charge conductivity.

Figure 5c gives information regarding the electrode cycling stability during tests conducted by charging/discharging in the potential range of 0.4–1.5 V at a constant current density of 1 A/g. The specific capacitances of all samples decreased slightly at the beginning of the test since initial current density was 0.1 A/g, and then maintained approximately 94% of the initial data over 6000 cycles of charging and discharging at 1 A/g. At the same time, the Coulombic efficiency of all samples was more than 99%, which indicated an excellent charge and discharge reversibility.

Figure 6 demonstrates the impedance spectra of the symmetrical coin cells that contained different activated carbons as the active material. All spectra contained semicircles in the high-frequency region, associated with charge transfer resistance ($R_{CT}$), and the Warburg line in the intermediate-frequency region with a slope of about 45°, which is attributed to the diffusion capability of electrolyte ions. Among all the samples, the wheat-bran-based electrodes demonstrated the lowest $R_{CT}$, reaching about 2.7 Ohm, while the $R_{CT}$ for the BS- and WhS-based electrodes was 4.2 and 9.1 Ohm, respectively. Despite the difference in the Warburg impedance, the WhB-based electrodes showed the highest energy density of 33 Wh/kg at 122.6 W/kg, while that of the barley-straw-based sample was 29.66 Wh/kg at the same power density. The lowest energy density of 16.2 Wh/kg at 98 W/kg was demonstrated by the WhS sample. At the highest power density of 8 kW/h, the WhB sample showed an energy density of 10.1 Wh/kg, followed by the BS (6.54 Wh/kg) and WhS (5.7 Wh/kg) samples at a power density of 7.3 kW/h. For the power and energy density calculations, the mass of the active material was used.

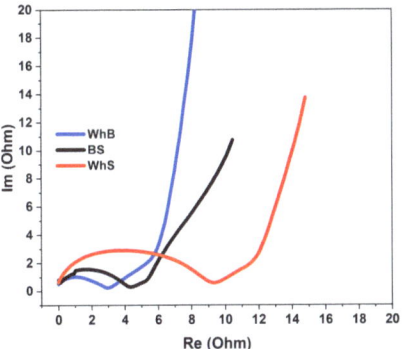

**Figure 6.** Nyquist plots of symmetrical coin cells with the electrodes based on activated carbons obtained from barley straw (BS), wheat straw (WhS), and wheat bran (WhB). The spectra were shifted to zero for clarity.

These results underscore the importance of selecting appropriate biomass sources to produce activated carbon to optimize the electrochemical performance of supercapacitor electrodes. The differences in specific surface area, pore volume, and crystalline structure directly affect the charge storage capabilities and retention properties of the electrodes under varying current conditions. Additionally, by comparing FTIR spectra, specific surface areas, pore distributions, and electrochemical characteristics, the impact of biomass composition on the structural and electrochemical properties of activated carbon can be adequately elucidated.

Finally, two-side coated electrodes with a total areal mass loading of about 7 mg/cm$^2$ were used in the pouch-cell-type supercapacitor prototyping. The wheat-bran-based activated carbon was used as the active electrode material. The electrode slurry content, separator, and electrolyte were the same as for the coin cells studied. The electrode area was 25 cm$^2$ (4.3 × 5.8 cm). The prototype was stacked by eight electrodes with opposite current collectors (Figure 7a). The mass of the pouch cell supercapacitor was 4.16 g.

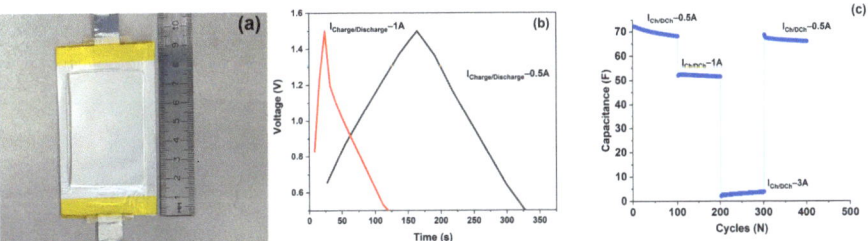

**Figure 7.** Image of the supercapacitor prototype (**a**), galvanostatic charge/discharge curves at different currents (**b**), C-rate performance (**c**).

Figure 7b demonstrates the galvanostatic charge/discharge curves in a voltage range of 0.5–1.5 V, and the C-rate performance at a different current is shown in Figure 7c. The discharge capacitance of the prototype was 72 F at a discharge current of 0.5 A. Considering the total mass of the prototype, its energy density was estimated as 4.8 Wh/kg. The results support the scalability of the described laboratory electrode technology, which indicates that the proposed activated carbon is potentially suitable for large-scale production.

## 3. Materials and Methods

### 3.1. Materials

The following materials were used: aluminum foil (99.99%, 20 μm thick, Goodfellow); argon gas (99.99%, Ikhsan Technogas Ltd., Almaty, Kazakhstan); methane (99.9%, Ikhsan Technogas Ltd., Almaty, Kazakhstan); oxygen (99.5%, Ikhsan Technogas Ltd., Almaty, Kazakhstan); barley straw, wheat straw, and wheat bran (from Turkistan region, Kazakhstan); potassium hydroxide (KOH, purity not <85%, Sigma Aldrich); nitrogen gas (99.6% Ikhsan Technogas Ltd., Almaty, Kazakhstan); conductive carbon black (Super C45, MTI Corporation); polyvinylidene fluoride (PVDF, ≥99.5, MTI Corporation); N-methyl-2-pyrrolidinone (NMP, ≥99.0%, Sigma Aldrich).

### 3.2. Synthesis of Activated Carbon from Biomass

Activated carbon was obtained from barley straw (BS), wheat straw (WhS), and wheat bran (WhB) by pyrolysis (carbonization) and subsequent thermochemical activation. Before pyrolysis, the initial samples were cleaned and ground. The cleaning process included washing with hot water using household chemicals and rinsing in distilled water, followed by drying in a drying oven at a temperature of 110 °C for 12 h. Drying time may vary depending on the amount of wet substance and the type of drying oven used. The pyrolysis process was carried out at a temperature of 550 °C for 100 min in a vertical tube furnace in a nitrogen gas atmosphere at a flow rate of 150 SCCM. Thermochemical activation was carried out in a stainless-steel reactor (AISI321), where the carbonized mass was mixed with potassium hydroxide in a ratio of 1:4. Next, the reactor was heated to a temperature of 850 °C at a heating rate of 7 °C/min with a supply of gaseous nitrogen (150 SCCM) and a holding time at a temperature of 850 °C for 120 min. The cooling process during both pyrolysis and chemical activation was carried out in a natural way.

### 3.3. Cell Fabrication and Electrochemical Measurements

The electrochemical characteristics of the electrodes containing highly porous activated carbon derived from barley straw, wheat straw, and wheat bran were assessed using a Neware BTS workstation (https://newarebattery.com/, China).

In order to prepare the electrode slurry, polymer binder PVDF Solef 5130 (TMax, China) was dissolved in N-methyl pyrrolidone for 2 h at 60 °C under stirring. After complete dissolution of the PVDF, a pre-mixed sample of the active material and the conductive additive Super C45 (TMax, China) was added and stirred on an overhead mixer for 20 h to form a homogeneous slurry.

Next, the obtained electrode slurry was stirred on a vacuum mixer for 20 min to remove gaseous substances. After that, the slurry was applied to aluminum foil using the Doctor Blade technique (Gelon, China) and dried at 100 °C for 12 h until the solvent completely evaporated.

After complete drying, the electrode tape was calendared at a temperature of 100 °C with a compression ratio of 20%. Furthermore, the electrodes were laser-cut on discs with an area of 1.77 cm$^2$ for 2032-coin cells.

The electrodes were weighed and vacuum-dried at a temperature of 120 °C for five hours to remove trace amounts of water and transferred to a glove box, where the coin cells were assembled in an argon atmosphere.

Symmetric supercapacitor coin cells were assembled with an organic electrolyte based on acetonitrile (1M TEATFB in AN), employing Celgard 2500 (TMax, China) as a separator.

Each electrode comprised 92 wt% of synthesized activated carbon as the active material, 3 wt% conductive additive, and 5 wt% binder. The total electrode areal mass loading was approximately $4.7 \pm 0.7$ mg/cm$^2$. Specific capacitance was determined from galvanostatic charge/discharge curves in a voltage range of 0.4–1.5 V at a current density of 1–10 A/g.

The electrode capacitance C was calculated based on the galvanostatic charge/discharge curves of coin cells according to the following equation:

$$C = 2 \times (I \times \Delta t)/\Delta V \qquad (2)$$

where I is the charge/discharge current, $\Delta t$ is the charge/discharge time, $\Delta V$ is the voltage window.

Gravimetric capacitance (F/g) was calculated by dividing the capacitance C by the mass fraction of the active material in the electrode layer.

*3.4. Characterization of Obtained Samples*

The carbon structures obtained on a catalytic nickel substrate were characterized using an NTEGRA Spectra Raman spectrometer (The Netherlands) operating at a wavelength of $\lambda$ = 473 nm. Surface morphology was examined via scanning electron microscopy (SEM) using a JEOL JSM-6490LA instrument (Japan), with magnifications ranging from ×5 to ×300,000 and an accelerating voltage from 0.1 to 30 kV. An elemental analysis of the carbon structures was performed using energy-dispersive X-ray (EDX) on the same SEM instrument. The specific surface area of the activated carbon was determined by nitrogen adsorption–desorption isotherms at 77 K using a gas sorption analyzer BSD-660S (China).

## 4. Conclusions

In conclusion, this research highlights the viability of using waste biomass to produce activated carbons with desirable properties for supercapacitor applications. The FTIR and Raman spectroscopic analyses reveal the structural transformations and functional group changes during carbonization and activation, which are critical for understanding the performance of the resultant activated carbons. The electrochemical evaluations show that the source of the biomass significantly influences the specific capacitance and energy density of the supercapacitors. Among the tested materials, wheat-bran-derived activated carbon exhibited the highest specific capacitance and energy density, making it a promising candidate for high-performance energy storage devices. The specific capacitance of the electrodes based on wheat-bran-derived activated carbon reached 143 F/g at 0.1 A/g.

At the same time, the activated carbons studied in this work demonstrated high cycling stability, reaching about 94% of the initial capacitance over 6000 cycles at 1 A/g.

These findings underscore the importance of selecting appropriate biomass sources and optimizing activation processes to enhance the electrochemical performance of supercapacitors. This study provides valuable insights into the sustainable production of advanced materials for energy storage, promoting the development of efficient and eco-friendly supercapacitors.

**Author Contributions:** Conceptualization, V.K.; Methodology, F.N.; Software, F.N.; Formal analysis, M.Y. (Meir Yerdauletov), M.Y. (Mukhtar Yeleuov), A.R., M.K. and A.Z.; Investigation, A.A., A.M. and A.Z.; Resources, M.Y. (Mukhtar Yeleuov); Data curation, M.Y. (Mukhtar Yeleuov), A.M. and A.R.; Writing—original draft, A.A.; Writing—review & editing, K.N. and M.Y. (Meir Yerdauletov); Visualization, M.Y. (Meir Yerdauletov) and M.K.; Supervision, V.K.; Project administration, K.N. All authors have read and agreed to the published version of the manuscript.

**Funding:** This research was funded by the Science Committee of the Ministry of Science and Higher Education of the Republic of Kazakhstan (grant No. AP19577080).

**Institutional Review Board Statement:** Not applicable.

**Informed Consent Statement:** Not applicable.

**Data Availability Statement:** The processed data required to reproduce the above findings are available on request.

**Acknowledgments:** The authors are grateful to O. O. Kapitanova and M. K. Atamanov for invaluable assistance in the analysis of IR and Raman spectra. V.K. and F.N. are grateful to Ministry of Science and Higher Education of the Russian Federation for the support (No. 1024011500004-2-1.4.5).

**Conflicts of Interest:** Authors Alisher Abdisattar and Mukhtar Yeleuov were employed by the company Bes Saiman Group. The remaining authors declare that the research was conducted in the absence of any commercial or financial relationships that could be construed as a potential conflict of interest.

## References

1. Yerdauletov, M.S.; Nazarov, K.; Mukhametuly, B.; Yeleuov, M.A.; Daulbayev, C.; Abdulkarimova, R.; Yskakov, A.; Napolskiy, F.; Krivchenko, V. Characterization of Activated Carbon from Rice Husk for Enhanced Energy Storage Devices. *Molecules* **2023**, *28*, 5818. [CrossRef] [PubMed]
2. Ahmed, S.; Ahmed, A.; Rafat, M. Supercapacitor performance of activated carbon derived from rotten carrot in aqueous, organic and ionic liquid based electrolytes. *J. Saudi Chem. Soc.* **2018**, *22*, 993–1002. [CrossRef]
3. Gorbounov, M.; Petrovic, B.; Ozmen, S.; Clough, P.; Soltani, S.M. Activated carbon derived from Biomass combustion bottom ash as solid sorbent for $CO_2$ adsorption. *Chem. Eng. Res. Des.* **2023**, *194*, 325–343. [CrossRef]
4. Taurbekov, A.; Abdisattar, A.; Atamanov, M.; Yeleuov, M.; Daulbayev, C.; Askaruly, K.; Kaidar, B.; Mansurov, Z.; Castro-Gutierrez, J.; Celzard, A.; et al. Biomass Derived High Porous Carbon via $CO_2$ Activation for Supercapacitor Electrodes. *J. Compos. Sci.* **2023**, *7*, 444. [CrossRef]
5. Lesbayev, B.; Rakhymzhan, N.; Ustayeva, G.; Maral, Y.; Atamanov, M.; Auyelkhankyzy, M.; Zhamash, A. Preparation of Nanoporous Carbon from Rice Husk with Improved Textural Characteristics for Hydrogen Sorption. *J. Compos. Sci.* **2024**, *8*, 74. [CrossRef]
6. Abdisattar, A.; Yeleuov, M.; Daulbayev, C.; Askaruly, K.; Tolynbekov, A.; Taurbekov, A.; Prikhodko, N. Recent advances and challenges of current collectors for supercapacitors. *Electrochem. Commun.* **2022**, *142*, 107373. [CrossRef]
7. Taurbekov, A.; Fierro, V.; Kuspanov, Z.; Abdisattar, A.; Atamanova, T.; Kaidar, B.; Mansurov, Z.; Atamanov, M.; Yeleuov, M.; Daulbayev, C.; et al. Nanocellulose and carbon nanotube composites: A universal solution for environmental and energy challenges. *J. Environ. Chem. Eng.* **2024**, *12*, 113262. [CrossRef]
8. Taurbekov, A.; Abdisattar, A.; Atamanov, M.; Kaidar, B.; Yeleuov, M.; Joia, R.; Amrousse, R.; Atamanova, T. Investigations of Activated Carbon from Different Natural Sources for Preparation of Binder-Free Few-Walled CNTs/Activated Carbon Electrodes. *J. Compos. Sci.* **2023**, *7*, 452. [CrossRef]
9. Correa, C.R.; Otto, T.; Kruse, A. Influence of the biomass components on the pore formation of activated carbon. *Biomass Bioenergy* **2017**, *97*, 53–64. [CrossRef]
10. Xu, F.; Wang, D. Chapter 2—Analysis of Lignocellulosic Biomass Using Infrared Methodology. In *Pretreat of Biomass*; Pandey, A., Negi, S., Binod, P., Larroche, C., Eds.; Elsevier: Amsterdam, The Netherland, 2015; pp. 7–25. [CrossRef]
11. Trache, D.; Hussin, M.H.; Chuin, C.T.H.; Sabar, S.; Fazita, M.N.; Taiwo, O.F.; Hassan, T.; Haafiz, M.M. Microcrystalline cellulose: Isolation, characterization and bio-composites application—A review. *Int. J. Biol. Macromol.* **2016**, *93*, 789–804. [CrossRef] [PubMed]
12. Akhinzhanova, A.; Sultahan, S.; Tauanov, Z.; Mansurov, Z.; Capobianchi, A.; Amrousse, R.; Atamanov, M.; Yan, Q.-L. Preparation and evaluation of effective thermal decomposition of tetraamminecopper (II) nitrate carried by graphene oxide. *Combust. Flame* **2023**, *250*, 112672. [CrossRef]
13. Abderrahim, B.; Abderrahman, E.; Mohamed, A.; Fatima, T.; Abdesselam, T.; Krim, O. Kinetic Thermal Degradation of Cellulose, Polybutylene Succinate and a Green Composite: Comparative Study. *World J. Environ. Eng.* **2015**, *3*, 95–110. [CrossRef]
14. Ong, H.C.; Yu, K.L.; Chen, W.-H.; Pillejera, M.K.; Bi, X.; Tran, K.-Q.; Pétrissans, A.; Pétrissans, M. Variation of lignocellulosic biomass structure from torrefaction: A critical review. *Renew. Sustain. Energy Rev.* **2021**, *152*, 111698. [CrossRef]
15. Salim, R.M.; Asik, J.; Sarjadi, M.S. Chemical functional groups of extractives, cellulose and lignin extracted from native *Leucaena leucocephala* bark. *Wood Sci. Technol.* **2021**, *55*, 295–313. [CrossRef]
16. Klecker, C.; Nair, L.S. Chapter 13—Matrix Chemistry Controlling Stem Cell Behavior. In *Biology and Engineering of Stem Cell Niches*; Vishwakarma, A., Karp, J.M., Eds.; Academic Press: Boston, MA, USA, 2017; pp. 195–213. [CrossRef]
17. Xu, L.; Zhang, J.; Ding, J.; Liu, T.; Shi, G.; Li, X.; Dang, W.; Cheng, Y.; Guo, R. Pore Structure and Fractal Characteristics of Different Shale Lithofacies in the Dalong Formation in the Western Area of the Lower Yangtze Platform. *Minerals* **2020**, *10*, 72. [CrossRef]
18. Thommes, M.; Kaneko, K.; Neimark, A.V.; Olivier, J.P.; Rodriguez-Reinoso, F.; Rouquerol, J.; Sing, K.S.W. Physisorption of gases, with special reference to the evaluation of surface area and pore size distribution (IUPAC Technical Report). *Pure Appl. Chem.* **2015**, *87*, 1051–1069. [CrossRef]
19. Wu, J.-B.; Lin, M.-L.; Cong, X.; Liu, H.-N.; Tan, P.-H. Raman spectroscopy of graphene-based materials and its applications in related devices. *Chem. Soc. Rev.* **2018**, *47*, 1822–1873. [CrossRef] [PubMed]
20. Claramunt, S.; Varea, A.; López-Díaz, D.; Velázquez, M.M.; Cornet, A.; Cirera, A. The Importance of Interbands on the Interpretation of the Raman Spectrum of Graphene Oxide. *J. Phys. Chem. C* **2015**, *119*, 10123–10129. [CrossRef]

21. Lee, A.Y.; Yang, K.; Anh, N.D.; Park, C.; Lee, S.M.; Lee, T.G.; Jeong, M.S. Raman study of D* band in graphene oxide and its correlation with reduction. *Appl. Surf. Sci.* **2020**, *536*, 147990. [CrossRef]
22. Nazhipkyzy, M.; Maltay, A.B.; Askaruly, K.; Assylkhanova, D.D.; Seitkazinova, A.R.; Mansurov, Z.A. Biomass-Derived Porous Carbon Materials for Li-Ion Battery. *Nanomaterials* **2022**, *12*, 3710. [CrossRef] [PubMed]

**Disclaimer/Publisher's Note:** The statements, opinions and data contained in all publications are solely those of the individual author(s) and contributor(s) and not of MDPI and/or the editor(s). MDPI and/or the editor(s) disclaim responsibility for any injury to people or property resulting from any ideas, methods, instructions or products referred to in the content.

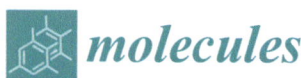 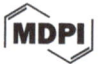

Review

# Bridging Materials and Analytics: A Comprehensive Review of Characterization Approaches in Metal-Based Solid-State Hydrogen Storage

Yaohui Xu [1,3], Yang Zhou [2,*], Yuting Li [4] and Yang Zheng [5,*]

1. Laboratory for Functional Materials, School of New Energy Materials and Chemistry, Leshan Normal University, Leshan 614000, China
2. State Key Laboratory of New Textile Materials and Advanced Processing Technology, School of Textile Science and Engineering, Wuhan Textile University, Wuhan 430200, China
3. Leshan West Silicon Materials Photovoltaic New Energy Industry Technology Research Institute, Leshan 614000, China
4. College of Materials Science and Engineering, National Engineering Research Center for Magnesium Alloys, Chongqing University, Chongqing 400044, China
5. The State Key Laboratory of Refractories and Metallurgy, Institute of Advanced Materials and Nanotechnology, Wuhan University of Science and Technology, Wuhan 430081, China
* Correspondence: yzhou@wtu.edu.cn (Y.Z.); yzheng@wust.edu.cn (Y.Z.)

**Abstract:** The advancement of solid-state hydrogen storage materials is critical for the realization of a sustainable hydrogen economy. This comprehensive review elucidates the state-of-the-art characterization techniques employed in solid-state hydrogen storage research, emphasizing their principles, advantages, limitations, and synergistic applications. We critically analyze conventional methods such as the Sieverts technique, gravimetric analysis, and secondary ion mass spectrometry (SIMS), alongside composite and structure approaches including Raman spectroscopy, X-ray diffraction (XRD), X-ray photoelectron spectroscopy (XPS), scanning electron microscopy (SEM), transmission electron microscopy (TEM), and atomic force microscopy (AFM). This review highlights the crucial role of in situ and operando characterization in unraveling the complex mechanisms of hydrogen sorption and desorption. We address the challenges associated with characterizing metal-based solid-state hydrogen storage materials discussing innovative strategies to overcome these obstacles. Furthermore, we explore the integration of advanced computational modeling and data-driven approaches with experimental techniques to enhance our understanding of hydrogen–material interactions at the atomic and molecular levels. This paper also provides a critical assessment of the practical considerations in characterization, including equipment accessibility, sample preparation protocols, and cost-effectiveness. By synthesizing recent advancements and identifying key research directions, this review aims to guide future efforts in the development and optimization of high-performance solid-state hydrogen storage materials, ultimately contributing to the broader goal of sustainable energy systems.

**Keywords:** solid-state hydrogen storage materials; characterization techniques; hydrogen storage performance; structure and composition

Citation: Xu, Y.; Zhou, Y.; Li, Y.; Zheng, Y. Bridging Materials and Analytics: A Comprehensive Review of Characterization Approaches in Metal-Based Solid-State Hydrogen Storage. *Molecules* 2024, 29, 5014. https://doi.org/10.3390/molecules29215014

Academic Editor: Maurizio Peruzzini

Received: 19 September 2024
Revised: 14 October 2024
Accepted: 17 October 2024
Published: 23 October 2024

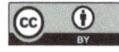

**Copyright:** © 2024 by the authors. Licensee MDPI, Basel, Switzerland. This article is an open access article distributed under the terms and conditions of the Creative Commons Attribution (CC BY) license (https://creativecommons.org/licenses/by/4.0/).

## 1. Introduction

The quest for clean and sustainable energy solutions has propelled the development of solid-state hydrogen storage materials to the forefront of scientific research [1–3]. These materials offer several advantages over traditional compressed or liquefied hydrogen storage methods, including higher storage capacities, improved safety, and ease of handling [4–6]. However, the complex nature of hydrogen storage mechanisms and the diverse range of materials being investigated present significant challenges in understanding their behavior and optimizing their performance [7–9].

To advance solid-state hydrogen storage materials from laboratory research to practical application, a comprehensive understanding of the microstructure, compositional changes, and dynamic behavior during hydrogenation/dehydrogenation processes is essential, and this is precisely where characterization techniques play a critical role [10,11]. For instance, techniques like the Sieverts method and gravimetric analysis are excellent for measuring the hydrogen storage capacity and kinetic behavior of materials, but when it comes to analyzing microstructural changes, they need to be complemented by optical and surface analysis techniques such as X-ray diffraction (XRD), Raman spectroscopy, and X-ray photoelectron spectroscopy (XPS). Additionally, neutron scattering is advantageous for studying the distribution and dynamic behavior of hydrogen atoms, while electrochemical methods are particularly effective in analyzing the electronic structure and surface reactivity of materials [12–18].

In recent years, with the continuous advancement of materials science, metal-based hydrogen storage materials have become a research hotspot due to their unique structures and excellent hydrogen storage performance [19–22]. These novel materials demonstrate outstanding potential for hydrogen storage, particularly in terms of increasing storage density and adsorption/desorption rates. However, the structural and performance complexity of these materials presents new challenges for characterization [23–26]. Traditional characterization techniques have certain limitations in terms of precision, sensitivity, and applicability, making it difficult to fully reveal the dynamic behavior of these new materials during the hydrogen storage process [27]. It is important to note that there is typically no "optimal" technique when selecting and applying characterization methods. Each technique has its strengths in revealing specific properties of materials, but they are also accompanied by limitations [28–30]. Thus, different characterization methods often complement and synergize with one another.

In summary, characterization techniques for solid-state hydrogen storage materials are key tools for understanding and optimizing their performance. We have conducted a comprehensive review of various characterization methods, aiming to provide researchers with a thorough technical reference that encompasses both traditional and emerging methods. By comparing the advantages and limitations of different techniques in their applications, we emphasize their complementarity and synergistic relationships, rather than seeking the so-called "optimal" testing method. Each characterization technique has its unique applicable scenarios and focal points, and no single method can fully elucidate all the mechanisms involved in hydrogen storage within solid-state materials. Therefore, this review particularly focuses on the unique demands of characterizing these novel materials and discusses how existing techniques can be improved or new methods developed to address these challenges. This review not only provides researchers with a comprehensive technical overview of the field of solid-state hydrogen storage characterization but also highlights the difficulties in characterizing emerging materials and the trends for future technological development. Through an in-depth analysis of various characterization techniques, we hope to provide a theoretical basis and technical support for achieving efficient and sustainable hydrogen storage solutions, thereby contributing to the continued development and application of clean energy technologies.

## 2. Hydrogen Storage Performance Characterization Techniques

Hydrogen storage materials are crucial for advancing hydrogen-based energy systems, and their performance is highly dependent on their physical and chemical properties [31]. To thoroughly understand these materials, several fundamental characterization techniques are employed. The Sieverts method, gravimetric analysis, secondary ion mass spectrometry, neutron scattering, and electrochemical methods represent some of the most essential tools in this domain. By leveraging these methods, researchers can systematically evaluate and optimize hydrogen storage materials to meet the demands of practical applications in energy storage and conversion. Table 1 briefly summarizes the pros and cons of each basic characterization technique.

Table 1. The advantages and limitations of essential characterization techniques.

| Method | Advantages | Limitations | Refs. |
|---|---|---|---|
| Sieverts method | Simplicity and reliability, measures hydrogen sorption isotherms, provides thermodynamic information | Sensitivity to volume calibration and leaks, limited information on kinetics, requires accurate temperature control | [26,30,32–40] |
| Gravimetric analysis | High sensitivity, real-time monitoring of hydrogen sorption, enables kinetic studies | Sensitivity to buoyancy effects, influence of impurities and adsorbed species, requires careful calibration and correction procedures | [39,40] |
| Thermogravimetric analysis Differential scanning calorimetry | Simultaneously measure changes in mass and heat flow, providing comprehensive information about thermal stability, decomposition, and phase transitions of materials in a single experiment | Limited sensitivity in detecting small mass changes and subtle thermal events, making them less suitable for analyzing materials with very low levels of thermal degradation or phase change | [41–48] |
| Secondary ion mass spectrometry | High spatial resolution, sensitive to low hydrogen concentrations, provides depth profiling information | Destructive technique, requires careful calibration for quantitative analysis, challenging data interpretation due to matrix effects | [49–58] |
| Electrochemical methods | Simulates real-world operating conditions, provides information on charge–discharge behavior and kinetics, enables the study of cycle stability and long-term performance | Sensitivity to electrode preparation and cell configuration, requires careful interpretation of electrochemical data, may not provide direct structural and chemical information | [59–71] |

## 2.1. Sieverts Method

The Sieverts method, also known as the volumetric method, is one of the most widely used techniques for characterizing hydrogen storage materials [32,33]. The core principle is based on the ideal gas law and the pressure changes during the gas absorption and desorption processes. The simplified schematic of the device is shown in Figure 1 [34]. When high-pressure gas comes into contact with a metal sample, the gas dissolves into the metal. According to Henry's law, the solubility of the gas in the metal is proportional to the partial pressure of the gas. By measuring the pressure changes before and after gas injection with a high-precision pressure sensor system, the amount of gas dissolved in the metal sample can be calculated.

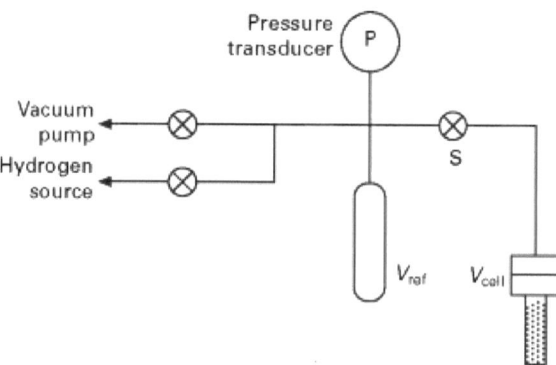

Figure 1. Schematic representation of a Sieverts apparatus [34].

The Sieverts method offers several advantages, including simplicity, reliability, and the ability to measure hydrogen sorption isotherms over a wide range of pressures and temperatures [35]. It provides essential thermodynamic information, such as the equilibrium pressure, enthalpy, and entropy of the hydrogen sorption reactions [36]. To overcome the limitations of the Sieverts method, researchers have developed advanced apparatus with improved temperature control, high-precision pressure sensors, and automated data acquisition systems. The Sieverts method is widely utilized in mainstream hydrogen testing and analysis instruments for analyzing hydrogen storage density in hydrogen storage materials. This technique provides essential measurements of hydrogen absorption and desorption capacities, critical for evaluating material performance in hydrogen storage applications [26,30]. Rigorous calibration procedures and error analysis methods have been implemented to enhance the accuracy and reliability of the measurements. The Sieverts method is particularly crucial for evaluating the hydrogen storage capacity and kinetics of metal hydrides.

Existing volumetric measurement instruments often suffer from low efficiency due to insufficient calibration techniques, temperature gradients, and limited automation. As shown in Figure 2a, the curve changes with the temperature of the sample. As the sample temperature increases, the line moves further from the sample cell, resulting in an increase in the apparent volume of the sample cell and a decrease in the apparent volume of the tube. The position of this line can be determined through calibration methods and is defined as a function of temperature. Zhu et al. [38] proposed a novel volumetric calibration and thermal gradient resistance method by introducing a continuous function to overcome temperature gradients across the entire test temperature range. This method was validated through TPD/TPA tests on MgH$_2$ powder, demonstrating automatic temperature control. Moreover, the new method enabled the completion of three PCT curves within 1.5 days. This innovative approach has the potential to make Sieverts instruments more effective, accurate, and reliable tools for characterizing hydrogen storage materials.

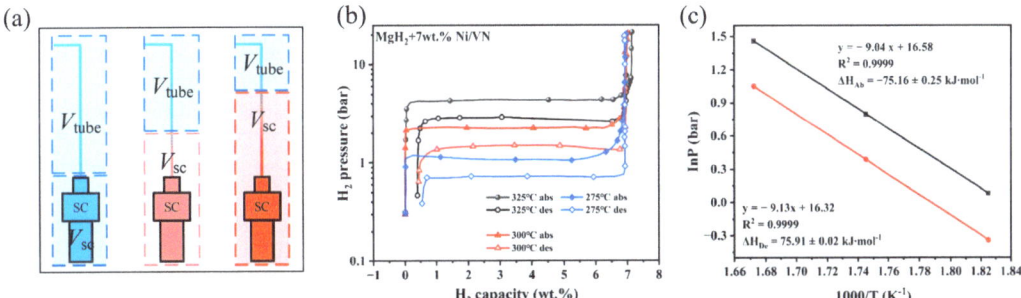

**Figure 2.** (a) Diagram of temperature gradients in the reactor [38]. The MgH$_2$ + 7 wt.% Ni/VN (b) PCT curves at 325 and 275 °C and (c) Van't Hoff plots [72].

The PCT curve is primarily used to describe the relationship between the composition of a chemical system and pressure under isothermal conditions, and it is commonly applied in the study of gas adsorption and metal hydrides for hydrogen storage. By analyzing the PCT curve, insights can be gained into the phase behavior of the system, adsorption or desorption processes, and the hydrogen storage capacity of the material. The van't Hoff equation $lnK = -\Delta H/RT + \Delta S/R$, where $K$ is the equilibrium constant, $\Delta H$ is the standard reaction enthalpy (kJ/mol), $\Delta S$ is the standard reaction entropy (J/mol·K), $R$ is the gas constant (J/mol·K), and $T$ is the temperature (K), reveals the relationship between the chemical equilibrium constant and temperature, forming the theoretical foundation for studying the effect of temperature on equilibrium in reaction thermodynamics. Wu et al. [72] measured the PCT curves of MgH$_2$-7 wt.% Ni/VN and ball-milled MgH$_2$ samples at different temperatures (Figure 2b). The results show that the plateau pressures for

MgH$_2$-7 wt.% Ni/VN during desorption at 548, 573, and 598 K were 0.72, 1.49, and 2.90 bar, respectively, and during absorption, the plateau pressures were 1.10, 2.25, and 4.20 bar, respectively. For ball-milled MgH$_2$, the desorption plateau pressures at 598, 623, and 648 K were 2.20, 4.12, and 7.40 bar, respectively, while the absorption pressures were 3.82, 7.00, and 12.20 bar. Using the van't Hoff equation to calculate the ΔH for hydrogen absorption and desorption of MgH$_2$-7 wt.% Ni/VN at different temperatures based on the plateau pressures, the values were found to be $-75.16 \pm 0.25$ and $75.91 \pm 0.02$ kJ·mol$^{-1}$ (Figure 2c), indicating no significant reduction compared to pure MgH$_2$.

By experimentally determining the changes in the equilibrium constant with temperature, thermodynamic parameters such as enthalpy and entropy changes can be obtained. The van't Hoff equation not only helps in understanding the influence of temperature on the direction and extent of chemical reactions but also has wide applications in material design, catalysis, and industrial process optimization. The combination of the PCT curve and the van't Hoff equation allows for in-depth study of thermodynamic behavior in multi-phase systems such as gas–solid and liquid–solid phases, providing reliable thermodynamic parameters to optimize material performance and understand reaction mechanisms.

## 2.2. Gravimetric Analysis

Gravimetric analysis is another fundamental technique for characterizing hydrogen storage materials. It involves measuring the mass change of a sample during hydrogen absorption or desorption processes [39]. One of the main advantages of gravimetric analysis is its high sensitivity, allowing for the detection of small mass changes associated with hydrogen sorption. It provides real-time monitoring of the hydrogen uptake and release, enabling the study of kinetics and the determination of the rate-limiting steps in the sorption processes [40]. Gravimetric analysis offers unique advantages in studying hydrogen storage materials, particularly for understanding sorption kinetics and cycling stability. However, due to the high cost of high-temperature magnetic levitation balances, this method is rarely used in the practical analysis of hydrogen storage materials.

Thermogravimetric analysis (TG) is a method used to measure changes in the mass of a sample as the temperature increases or under isothermal conditions [42,44]. TG is usually combined with differential scanning calorimetry (DSC), which detects the heat flow difference between the sample and a reference during heating or cooling, revealing the endothermic or exothermic behavior of the material and the thermal decomposition process [45,47]. The advantage of TG-DSC technology lies in its ability to simultaneously acquire both mass changes and heat flow information, offering a more comprehensive view of the material's physical and chemical behavior at various temperatures [41,43,46]. TG-DSC precisely characterizes the decomposition temperature and exothermic or endothermic properties of composite materials, helping to determine thermal stability and processing parameters. For hydrogen storage materials, by applying the Kissinger equation ($\ln(\beta/T_p^2) = \ln(AR/E_a) - E_a/(RT_p)$), where β is the heating rate (K/min), $T_p$ is the desorption peak temperature (K), R is the gas constant (J/mol·K), $E_a$ is active energy (kJ/mol), and A is the frequency factor, to fit the TG-DSC results, the activation energy of hydrogen desorption can be analyzed, providing insights into the kinetic properties of the material. Xiao et al. [48] measured the DSC curve of samples and found that after doping MgH$_2$ with Ce$_{0.6}$Zr$_{0.4}$O$_2$, the desorption peak temperature decreased compared to that of ball-milled MgH$_2$ alone (Figure 3a). Two adjacent endothermic peaks appeared on the DSC curve: the first lower-temperature desorption peak was attributed to the activation of MgH$_2$ catalyzed by Ce$_{0.6}$Zr$_{0.4}$O$_2$, while the second higher-temperature peak was due to non-activated MgH$_2$. The Kissinger equation (Figure 3b) was used to calculate the activation energy for the first low-temperature desorption peak of MgH$_2$-7CeZrO, which was approximately 66.85 kJ/mol, about 45% lower than that of ball-milled MgH$_2$ 121.07 kJ/mol. In addition, the activation energy De-E$_a$ of MgH$_2$-7CeZrO was 116.06 kJ/mol by fitting the second dehydrogenation peak of MgH$_2$-7CeZrO, indicating that De-Ea was close to De-Ea after MgH$_2$ grinding, confirming the explanation that the second peak was inactive MgH$_2$.

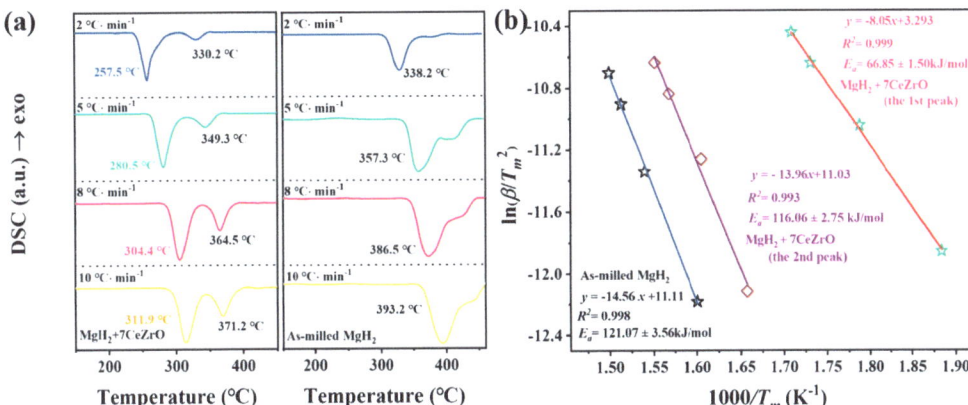

**Figure 3.** (**a**) The DSC profiles at 2, 5, 8, and 10 °C·min$^{-1}$ of MgH$_2$-7CeZrO and ball-milled MgH$_2$; (**b**) the apparent dehydrogenation activation energy of MgH$_2$-7CeZrO and undoped MgH$_2$ by Kissinger equation.

Although TG-DSC is highly effective in analyzing the hydrogen desorption kinetics of hydrogen storage materials, it should be noted that this method cannot monitor the hydrogen absorption process.

## 2.3. Secondary Ion Mass Spectrometry

Secondary ion mass spectrometry (SIMS) is a powerful surface characterization technique that provides detailed information about the elemental composition and distribution of hydrogen in storage materials [49,50]. As illustrated in Figure 4, SIMS involves bombarding the sample surface with a high-energy ion beam, producing secondary ions. These secondary ions are separated and detected by a mass spectrometer based on their mass-to-charge ratio (*m/z*), providing information about the composition and structure of the sample surface (Figure 4a). The primary ions (such as Cs$^+$ or O$^{2+}$) bombard the sample surface, causing sputtering of the surface material and generating secondary ions [51]. The production rate of secondary ions depends on the surface concentration of the sample and the sputtering yield of the primary ions (Figure 4b). By separating and detecting the secondary ions with a mass spectrometer, the composition and structure of the sample surface elements can be determined (Figure 4c).

The different binding energies of hydrogen atoms make the analysis of hydrogen storage processes in carbon-containing materials extremely complex. To differentiate between surface atoms and atoms embedded in the sample, Madroñero et al. [52] used a SIMS spectrometer with periodic ion beam interruption, observing some outgassing phenomena of surface hydrogen under room temperature and high-vacuum conditions. SIMS has proven invaluable in studying the spatial distribution of hydrogen and other elements in complex storage materials. For example, D. Andersen et al. [53] combined SIMS with dual-beam focused ion beam scanning electron microscopy to obtain high-resolution imaging of hydrogen and deuterium in Mg$_2$Ni/Mg$_2$NiH$_4$ hydrogen storage films. This allowed successful characterization of the formation process of hydrides at different depths in the films, providing valuable insights into the hydrogen storage mechanisms of the materials. When the grains exhibit an equiaxed structure (Figures 4c and 5a), hydrides mainly form on the film surface, evidenced by an enhanced $^1$H signal in the surface "hydride" local depth profile. In contrast, when the grains exhibit a columnar structure (Figure 5b,d), the hydrides extend toward the substrate, forming a continuous region. The local depth profile shows that the fully hydride layer is confined near the substrate and is surrounded by a sub-hydride layer.

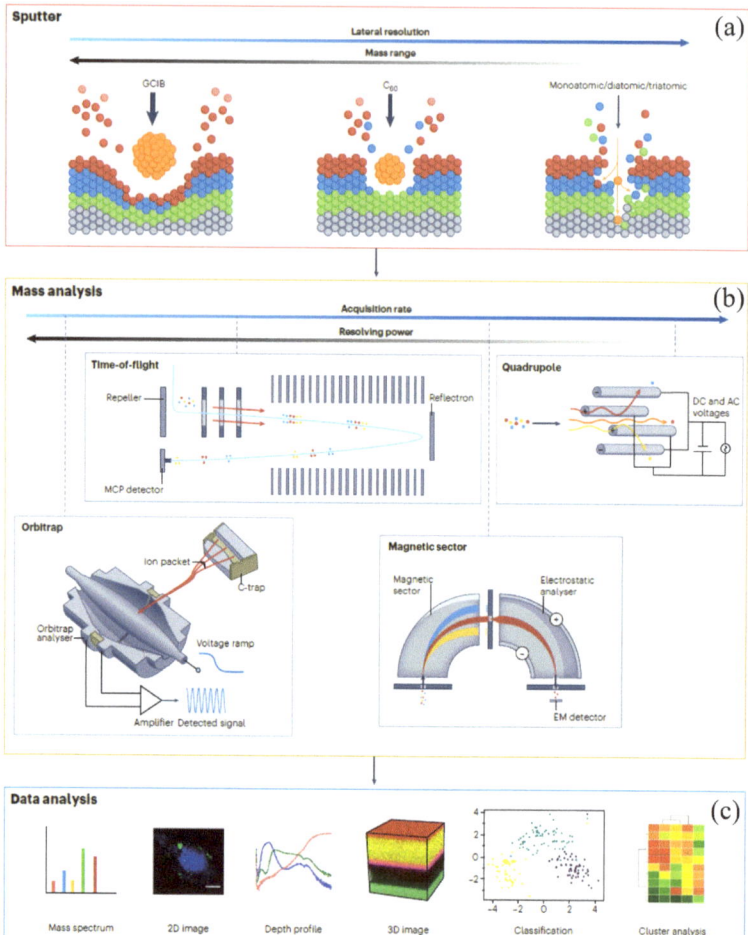

**Figure 4.** A schematic overview of the secondary ion mass spectrometry experiment [51]. (**a**) A surface is bombarded with a primary ion resulting in the sputtering of secondary ions characteristic of surface chemistry. Secondary ions are detected and measured by mass spectrometry. The bombardment is by primary ions, ranging from atomic ions offering the highest lateral resolution to massive gas cluster ion beams that liberate surface species up to several thousand mass units. (**b**) Mass analysis of secondary ions is generally by quadrupole magnetic sector, time-of-flight, or Orbitrap instruments. (**c**) Outputs from the analysis include mass spectra, 2D or 3D images, and depth profiles, which can be further processed using machine learning. EM, electromagnetic; MCP, microchannel plate [51].

Although SIMS technology is not extensively employed currently in the analysis of solid-state hydrogen storage materials, its unique advantages, including high spatial resolution, sensitivity to hydrogen concentrations as low as parts per million (ppm), and capability to provide depth profile information, offer significant potential. In the future, SIMS could play a crucial role in supplementing the characterization of hydrogen storage materials, addressing existing gaps in understanding various aspects of these materials [54,55]. To overcome the limitations of SIMS, advanced instrumentation with improved mass resolution and sensitivity has been developed [56]. The use of multi-modal SIMS, combining different primary ion beams and detection modes, has enhanced the capabilities of the technique [57]. Careful sample preparation and the use of appropriate reference materials are essential for accurate quantification [58].

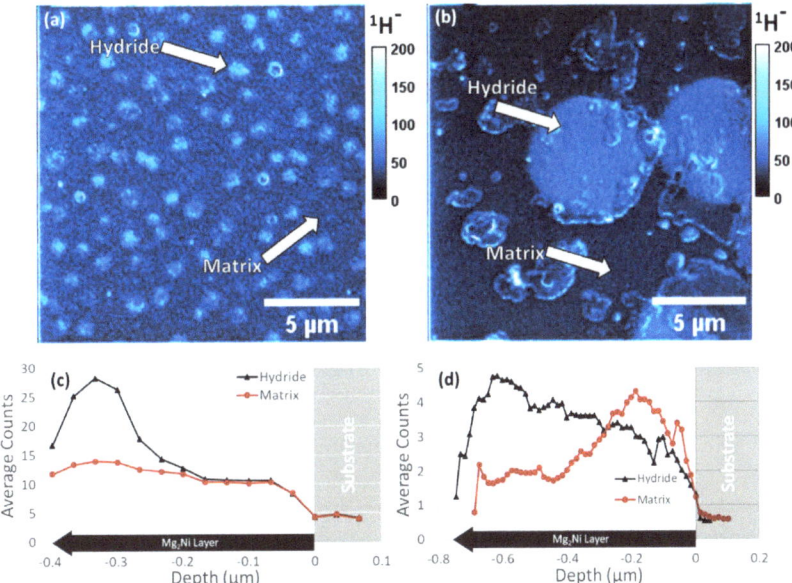

**Figure 5.** SIMS images from a hydrogenated sample with (**a**) equiaxed microstructure (*Batch A—Sample 1*) showing the summed signal over 3 slices and (**b**) columnar microstructure (*Batch B—Sample 2*) showing the summed signal over 14 slices. SIMS localized depth profiles from regions inside and outside of the surface-visible hydride areas for (**c**) *Sample 1* and (**d**) *Sample 2*. Note that for (**d**), the "hydride" data have been shifted to correct its depth so that both curves agree on the depth of the substrate (zero on the *x*-axis), since the hydrides stick above the surface (discussed below). For (**a**,**c**), 15 total slices were captured with an average slice thickness of 33 nm. Beam current of 50 pA and a dwell time of 4 ms per pixel. Image resolution of 256 × 256 pixels for FOV of 17 × 17 µm. For (**b**,**d**), 56 slices total were collected with an average slice thickness of 14.3 nm. Beam current of 100 pA and a dwell time of 1 ms per pixel. Image resolution of 256 × 256 pixels for FOV of 17 × 17 µm [53].

## 2.4. Electrochemical Characterization Methods

Electrochemical methods, including cyclic voltammetry, chronopotentiometry, and electrochemical impedance spectroscopy, are valuable tools for characterizing the electrochemical hydrogen storage properties of materials [59,60]. These techniques provide insights into the charge–discharge behavior, kinetics, and reversibility of hydrogen sorption processes in electrochemical systems, such as metal hydride batteries [61–63].

Cyclic voltammetry involves sweeping the potential of the working electrode containing the hydrogen storage material and measuring the resulting current. Chronopotentiometry applies a constant current to the electrode and monitors the potential response over time [64]. Electrochemical impedance spectroscopy (EIS) measures the impedance of the electrochemical system over a wide range of frequencies [65]. To overcome the limitations of electrochemical methods, researchers have developed advanced electrochemical cell designs and measurement protocols. The use of reference electrodes and optimized electrolyte compositions can improve the accuracy and reliability of the measurements [66]. Combining electrochemical methods with other characterization techniques, such as XRD and Raman spectroscopy, can provide a more comprehensive understanding of the electrochemical hydrogen storage behavior. The operational principle of nickel–metal hydride (NiMH) batteries fundamentally involves the absorption and desorption of hydrogen by metal hydrides. This principle can be similarly exploited through electrochemical methods to swiftly assess the performance characteristics of solid-state hydrogen storage materials [67–70]. Edalati et al. [71] discovered that Ti$_x$Zr$_{2-x}$CrMnFeNi alloys, benefiting from the Ti/Zr ratio of the C14 Laves structure, exhibit good room-temperature hydrogenation/dehydrogenation capabilities. Electrochemical tests on their discharge potential, discharge capacity, and discharge capacity versus cycle number showed that this high-entropy alloy (HEA) successfully functions as the negative electrode of a nickel–metal hydride battery, with excellent charge–discharge cycling performance. The optimal Ti/Zr ratio achieved the highest storage capacity and fastest activation.

## 3. Structure and Composition Characterization Techniques

As the field of hydrogen storage materials evolves, advanced spectroscopic and microscopic techniques have become indispensable for detailed characterization at the molecular and atomic levels [73]. Techniques such as Raman spectroscopy, X-ray diffraction, and X-ray photoelectron spectroscopy offer unparalleled capabilities in probing the structural, electronic, and chemical properties of hydrogen storage materials. These advanced techniques enable researchers to achieve a deeper understanding of the interactions and mechanisms at play within these materials, facilitating the development of more efficient and robust hydrogen storage solutions. By employing these sophisticated methods, scientists can gain comprehensive insights that drive innovation and optimization in the design and application of hydrogen storage materials. Table 2 briefly summarizes the pros and cons of various spectroscopic and microscopic techniques.

Table 2. The advantages and limitations of advanced spectroscopic and microscopic techniques.

| Method | Advantages | Limitations | Refs. |
| --- | --- | --- | --- |
| Raman spectroscopy | Non-destructive and non-contact technique, high spectral resolution, identifies different hydrogen-bonding configurations | Sensitivity to sample surface and orientation, challenging interpretation for complex materials, may not provide quantitative hydrogen content information | [74–85] |
| Fourier transform infrared spectroscopy | Rapid, non-destructive detection with high sensitivity to low-concentration molecular vibrations; wide range of organic and inorganic materials; excels in identifying functional groups and chemical bonds | It is sensitive to moisture, with water absorption peaks potentially interfering with analysis. It only detects infrared-active functional groups, making non-polar bond vibrations difficult to observe. | [37,86–91] |
| X-ray diffraction | Crystalline Structure Determination, wide range of materials, Phase Identification | Limited to Crystalline Materials, Penetration Depth, Size Limitation | [92–105] |
| Neutron scattering techniques | Non-destructive technique, provides bulk structural and dynamic information, sensitive to light elements like hydrogen | Requires access to specialized neutron sources, complex data interpretation, challenging sample preparation | [106–112] |
| X-ray photoelectron spectroscopy | Surface-sensitive technique, provides elemental composition and chemical state information, investigates surface catalysts and coatings | Limited information on bulk properties, requires clean and well-defined sample surface, may not provide direct hydrogen content information | [113–123] |
| Scanning electron microscopy | High-resolution surface imaging, large depth of focus, suitable for three-dimensional topography observation, simple sample preparation | Can only observe surface structures; cannot provide internal structural information; may require metal coating, which affects the true morphology | [124–132] |

Table 2. *Cont.*

| Method | Advantages | Limitations | Refs. |
|---|---|---|---|
| Atomic force microscopy | Ultra-high resolution, reaching atomic level; does not require a vacuum environment, allowing for observation of live samples; capable of measuring mechanical and electrical properties of materials | Slow scanning speed, suitable for small area samples; influenced by probe shape, which may cause artifacts; requires surface flattening treatment of the sample | [133–138] |
| Transmission and scanning transmission electron microscopy | Extremely high resolution, capable of observing atomic-level structures; can provide internal structural information of samples; able to perform compositional and phase analysis | Samples must be very thin; complex sample preparation, which may introduce artifacts; requires a vacuum environment, potentially causing sample damage | [139–148] |

*3.1. Composition Characterization Techniques*

3.1.1. Raman and Fourier Transform Infrared Spectroscopy

Raman spectroscopy has emerged as a powerful technique for investigating the local structure, bonding, and vibrational properties of hydrogen in storage materials [74,75]. When monochromatic light (usually a laser) illuminates a sample, photons interact with molecules, producing scattered light. A portion of this scattered light undergoes a frequency shift (Raman scattering), which provides information on molecular vibrations and rotations. When the laser illuminates the sample, most photons undergo Rayleigh scattering (elastic scattering with no frequency shift), but a small number of photons undergo Raman scattering (inelastic scattering), with their frequencies shifted due to changes in molecular vibrational or rotational energy levels. Raman-active molecules located near waveguides can be excited through either in-plane coupling (waveguide mode) or out-of-plane coupling (as depicted in Figure 6a). In "classical" Raman scattering, emission typically occurs in the reverse direction to eliminate background interference from the excitation light (as illustrated in Figure 6b). This technique is particularly vital for studying amorphous hydrogen storage materials, providing crucial insights into their structural properties [76].

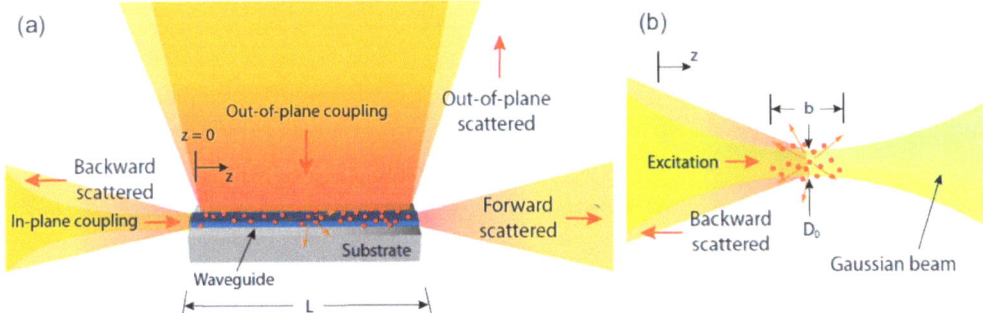

**Figure 6.** (**a**) Schematic of different configurations of laser excitation and Raman scattered light collection. (**b**) Schematic of laser excitation and Raman scattered light collection in free space [76].

Raman spectroscopy offers several advantages for characterizing hydrogen storage materials, including its non-destructive and non-contact nature, high spectral resolution, and the ability to identify different hydrogen-bonding configurations [77]. It is particularly useful for studying the interactions between hydrogen and the host material, such as the formation of metal–hydrogen bonds [78]. This technique is particularly vital for studying amorphous hydrogen storage materials, providing crucial insights into their structural properties [79–81]. Raman spectroscopy has proven invaluable in studying the local structure and bonding in complex hydrides. Ross et al. [74] used this technique to investigate the decomposition pathway of sodium aluminum hydride (NaAlH$_4$), a promising hydrogen storage material. Their study revealed distinct Raman shifts associated with different Al-H bond configurations, providing insights into the dehydrogenation mechanism. Pedraza et al. [82] studied the mechanism of hydrogen release from ammonia borane within mesoporous materials using Raman spectroscopy and mass spectrometry. Figure 6a,b show that, at the point of maximum hydrogen evolution, the deformation mode of -NH$_3$ at 1601 cm$^{-1}$ disappears, while two new modes emerge at 1565 cm$^{-1}$ and 1085 cm$^{-1}$, indicating the formation of polymeric aminoborane (PAB). When the temperature reaches around 101 °C, the intensity of these modes decreases significantly, along with other vibrational modes such as B-H, H-B-H, B-N, and N-B-H. At 50 °C, the B-N stretching modes of $^{10}$B and $^{11}$B at 799 cm$^{-1}$ and 783 cm$^{-1}$ show a slight redshift (see inset in Figure 7), and around 106 °C, they merge and diminish sharply, almost disappearing at 109 °C. However, the mode near 783 cm$^{-1}$ persists at higher temperatures and is associated with the B-N vibrational mode in polyaminoborane (-[BH$_2$NH$_2$]$^{n-}$), indicating the formation of this phase. Additionally, above 100 °C and with Raman shifts higher than 3150 cm$^{-1}$, strong noise appears in the signal. The entire Raman spectrum undergoes significant changes around 106 °C, with all vibrational modes weakening, while hydrogen release becomes highly significant in the online mass spectrometry analysis (Figure 7c).

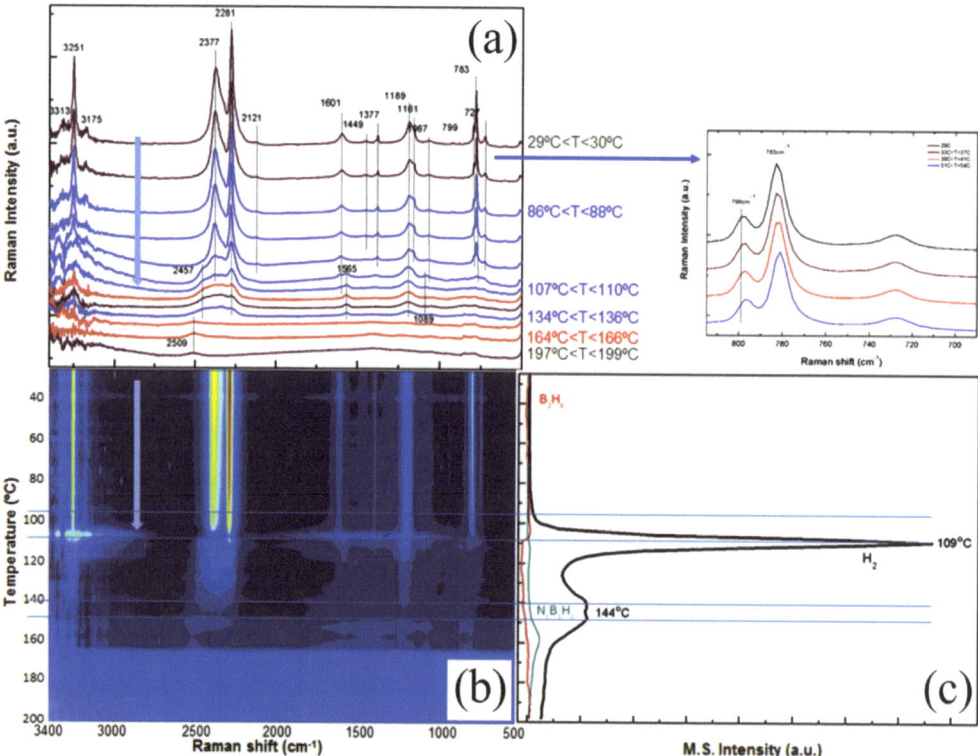

Figure 7. (a) Representative Raman spectra. (b) In situ Raman profile of materials under heating conditions (from room temperature to 200 °C) and (c) simultaneous mass spectrometry profiles for H$_2$ and other volatile components evolved during thermal decomposition of neat AB under a ramp of 1 °C·min$^{-1}$ [82].

Fourier transform infrared spectroscopy (FTIR) is an analytical technique that studies the molecular composition and chemical structure of a sample by measuring the absorption or transmission of infrared spectra [89,91]. Different molecular functional groups exhibit specific absorption characteristics for particular wavelengths of infrared light [88,90]. FTIR identifies these characteristic absorption peaks, allowing for rapid, sensitive, and non-destructive qualitative and semi-quantitative analysis [86,87]. It is widely applied in fields such as chemistry, materials science, environmental monitoring, and pharmaceuticals.

In the study of coordination hydrides, FTIR plays a key role as it can accurately detect changes in molecular structure and chemical bonds. Coordination hydrides undergo dynamic changes in metal–hydrogen coordination bonds or hydride groups during hydrogen storage and release processes. FTIR can reveal the mechanisms of hydrogenation and dehydrogenation by monitoring the characteristic absorption peaks of these chemical bonds. By tracking the changes in M–H (metal–hydrogen) bond vibration frequencies, FTIR can directly follow the interactions between metal centers and hydrogen in coordination hydrides during hydrogen absorption and desorption. Different metal coordination centers (e.g., transition metals or rare-earth elements) and hydride combinations produce unique infrared absorption peaks, allowing FTIR to distinguish these changes and identify different hydrogen storage mechanisms. Ding et al. [37] utilized FTIR to investigate the hydrogen storage mechanism of the $LiBH_4$-$MgH_2$ system prepared via ball milling aerosol spraying (BMAS), as shown in Figure 8. Although the characteristic absorption of LiH at 1030 $cm^{-1}$ overlaps with the absorption band of α-$Mg(BH_4)_2$, the absorption bands of $Mg(BH_4)_2$ at 1262 and 1375 $cm^{-1}$ almost disappeared in the 8R sample, while the absorption band at 1030 $cm^{-1}$ remained visible, indicating the presence of LiH during the reaction process. This observation suggests that $Mg(BH_4)_2$ gradually decomposes over several dehydrogenation cycles, while LiH is formed through the reactions as follows: $12LiBH_4(s) = Li_2B_{12}H_{12}(s) + 10LiH(s) + 13H_2(g)$ and $Li_2B_{12}H_{12}(s) + 6MgH_2(s) = 6MgB_2(s) + 2LiH(s) + 11H_2(g)$. The gradual increase in the intensity of $MgB_2$ and LiH in the samples after cycling reflects the partial reversibility of the above reactions and further explains the gradual decline in hydrogen capacity of the BMAS powders during the cycling process.

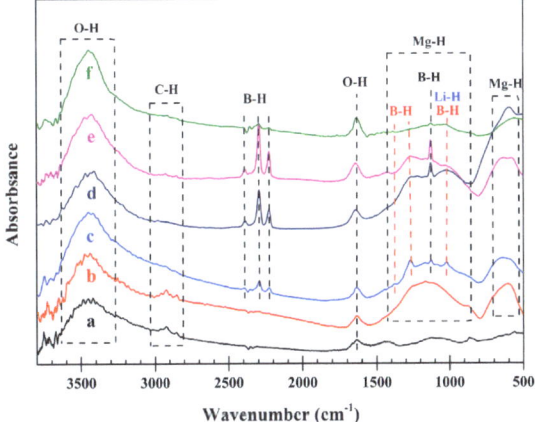

Figure 8. FTIR spectra of (a) the commercially purchased bulk KBr powder, (b) hand-mixed $MgH_2$ + 5 vol% C, (c) BMAS powder, (d) BMAS powder after one dehydrogenation (1R) powder, (e) BMAS powder after one dehydrogenation and then re-hydrogenation (1S) powder, and (f) BMAS powder after 7 cycles of dehydrogenation and re-hydrogenation and then dehydrogenation again (8R) powder [37].

Raman spectroscopy is a key tool for studying the hydrogenation and dehydrogenation mechanisms of metal hydrides. By monitoring changes in Raman spectra during hydrogen adsorption, insights into phase transitions, structural changes, and kinetics can be obtained. To fully exploit the potential of Raman spectroscopy, researchers have developed advanced instruments and data analysis methods, such as confocal Raman microscopy for high-resolution spatial mapping and in situ Raman spectroscopy for real-time monitoring of hydrogen adsorption processes. Alongside Raman spectroscopy, FTIR also plays an important role in hydrogen storage studies by detecting changes in chemical bonds between hydrogen and metal or metal oxide matrices, providing molecular vibrational information during hydrogen absorption and desorption.

These two techniques complement each other, with FTIR being particularly advantageous for detecting X-H (such as M-H or O-H) stretching vibrations in hydrides. In combination, Raman and FTIR spectroscopy provide a comprehensive analysis of material structures, chemical bond vibrations, and phase transitions, offering powerful tools for the design and optimization of hydrogen storage materials.

3.1.2. X-Ray Diffraction and Neutron Scattering

X-ray diffraction (XRD) is a fundamental technique for characterizing the crystallographic structure, phase composition, and structural changes in hydrogen storage material, and the schematic diagram is shown in Figure 9. Its fundamental equation is Bragg's law, which describes the conditions for XRD in a crystal. When X-rays illuminate a crystal, the atomic planes within the crystal cause the XRD [92,93]. By measuring the diffraction angles and intensities, one can determine the lattice parameters and atomic arrangement of the crystal [104,105]. Bragg's law reveals the relationship between the crystal structure and the X-ray wavelength, enabling the inference of the crystal's three-dimensional structure from its diffraction pattern [103].

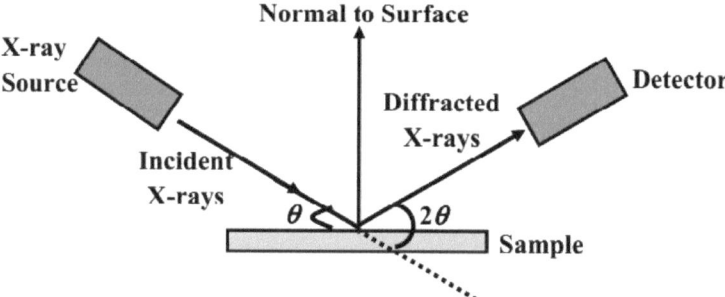

**Figure 9.** Schematic diagram of the XRD principle.

XRD is widely used in hydrogen storage research to investigate the structural properties of metal hydrides, complex hydrides, and other crystalline storage materials [94–96]. It allows for the identification of the hydrogen storage phases, the determination of the phase abundances, and the study of phase transitions during the hydrogen sorption processes. One of the advantages of XRD is its non-destructive nature, allowing for the characterization of the bulk properties of the material [97]. It provides statistical information about the average structure, complementing local probe techniques like Raman spectroscopy. In situ XRD has emerged as a powerful tool for studying the structural evolution of hydrogen storage materials during absorption and desorption cycles. Zlotea et al. [98] used in situ XRD to analyze the hydrogen release and absorption process of the TiZrNbHfTa high-entropy alloy. Through in situ XRD (Figure 10a,b), the phase transformations between the alloy, monohydride, and dihydride were observed clearly, greatly aiding researchers in understanding the dynamic hydrogen absorption and desorption processes of the alloy materials.

Furthermore, the advent of high-energy synchrotron X-ray sources has enabled rapid, time-resolved XRD measurements. Jensen et al. [99] leveraged this capability to study the dehydrogenation kinetics of $NaAlH_4$, a promising complex hydride. Their millisecond-resolution measurements uncovered transient phases that play a critical role in the hydrogen release process, demonstrating the power of advanced XRD techniques in elucidating complex reaction mechanisms.

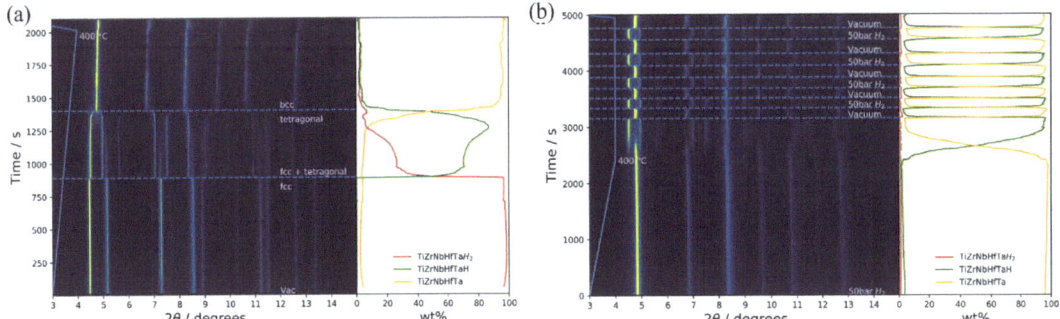

Figure 10. In situ SR-XRD and phase content at 400 °C during (a) hydrogen desorption in dynamic vacuum and (b) cycling between 50 bar $H_2$ and dynamic vacuum [98].

Neutron scattering techniques, including neutron diffraction and inelastic neutron scattering, are powerful tools for investigating the structural and dynamic properties of hydrogen in storage materials [100,101]. Neutron scattering involves the interaction of neutrons with the atomic nuclei in the material to study the structure and dynamics of the material. Neutron scattering includes elastic scattering (such as neutron diffraction) and inelastic scattering. When a neutron beam irradiates a sample, neutrons scatter off the sample's atomic nuclei, and the scattered neutrons are collected by detectors, as illustrated in Figure 11 [102]. By analyzing the angle and energy distribution of the scattered neutrons, information about the atomic structure and dynamics of the sample can be obtained.

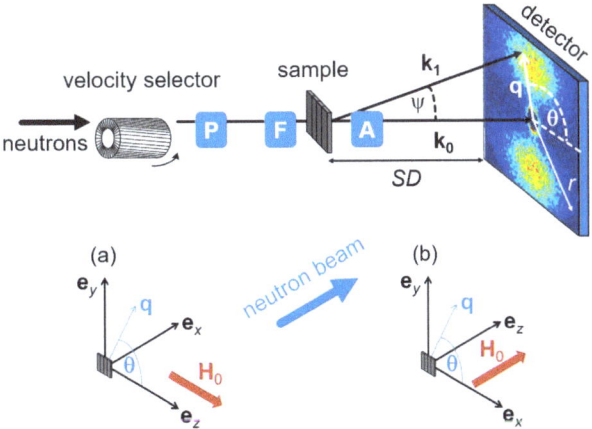

Figure 11. Schematic diagram of a neutron scattering device [102].

By measuring and analyzing the scattering cross-section and momentum transfer, the atomic structure and dynamics of the sample can be inferred. Neutrons have unique advantages for studying hydrogen, as they can penetrate deep into the material and have high sensitivity to light elements like hydrogen [106]. In situ neutron scattering can determine the reaction process of Mg-based hydrides by tracking phase changes and distributions during $H_2$ desorption and absorption reactions. Ponthieu et al. [107] studied the reversible deuterium absorption of $MgD_2$-$TiD_2$ nanocomposites using this technique. By examining the in situ $H_2$ desorption process, they found that the dehydrogenation peak of $0.3TiH_2$-$0.7MgH_2$ appeared at 520 K, approximately 30 K lower than that of pure $MgD_2$, and the desorption kinetics were significantly faster. They discovered that the transformation of β-$MgD_2$ to Mg is the only reversible loading path for deuterium at moderate pressure and temperature (i.e., $p < 1$ MPa, T < 600 K). The addition of $TiD_2$ not only restricted grain growth of the Mg and $MgD_2$ phases but also induced lattice distortion in β-$MgD_2$. The $TiD_2$ phase facilitated hydrogen migration through the sub-stoichiometric $MgD_2$-η phase and $TiD_2$-η phase, as well as the coherent interface between $TiD_2$ and Mg/$MgD_2$ phases. As shown in Figure 12a, XRD can clearly characterize the phase composition of the composite material but struggles to distinguish its crystal structure. Therefore, neutron diffraction becomes crucial for analysis. In Figure 12b, the signal intensity of γ-$MgD_2$ is significantly stronger than in the XRD results. The combination of these results confirms the coexistence of both β-$MgD_2$ and γ-$MgD_2$ phases in the composite material. It is worth noting that, in neutron scattering analysis, different hydrogen isotopes may occupy different interstitial sites within the metal lattice and have varying activation diffusion barriers, which could impact the performance analysis of hydrogen storage materials. Thus, ensuring the accuracy of the research is another challenge that must be addressed when using this method in hydrogen storage material studies.

Neutron diffraction provides detailed information about the crystal structure, phase composition, and hydrogen occupancy in storage materials [108–110]. Inelastic neutron scattering, on the other hand, probes the vibrational and rotational dynamics of hydrogen within the material [111]. To harness the full potential of neutron scattering techniques, researchers have developed advanced instrumentation and data analysis methods [106]. The use of high-intensity neutron sources and optimized sample environments has enhanced the capabilities of these techniques [112]. Combining neutron scattering with complementary characterization methods, such as XRD and Raman spectroscopy, provides a comprehensive understanding of the structural and dynamic aspects of hydrogen storage materials.

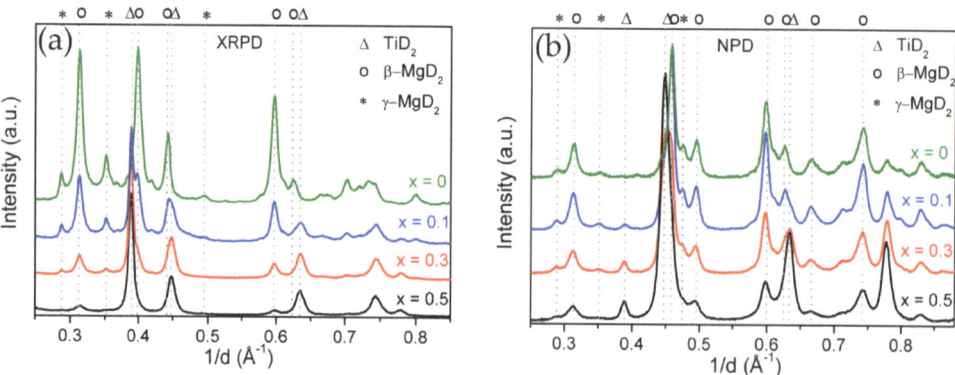

**Figure 12.** (a) X-ray and (b) neutron diffraction patterns of deuterated $(1-x)MgD_2$–$xTiD_2$ nanocomposites for x = 0, 0.1, 0.3, and 0.5 [107].

### 3.1.3. X-Ray Photoelectron Spectroscopy

X-ray photoelectron spectroscopy (XPS) is a surface-sensitive technique that provides valuable information about the elemental composition, chemical states, and electronic structure of hydrogen storage materials [113]. This method is based on the excitation of photoelectrons from a sample by X-rays and the measurement of the photoelectrons' kinetic energy to determine the elemental composition and chemical states of the sample. When X-rays illuminate a sample, the atoms in the sample absorb the X-ray energy and emit photoelectrons (Figure 13). The kinetic energy of these photoelectrons is related to the energy of the incident X-rays and the binding energy of the atomic nucleus. By analyzing the photoelectron spectrum, one can obtain binding energy information for the elements on the sample surface, thereby determining the sample's elemental composition and chemical state [114].

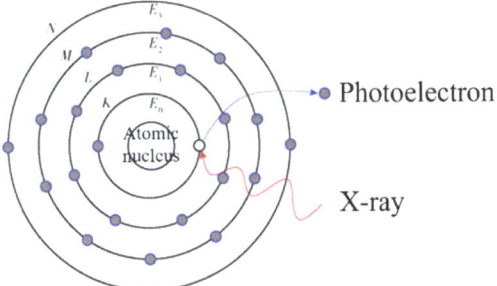

**Figure 13.** Schematic diagram of the XPS principle. $E$ is the binding energy [113].

XPS is particularly useful for studying the surface chemistry of hydrogen storage materials, as it can probe the top few nanometers of the sample [115]. It can provide insights into the surface oxidation states, contamination levels, and chemical bonding between hydrogen and the host material [116,117]. XPS has been widely used to investigate the surface properties of metal hydrides, complex hydrides, and nanostructured storage materials [118,119].

Selvam et al. [120] utilized XPS to analyze $Mg_2Cu$ and $Mg_2Ni$ alloys exposed to air, finding that they undergo surface decomposition and preferential segregation of magnesium in the presence of oxygen and moisture. The segregated magnesium primarily existed as oxides and hydroxides on the surface, while Ni or Cu also appeared in oxidized states. The passivation of the alloys was caused by the oxidation of the transition metal components, and the researchers believed that the activation of these alloys involved the reduction of the oxidized three-dimensional elements and the formation of metal clusters. To investigate the influence of $TiO_x$ on $MgH_2$ in greater depth, Zhang et al. [123] analyzed the internal chemical states of the samples using X-ray photoelectron spectroscopy (XPS). As shown in Figure 14a,b, compared to the single $Ti^{4+}$ state in $TiO_2$, the Ti in the $Ni_{0.034}@TiO_2$ catalyst exhibits a mixed valence state of $Ti^{4+}$ and $Ti^{3+}$. During the dehydrogenation process, the content of $Ti^{4+}$ and $Ti^{3+}$ decreases, while the proportion of $Ti^{2+}$ and $Ti^0$ increases. Meanwhile, due to the electronegativity of Ti (1.54), which lies between that of Mg (1.31) and H (2.20), it helps to weaken the Mg-H bond, thereby accelerating the dehydrogenation reaction. Throughout the evolution of Ti valence states, the valence state of oxygen (O) also changes. The O 1s XPS spectra of $TiO_2$ show two peaks located at 529.18 eV and 530.98 eV, corresponding to the Ti-O-Ti oxygen lattice (OL) and oxygen vacancies (OVs), respectively. The OL/OV ratio in $TiO_2$ is 87/13, while the OL/OV ratio in the $Ni_{0.034}@TiO_2$ catalyst is 71/29, significantly lower than that of $TiO_2$. This indicates that the presence of single-atom Ni promotes the formation of oxygen vacancies. Additionally, the OL/OV ratio in the $Ni_x@TiO_2$ sample is also lower than that in $TiO_2$, further proving that Ni facilitates the generation of oxygen vacancies. Combined with X-ray absorption spectroscopy data, the Ni in the $Ni_{0.034}@TiO_2$ catalyst exhibits a mixed positive valence state, with a strong electron-accepting capability. In this case, Ni attracts O ions, promoting the formation of oxygen vacancies in $TiO_2$, resulting in a higher number of oxygen vacancies compared to that of pure $TiO_2$. This is also consistent with recent findings on the influence of metal particles on oxygen vacancies. Figure 14c illustrates the catalytic mechanism during hydrogenation and dehydrogenation. Single-atom Ni can promote the formation of OVs and multivalent $Ti^{x+}$ species around $TiO_2$ units. Oxygen vacancies serve as active sites that accelerate electron transfer, while Ti$^{x+}$ facilitates transitions between valence states via electron mediation, thus avoiding the high energy required to directly break the Mg-H bond. The atomic interface formed between isolated Ni atoms and Ti$^{x+}$ constitutes dispersed Ni-O-Ti$^{x+}$ active centers, thereby enhancing catalytic performance. Overall, the synergistic interaction between single-atom Ni and the TiO$_2$ support significantly improves the catalytic effect.

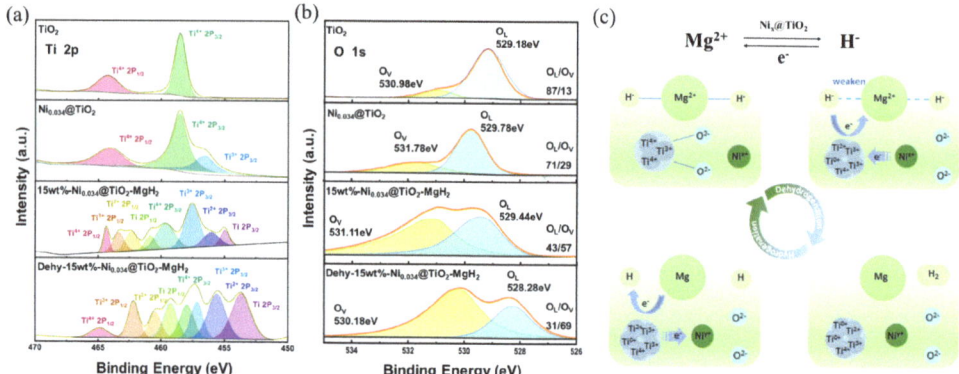

**Figure 14.** High-resolution XPS spectra of (**a**) Ti 2p and (**b**) O 1s, as well as (**c**) valence changes during the hydrogenation and dehydrogenation processes.

One of the key applications of XPS in hydrogen storage research is the study of surface catalysts and coatings that enhance the hydrogen sorption kinetics [121,122]. By analyzing the chemical composition and oxidation states of the surface species, the role of catalysts in promoting hydrogen dissociation, diffusion, and recombination can be elucidated. To overcome the limitations of XPS, researchers have developed advanced instrumentation and data analysis methods, such as synchrotron-based XPS for high-resolution measurements and in situ XPS studies for real-time monitoring of surface chemical changes. Combining XPS with other surface characterization techniques, such as scanning tunneling microscopy (STM) and atomic force microscopy (AFM), has provided a comprehensive understanding of the surface morphology and chemical properties of hydrogen storage materials. XPS has been crucial in understanding surface phenomena in hydrogen storage materials, particularly catalytic effects and degradation mechanisms.

### 3.2. Structure Characterization Techniques

#### 3.2.1. Scanning Electron Microscopy

Scanning electron microscopy (SEM) is an ideal tool for studying the microstructure and surface characteristics of hydrogen storage materials due to its high-resolution imaging capabilities [125]. SEM can reveal detailed morphological features of materials, helping scientists understand the interactions between hydrogen and these materials, which is crucial for designing more efficient hydrogen storage systems [126,127]. The microstructure of materials, such as pore size, distribution, and surface roughness, directly affects the adsorption and diffusion rates of hydrogen.

Through SEM, researchers can clearly see these structural features and evaluate their specific impact on hydrogen storage performance. For example, larger pores may promote rapid hydrogen diffusion, while higher surface roughness can increase the surface area, providing more active sites for hydrogen adsorption. Additionally, SEM analysis can reveal potential defects on material surfaces, such as cracks, fractures, or other irregular shapes, which could affect the long-term stability and hydrogen storage efficiency of the materials. By regularly using SEM to monitor these materials, scientists can track performance changes during long-term use and adjust preparation processes or select more suitable materials accordingly. Silva et al. [124] used SEM to observe the surface morphology of

$Ti_{11}V_{30}Nb_{28}Cr_{31}$ at different stages of hydrogenation, finding that during laser processing, the surface of the debris particles melted, increasing the proportion of oxides near the surface. The manual grinding process leads to random particle size distribution, as shown in Figure 15a,d,g,j. Figure 15b,c illustrate that the surface of the particles after breaking the original alloy remains smooth with sharp edges, consistent with the brittle characteristics of the alloy. Figure 15e,f show that laser treatment significantly alters the particle surface, where rounded edges and a smooth surface suggest that the particles underwent remelting and rapid solidification. The inset in Figure 15f reveals microcracks on the remelted surface, which may contribute to the activation of the sample. Additionally, the remelted surface could restore the hydrogenation ability of the aged sample. Figure 15h,i,k,l display the similar behavior of both original and aged samples during hydrogenation. Surface cracks caused by volume expansion during the hydrogenation process were observed in particles analyzed under both conditions. These changes enhanced the alloy's hydrogen storage capacity. Therefore, surface remelting, oxide layer formation, and crack formation were confirmed to be factors influencing the hydrogen storage capacity of the pulse laser-activated $Ti_{11}V_{30}Nb_{28}Cr_{31}$ alloy.

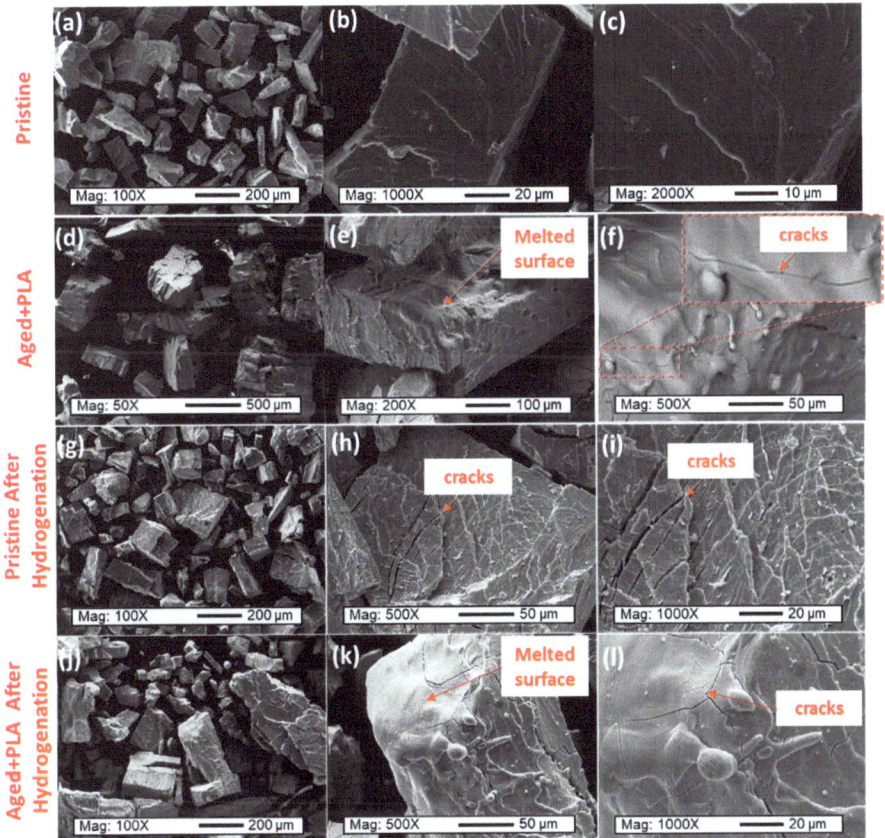

**Figure 15.** SEM analyses of the (**a–c**) pristine sample, (**d–f**) aged + PLA sample, (**g–i**) pristine sample after hydrogenation, and (**j–l**) aged + PLA sample after hydrogenation [124].

In recent years, the development of environmental scanning electron microscopy (ESEM) has brought revolutionary advancements to hydrogen storage research [128,131]. Unlike traditional SEM, ESEM allows for sample observation under near-natural conditions without requiring high vacuum or complex sample preparation [130,132]. This enables researchers to directly monitor and record changes in material surfaces and microstructures during hydrogen absorption and desorption processes in real time. ESEM is particularly suitable for studying the interactions between hydrogen and materials. During hydrogen absorption, ESEM can capture morphological changes on the material surface, such as surface expansion, crack formation, or other structural deformations, in real time. These observations provide valuable information for optimizing material design and improving reaction speed and hydrogen storage capacity. Similarly, during hydrogen release, ESEM can offer crucial visual evidence to help scientists understand the material's regeneration capability and long-term stability.

### 3.2.2. Transmission and Scanning Transmission Electron Microscopy

Advanced electron microscopy techniques, particularly transmission electron microscopy (TEM), have revolutionized our understanding of hydrogen storage materials at the atomic scale [140]. With its superior resolution and accuracy, TEM allows researchers to observe the atomic and molecular structure of materials in unprecedented detail. This unique perspective provides scientists with critical insights into how these materials behave during hydrogen storage [142].

Through TEM, scientists can directly observe the atomic arrangement and molecular configuration within materials [141]. This capability not only helps reveal the fundamental structural characteristics of materials but also allows researchers to see subtle changes in the internal structure during hydrogen adsorption and desorption [143]. For example, researchers can observe how hydrogen atoms bond with specific sites within the material or how the lattice structure of the material deforms during hydrogen absorption. These detailed observations provide valuable information for understanding the behavior of hydrogen storage materials. By analyzing these microstructural changes, scientists can better comprehend the mechanisms of hydrogen adsorption and the key factors influencing storage capacity and release rate [149]. This in-depth understanding aids in developing new materials and optimizing the chemical composition and microstructure of existing materials to enhance their hydrogen storage performance. Furthermore, TEM's high-resolution imaging allows researchers to identify small defects within materials, such as dislocations, vacancies, and interfacial mismatches. These defects significantly impact the overall performance of materials, especially during repeated cycles of hydrogen adsorption and desorption. Therefore, accurately identifying and analyzing these defects is crucial for designing more durable and efficient hydrogen storage materials. Wu et al. [150] prepared $LiBH_4$ composites confined within bilayer carbon nanobowls through a strong capillary effect under 100 bar $H_2$ pressure. TEM analysis confirmed the gradual formation of bilayer carbon nanobowls. Benefiting from the nanoscale confinement and catalytic functions of carbon, the composite released hydrogen from 225 °C, peaking at 353 °C, with a hydrogen release amount of up to 10.9 wt.%. Compared to bulk $LiBH_4$, the peak dehydrogenation temperature decreased by 112 °C. More importantly, the composite absorbed about 8.5 wt.% $H_2$ at 300 °C and 100 bar $H_2$, demonstrating significant reversible hydrogen storage capability. Ren et al. [133] investigated the dehydrogenation mechanism of the $MgH_2$/Ni@pCNF composite using in situ high-resolution transmission electron microscopy (HRTEM) to observe the microstructural evolution under electron-beam irradiation. Figure 16a–c show HAADF, BF, and corresponding element mapping images of hydrogenated $MgH_2$/Ni@pCNF, with the red dashed box indicating the irradiated area. Figure 16d–g present the HRTEM images of the composite material during the hydrogen release process, where the lattice fringes observed in the selected area electron-diffraction patterns in each subfigure correspond to the phase changes of the material throughout the reaction. Before irradiation, lattice fringes were used to identify $MgH_2$ (101) (Figure 16(d1)), $Mg_2NiH_4$ (311) (Figure 16(d2)), and MgO (200) (Figure 16(d3)). Additionally, amorphous carbon frameworks of pCNF, acting as scaffolds for the nanoconfined $MgH_2$, were observed in all HRTEM images (Figure 16d–g). After 3 min of irradiation, part of the $Mg_2NiH_4$ began to decompose, converting into $Mg_2Ni$

(Figure 16(e2)). A 0.246 nm plane spacing was observed between MgH$_2$ (Figure 16(e3)) and Mg$_2$NiH$_4$ (Figure 16(e4)), corresponding to Mg (101) (Figure 16(e1)), indicating that MgH$_2$ near MgH$_2$NiH$_4$ was also starting to decompose. The desorption of Mg$_2$NiH$_4$ induced lattice volume changes, which introduced internal stress and defects at the Mg$_2$NiH$_4$/MgH$_2$ interface, promoting MgH$_2$ desorption. Furthermore, the interface between the catalyst (Mg$_2$NiH$_4$/Mg$_2$Ni) and the matrix (MgH$_2$) facilitated rapid hydrogen diffusion, accelerating MgH$_2$ desorption. After 6 min of irradiation, only Mg$_2$Nif (Figure 16(f2)), Mg (Figure 16(f1)), and MgH$_2$ (Figure 16(f3)) remained, indicating that Mg$_2$NiH$_4$ completely decomposed earlier than MgH$_2$. After 10 min of electron-beam irradiation, the hydrogen in the irradiated area was fully released and transferred to Mg (Figure 15(g1)) and Mg$_2$Ni (Figure 15(g2)). Moreover, due to the confinement of pCNF, the Mg-based nanoparticles did not experience significant growth or agglomeration.

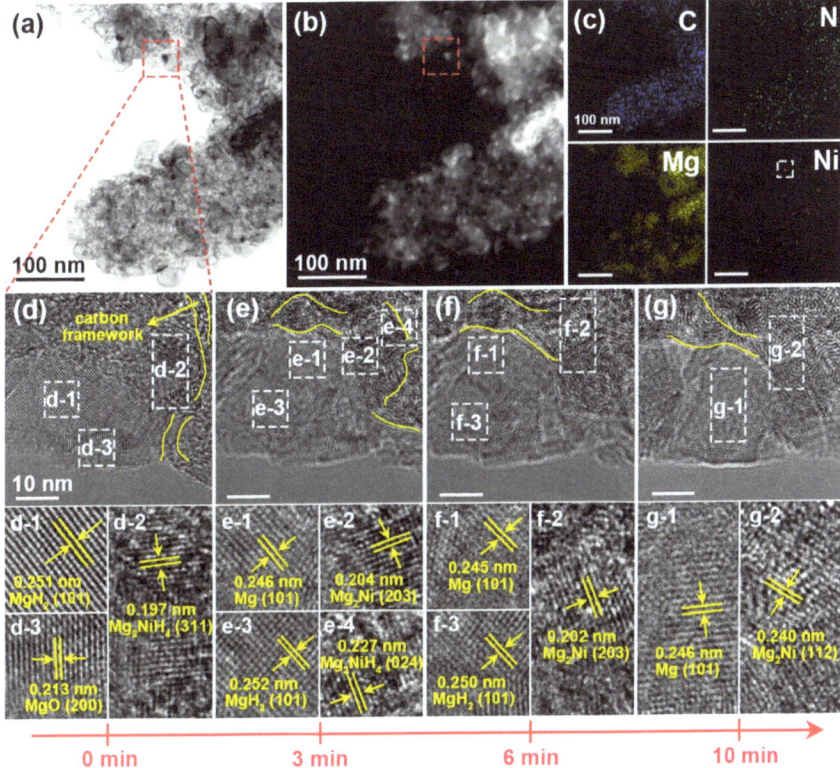

**Figure 16.** In situ TEM analysis of the hydrogenated MgH$_2$/Ni@pCNF composites: (**a**) HAADF image (the square marked by red dotted line indicates the irradiated area). (**b**) BF image. (**c**) The corresponding elemental mapping of C, N, Mg, and Ni. (**d–g**) HRTEM images and selective electron diffraction at random points showing the evolution of microstructure upon hydrogen desorption induced by the electron-beam irradiation. (**d1–d3**) Initial microstructure showing lattice fringes of MgH$_2$ (101), Mg$_2$NiH$_4$ (311), and MgO (200), respectively, before irradiation. (**e1–e4**) After 3 min, partial decomposition of Mg$_2$NiH$_4$ into Mg$_2$Ni begins, with defects forming at the Mg$_2$NiH$_4$/MgH$_2$ interface, promoting hydrogen desorption, while some MgH$_2$ remains stable. (**f1–f3**) At 6 min, complete decomposition of Mg$_2$NiH$_4$ is observed, while MgH$_2$ remains partially stable, and Mg nanoparticles become visible. (**g1,g2**) After 10 min, hydrogen is fully released and transferred to Mg and Mg$_2$Ni [133].

Additionally, the development of in situ environmental transmission electron microscopy (E-TEM) has made it possible to observe materials directly under dynamic, real-world conditions, which is crucial for studying hydrogen storage materials [147,148]. Traditional TEM requires vacuum conditions, limiting the observation of material behavior under actual operating conditions [145,146]. In contrast, E-TEM allows for the observation of materials in a gaseous environment, which can include hydrogen, thus providing genuine insights into the behavior of these materials during hydrogen adsorption and desorption [144]. Through E-TEM, researchers can observe structural changes during the hydrogen cycling process in real time [151,152]. This includes observing how atoms rearrange, how defects in the material evolve, and how the crystal structure of the material changes during hydrogen adsorption and release. These observations are critical for understanding the mechanisms of hydrogen adsorption and the factors influencing the efficiency and durability of storage materials. Future rational use of E-TEM can help identify the best materials and designs for hydrogen storage, allowing scientists to conduct experiments on different materials and under various environmental conditions.

### 3.2.3. Atomic Force Microscopy

Atomic force microscopy (AFM), as a precise surface analysis tool, has provided valuable insights into the surface morphology and mechanical properties of hydrogen storage materials [135,137]. AFM measures forces through interactions between the probe and the sample surface, allowing for nanoscale mapping of material surfaces [136,138]. This detailed surface characterization is crucial for understanding and optimizing the performance of hydrogen storage materials [134]. AFM's high-resolution imaging capabilities enable it to reveal the microstructure of materials, such as nanoparticles, pores, and cracks, which are key factors in evaluating the adsorption capacity of materials. Furthermore, AFM can measure mechanical properties such as hardness and elastic modulus, which are critical for designing hydrogen storage systems that maintain structural stability under various operating conditions.

Kalisvaart et al. [139] used AFM to analyze the surface changes of Mg and Mg-10%Cr-10%V films in both deposited and hydrogenated states. As shown in Figure 17, the surface of the deposited palladium (Pd) film is extremely smooth, with a root-mean-square (RMS) roughness of only 5 Å. In the hydrogenated state, the Pd layer appears to break into small particles with diameters of approximately 20 nm, leading to a 2- to 13-fold increase in the measured RMS roughness. Due to the tip effect, atomic force microscopy (AFM) often underestimates roughness. In fact, because of the close spacing of Pd particles, the relatively large tip radius of the AFM (6 nm) almost certainly leads to a significant underestimation of roughness, especially in hydrogenated samples. Therefore, the increase in surface roughness observed after combining neutron reflectometry (NR) data are primarily attributed to the fragmentation of the Pd layer into small particles.

Recent advancements in high-speed atomic force microscopy (high-speed AFM) technology have enabled scientists to observe dynamic processes at the nanoscale in real time [153,154]. High-speed AFM significantly improves imaging speed, allowing researchers to observe and record changes in material surfaces during hydrogen adsorption and desorption almost in real time [155,156]. This capability is particularly important for understanding the dynamic characteristics of hydrogen–material interactions [157]. For example, through high-speed AFM, researchers can directly observe changes in surface morphology caused by hydrogen adsorption, such as slight expansion or contraction of the surface. These changes might be difficult to capture with traditional AFM due to their rapid occurrence. Additionally, this technology can be used to study the fatigue behavior of materials during multiple cycles of hydrogen adsorption and desorption, providing direct experimental data for assessing the long-term stability and reusability of materials.

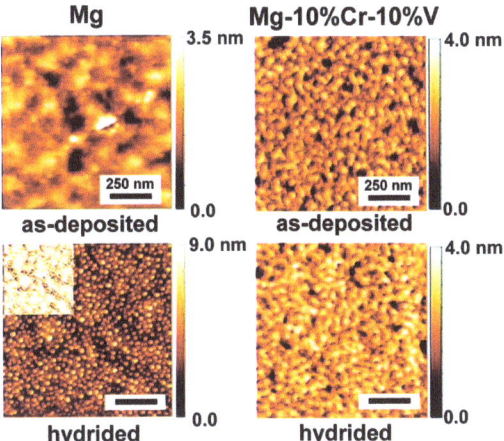

**Figure 17.** AFM micrographs of Ta/Mg/CrV/Pd and Ta/Mg-10%Cr-10%V/CrV/Pd in the as-deposited and hydrogenated state. The Ta/Mg/CrV/Pd was hydrogenated at 50 mbar for 14 h and Ta/Mg-10%Cr-10%V/CrV/Pd at 10 mbar for 20 h. The inset shows the micrograph of the hydrided film on the same brightness scale as the as-deposited state for Ta/Mg/CrV/Pd [139].

## 4. Challenges and Limitations

### 4.1. Obstacles and Limitations in Hydrogen Storage Performance Characterization

The characterization of hydrogen storage performance faces multifaceted challenges that significantly impact the accuracy, reliability, and interpretability of experimental data.

Volumetric measurements, particularly the Sieverts method, are susceptible to systematic errors arising from thermal gradients, pressure sensor drift, and gas impurities. Zhou et al. [21] highlighted the critical impact of temperature gradients on volumetric measurements, demonstrating how even minor thermal fluctuations can lead to substantial errors in calculated hydrogen uptake. This issue is particularly pronounced for materials with low storage capacities or slow kinetics, where small measurement errors can lead to significant overestimation or underestimation of storage performance.

The challenge of achieving true equilibrium conditions during measurements is exacerbated by the slow kinetics of many advanced storage materials. Complex hydrides and nanostructured composites often exhibit multi-step absorption/desorption processes with varying time scales, making it difficult to determine when true equilibrium has been reached. This kinetic limitation can lead to underestimation of storage capacities and misinterpretation of thermodynamic parameters, particularly when fixed measurement times are used across different materials.

The discrepancy between laboratory-scale measurements and real-world performance remains a significant hurdle. Factors such as heat and mass transfer limitations, which are often negligible in small-scale experiments, become critical in larger systems. The work of Ding et al. [28] on nanostructured $LiBH_4$-$MgH_2$ systems exemplifies this challenge, where the excellent performance observed in laboratory tests may not directly translate to practical storage systems due to scaling effects on heat transfer and reaction kinetics.

### 4.2. Challenges and Constraints in Structure and Composition Characterization

The structural and compositional characterization of hydrogen storage materials presents unique challenges that limit our ability to fully understand storage mechanisms and material properties.

In situ characterization, which observes materials in their "native environment", and operando characterization, which captures real-time data under "actual working conditions", can provide researchers with deep insights into the structural and functional changes of materials. Although in situ and operando characterization techniques are highly powerful, they often require certain compromises in experimental conditions, such as reduced resolution, decreased sensitivity, or simplified setups, to meet the demands of real-time monitoring. In situ TEM, for instance, allows real-time observation of structural changes during hydrogen absorption/desorption but typically operates at lower pressures than those used in practical storage systems. This pressure gap can lead to observations that may not accurately represent material behavior under realistic conditions. The study by Ren et al. [133] on $MgH_2$/Ni@pCNF composites using in situ HRTEM illustrates both the power and limitations of these techniques in studying the dehydrogenation mechanism of complex nanostructured materials.

Raman spectroscopy, while sensitive to hydrogen-containing bonds, faces challenges in quantitative analysis due to variations in scattering cross-sections and the potential for laser-induced sample heating. The work of Pedraza et al. [82] on ammonia borane decomposition demonstrates both the power and limitations of Raman spectroscopy in studying hydrogen storage materials, highlighting the need for careful experimental design and data interpretation.

The characterization of multi-component and nanostructured materials presents additional complexities. Techniques like XPS and SIMS offer high surface sensitivity but may not accurately represent bulk compositions. Conversely, bulk techniques may overlook critical surface phenomena that govern hydrogen uptake and release. The study by Xing et al. [121] on carbon-coated CoNi nanocatalysts illustrates the challenge of characterizing complex nanostructured materials, where the distribution and chemical state of catalytic components play crucial roles in enhancing storage performance.

Addressing these challenges requires continued development of advanced characterization tools, improved experimental protocols, and sophisticated data analysis methods. Emerging approaches, such as machine learning-assisted data interpretation and multi-modal characterization platforms [158], offer promising avenues for overcoming current limitations. However, realizing the full potential of these advanced characterization approaches will require close collaboration between experimentalists, theorists, and instrument developers to ensure that the data obtained accurately reflects the intrinsic properties and behavior of hydrogen storage materials under realistic operating conditions.

## 5. Conclusions and Perspective

The field of solid-state hydrogen storage materials has made significant strides in recent years, with the development of advanced characterization techniques and the emergence of novel materials. However, ongoing challenges in understanding the complex hydrogen storage mechanisms and optimizing material performance necessitate continued research and innovation.

This comprehensive review has provided an overview of the key characterization techniques employed in the field of solid-state hydrogen storage, discussing their principles, advantages, limitations, and synergistic applications. Conventional techniques such as Sieverts method, gravimetric analysis, SIMS, TDS, neutron scattering, and electrochemical methods have been discussed in detail, highlighting their roles in unraveling the intricate relationship between the structure, composition, and properties of hydrogen storage materials. Emerging optical characterization techniques, including Raman spectroscopy, XRD, and XPS, have been explored, emphasizing their potential in providing insights into the local structure, bonding, and surface chemistry of these materials.

Practical considerations, such as equipment availability, sample preparation, and cost-effectiveness, have been addressed to provide a pragmatic guide for researchers in the field. The challenges associated with characterizing novel hydrogen storage materials, such as nanoconfined hydrides, MOFs, and graphene-related materials, have been highlighted, and innovative approaches to tackle these challenges have been discussed.

Looking ahead, the integration of in situ and operando characterization techniques, computational modeling, and data-driven approaches will be crucial for accelerating the discovery and optimization of high-performance hydrogen storage materials. Collaborative efforts among researchers from diverse disciplines and the establishment of standardized characterization protocols and databases will be essential for advancing the field towards practical applications.

As the world transitions towards a sustainable energy future, the development of efficient and reliable hydrogen storage solutions will play a critical role in enabling the widespread adoption of clean energy technologies. By addressing the characterization challenges and embracing innovative approaches, the scientific community can unlock the full potential of solid-state hydrogen storage materials and contribute to the realization of a hydrogen-based energy economy.

**Funding:** This study was financially supported by the Opening Project of Crystalline Silicon Photovoltaic New Energy Research Institute (2022CHXK002), and the Leshan Normal University Research Program (KYPY2023-0001).

**Conflicts of Interest:** The authors declare no conflicts of interest.

## References

1. Cheng, H.; Chen, L.; Cooper, A.C.; Sha, X.; Pez, G.P. Hydrogen spillover in the context of hydrogen storage using solid-state materials. *Energy Environ. Sci.* **2008**, *1*, 338–354. [CrossRef]
2. Broom, D.P.; Hirscher, M. Irreproducibility in hydrogen storage material research. *Energy Environ. Sci.* **2016**, *9*, 3368–3380. [CrossRef]
3. Gupta, A.; Baron, G.V.; Perreault, P.; Lenaerts, S.; Ciocarlan, R.-G.; Cool, P.; Mileo, P.G.M.; Rogge, S.; Van Speybroeck, V.; Watson, G.; et al. Hydrogen Clathrates: Next Generation Hydrogen Storage Materials. *Energy Storage Mater.* **2021**, *41*, 69–107. [CrossRef]
4. Cho, E.S.; Ruminski, A.M.; Liu, Y.S.; Shea, P.T.; Kang, S.; Zaia, E.W.; Park, J.Y.; Chuang, Y.D.; Yuk, J.M.; Zhou, X.; et al. Hierarchically Controlled Inside-Out Doping of Mg Nanocomposites for Moderate Temperature Hydrogen Storage. *Adv. Funct. Mater.* **2017**, *27*, 1704316. [CrossRef]
5. Wang, Y.; Xue, Y.; Züttel, A. Nanoscale engineering of solid-state materials for boosting hydrogen storage. *Chem. Soc. Rev.* **2024**, *53*, 972–1003. [CrossRef]
6. Schneemann, A.; White, J.L.; Kang, S.; Jeong, S.; Wan, L.F.; Cho, E.S.; Heo, T.W.; Prendergast, D.; Urban, J.J.; Wood, B.C.; et al. Nanostructured Metal Hydrides for Hydrogen Storage. *Chem. Rev.* **2018**, *118*, 10775–10839. [CrossRef]
7. Gao, Y.; Li, Z.; Wang, P.; Li, C.; Yue, Q.; Cui, W.G.; Wang, X.; Yang, Y.; Gao, F.; Zhang, M.; et al. Solid-State Hydrogen Storage Origin and Design Principles of Carbon-Based Light Metal Single-Atom Materials. *Adv. Funct. Mater.* **2024**, *34*, 2316368. [CrossRef]
8. Li, Y.; Guo, Q.; Ding, Z.; Jiang, H.; Yan, H.; Du, W.; Zheng, Y.; Huo, K.; Shaw, L.L. MOFs-Based Materials for Solid-State Hydrogen Storage: Strategies and Perspectives. *Chem. Eng. J.* **2024**, *485*, 149665. [CrossRef]
9. Allendorf, M.D.; Hulvey, Z.; Gennett, T.; Ahmed, A.; Autrey, T.; Camp, J.; Seon Cho, E.; Furukawa, H.; Haranczyk, M.; Head-Gordon, M.; et al. An assessment of strategies for the development of solid-state adsorbents for vehicular hydrogen storage. *Energy Environ. Sci.* **2018**, *11*, 2784–2812. [CrossRef]
10. Wei, T.Y.; Lim, K.L.; Tseng, Y.S.; Chan, S.L.I. A review on the characterization of hydrogen in hydrogen storage materials. *Renew. Sustain. Energy Rev.* **2017**, *79*, 1122–1133. [CrossRef]
11. Sun, C.; Wang, C.; Ha, T.; Lee, J.; Shim, J.H.; Kim, Y. A brief review of characterization techniques with different length scales for hydrogen storage materials. *Nano Energy* **2023**, *113*, 108554. [CrossRef]
12. Afanasev, A.V.; Karlovets, D.V.; Serbo, V.G. Elastic scattering of twisted neutrons by nuclei. *Phys. Rev. C* **2021**, *103*, 054612. [CrossRef]
13. Aguilar, V.; Ruvalcaba-Sil, J.L.; Bucio, L.; Rivera-Muñoz, E.M. Characterization and setting protocol for a simultaneous X-ray Diffraction-X-ray Fluorescence system (XRD/XRF) for in situ analysis. *Eur. Phys. J. Plus* **2019**, *134*, 286. [CrossRef]
14. Hannon, A.C.; Gibbs, A.S.; Takagi, H. Neutron scattering length determination by means of total scattering. *J. Appl. Crystallogr.* **2018**, *51*, 854–866. [CrossRef]
15. Korolkovas, A. Fast X-ray diffraction (XRD) tomography for enhanced identification of materials. *Sci. Rep.* **2022**, *12*, 19097. [CrossRef]
16. Kumar, P.; Singh, S.; Hashmi, S.A.R.; Kim, K.H. MXenes: Emerging 2D materials for hydrogen storage. *Nano Energy* **2021**, *85*, 105989. [CrossRef]
17. Tan, W.L.; McNeill, C.R. X-ray diffraction of photovoltaic perovskites: Principles and applications. *Appl. Phys. Rev.* **2022**, *9*, 021310. [CrossRef]
18. Xia, Y.; Yang, Z.; Zhu, Y. Porous carbon-based materials for hydrogen storage: Advancement and challenges. *J. Mater. Chem. A* **2013**, *1*, 9365–9381. [CrossRef]
19. Kittner, N.; Lill, F.; Kammen, D.M. Energy storage deployment and innovation for the clean energy transition. *Nat. Energy* **2017**, *2*, 17125. [CrossRef]

20. Gao, Y.; Li, Z.; Wang, P.; Cui, W.G.; Wang, X.; Yang, Y.; Gao, F.; Zhang, M.; Gan, J.; Li, C.; et al. Experimentally validated design principles of heteroatom-doped-graphene-supported calcium single-atom materials for non-dissociative chemisorption solid-state hydrogen storage. *Nat. Commun.* **2024**, *15*, 928. [CrossRef]
21. Liu, Y.; Du, H.; Zhang, X.; Yang, Y.; Gao, M.; Pan, H. Superior catalytic activity derived from a two-dimensional $Ti_3C_2$ precursor towards the hydrogen storage reaction of magnesium hydride. *Chem. Commun.* **2016**, *52*, 705–708. [CrossRef] [PubMed]
22. Pan, H.; Liu, Y.; Gao, M.; Zhu, Y.; Lei, Y.; Wang, Q. An investigation on the structural and electrochemical properties of $La_{0.7}Mg_{0.3}(Ni_{0.85}Co_{0.15})_x$ ($x = 3.15 - 3.80$) hydrogen storage electrode alloys. *J. Alloys Compd.* **2003**, *351*, 228–234. [CrossRef]
23. Ding, Z.; Li, Y.; Jiang, H.; Zhou, Y.; Wan, H.; Qiu, J.; Jiang, F.; Tan, J.; Du, W.; Chen, Y.; et al. The integral role of high-entropy alloys in advancing solid-state hydrogen storage. *Interdiscip. Mater.* **2024**, 1–34. [CrossRef]
24. Liu, Y.; Pan, H.; Gao, M.; Wang, Q. Advanced hydrogen storage alloys for Ni/MH rechargeable batteries. *J. Mater. Chem.* **2011**, *21*, 4743–4755. [CrossRef]
25. Zhang, X.; Liu, Y.; Ren, Z.; Zhang, X.; Hu, J.; Huang, Z.; Lu, Y.; Gao, M.; Pan, H. Realizing 6.7 wt% reversible storage of hydrogen at ambient temperature with non-confined ultrafine magnesium hydrides. *Energy Environ. Sci.* **2021**, *14*, 2302–2313. [CrossRef]
26. Yang, H.; Ding, Z.; Li, Y.-T.; Li, S.-Y.; Wu, P.-K.; Hou, Q.-H.; Zheng, Y.; Gao, B.; Huo, K.-F.; Du, W.-J.; et al. Recent advances in kinetic and thermodynamic regulation of magnesium hydride for hydrogen storage. *Rare Met.* **2023**, *42*, 2906–2927. [CrossRef]
27. Ding, Z.; Li, H.; Yan, G.; Yang, W.; Gao, Z.; Ma, W.; Shaw, L. Mechanism of hydrogen storage on $Fe_3B$. *Chem. Commun.* **2020**, *56*, 14235–14238. [CrossRef]
28. Liu, Y.; Zhong, K.; Luo, K.; Gao, M.; Pan, H.; Wang, Q. Size-Dependent Kinetic Enhancement in Hydrogen Absorption and Desorption of the Li−Mg−N−H System. *J. Am. Chem. Soc.* **2009**, *131*, 1862–1870. [CrossRef]
29. Pang, Y.; Liu, Y.; Gao, M.; Ouyang, L.; Liu, J.; Wang, H.; Zhu, M.; Pan, H. A mechanical-force-driven physical vapour deposition approach to fabricating complex hydride nanostructures. *Nat. Commun.* **2014**, *5*, 3519. [CrossRef]
30. Ding, Z.; Li, Y.; Yang, H.; Lu, Y.; Tan, J.; Li, J.; Li, Q.; Chen, Y.a.; Shaw, L.L.; Pan, F. Tailoring $MgH_2$ for hydrogen storage through nanoengineering and catalysis. *J. Magnes. Alloys* **2022**, *10*, 2946–2967. [CrossRef]
31. Usman, M.R. Hydrogen storage methods: Review and current status. *Renew. Sustain. Energy Rev.* **2022**, *167*, 112743. [CrossRef]
32. Zhou, D.; Ye, Y.; Zhu, H.; Cheng, H. Thermal analysis and performance improvement of heat transfer in sample cell of Sieverts apparatus. *Int. J. Hydrog. Energy* **2024**, *50*, 61–70. [CrossRef]
33. Charbonnier, V.; Asano, K.; Kim, H.; Sakaki, K. How to evaluate hydrogen storage properties by Sieverts' method in the pressure range up to 100 MPa. *J. Alloys Compd.* **2023**, *960*, 170860. [CrossRef]
34. Gray, E.M. 7-Reliably measuring hydrogen uptake in storage materials. In *Solid-State Hydrogen Storage*; Walker, G., Ed.; Woodhead Publishing: Cambridge, UK, 2008; pp. 174–204. [CrossRef]
35. Webb, C.J.; Gray, E.M. The effect of inaccurate volume calibrations on hydrogen uptake measured by the Sieverts method. *Int. J. Hydrog. Energy* **2014**, *39*, 2168–2174. [CrossRef]
36. Webb, C.J.; Gray, E.M. Analysis of the uncertainties in gas uptake measurements using the Sieverts method. *Int. J. Hydrog. Energy* **2014**, *39*, 366–375. [CrossRef]
37. Ding, Z.; Li, H.; Shaw, L. New insights into the solid-state hydrogen storage of nanostructured $LiBH_4$-$MgH_2$ system. *Chem. Eng. J.* **2020**, *385*, 123856. [CrossRef]
38. Zhu, H.; Zhou, D.; Chen, D.; Cheng, H. Design of ultra-efficient and automatically temperature-variable cycle (TVC) Sieverts apparatus for testing sorption properties of hydrogen storage materials. *Int. J. Hydrog. Energy* **2024**, *62*, 172–185. [CrossRef]
39. Kadono, J.; Maruoka, T.; Nakazawa, D.; Hoshiyama, Y.; Miyake, H. Measuring the effects of boron mass addition to V–Fe hydrogen storage alloys on their hydrogen absorbing–desorbing characteristics and loss of boron by hydrogenation by employing new analysis methods; hybrid of Sieverts' method, inert gas fusion method, and gravimetric method. *Int. J. Hydrog. Energy* **2017**, *42*, 996–1003. [CrossRef]
40. Hurst, K.E.; Gennett, T.; Adams, J.; Allendorf, M.D.; Balderas-Xicohténcatl, R.; Bielewski, M.; Edwards, B.; Espinal, L.; Fultz, B.; Hirscher, M.; et al. An International Laboratory Comparison Study of Volumetric and Gravimetric Hydrogen Adsorption Measurements. *ChemPhysChem* **2019**, *20*, 1997–2009. [CrossRef]
41. Alomairy, S. Dissolution mechanism and kinetics of β(Mg17Al12) phases in AZ91 magnesium alloy. *J. Magnes. Alloys* **2024**, *12*, 1581–1592. [CrossRef]
42. Baird, J.A.; Taylor, L.S. Evaluation of amorphous solid dispersion properties using thermal analysis techniques. *Adv. Drug Deliv. Rev.* **2012**, *64*, 396–421. [CrossRef] [PubMed]
43. Demers, V.; Turenne, S.; Scalzo, O. Segregation measurement of powder injection molding feedstock using thermogravimetric analysis, pycnometer density and differential scanning calorimetry techniques. *Adv. Powder Technol.* **2015**, *26*, 997–1004. [CrossRef]
44. Drzeżdżon, J.; Jacewicz, D.; Sielicka, A.; Chmurzyński, L. Characterization of polymers based on differential scanning calorimetry based techniques. *TrAC Trends Anal. Chem.* **2019**, *110*, 51–56. [CrossRef]
45. Green, S.P.; Wheelhouse, K.M.; Payne, A.D.; Hallett, J.P.; Miller, P.W.; Bull, J.A. On the Use of Differential Scanning Calorimetry for Thermal Hazard Assessment of New Chemistry: Avoiding Explosive Mistakes. *Angew. Chem. Int. Ed.* **2020**, *59*, 15798–15802. [CrossRef]
46. Saadatkhah, N.; Carillo Garcia, A.; Ackermann, S.; Leclerc, P.; Latifi, M.; Samih, S.; Patience, G.S.; Chaouki, J. Experimental methods in chemical engineering: Thermogravimetric analysis—TGA. *Can. J. Chem. Eng.* **2019**, *98*, 34–43. [CrossRef]

47. Sanchez-Ruiz, J.M. Probing free-energy surfaces with differential scanning calorimetry. *Annu. Rev. Phys. Chem.* **2011**, *62*, 231–255. [CrossRef]
48. Xiao, H.; Qian, F.; Zhang, X.; Hu, H.; Tang, R.; Hu, C.; Zhou, W.; He, X.; Pu, Z.; Ma, C.; et al. Effect of $Ce_{0.6}Zr_{0.4}O_2$ nanocrystals on boosting hydrogen storage performance of $MgH_2$. *Chem. Eng. J.* **2024**, *494*, 153203. [CrossRef]
49. Benninghoven, A.; Huber, A.M.; Werner, H.W. Secondary ion mass spectrometry (SIMS VI): Wiley, Chichester, 1988 (ISBN 0-471-91832-6). xxvii + 1078 pp. Price £75.00. *Anal. Chim. Acta* **1988**, *215*, 366. [CrossRef]
50. Benninghoven, A. Surface analysis by Secondary Ion Mass Spectrometry (SIMS). *Surf. Sci.* **1994**, *299*, 246–260. [CrossRef]
51. Lockyer, N.P.; Aoyagi, S.; Fletcher, J.S.; Gilmore, I.S.; van der Heide, P.A.W.; Moore, K.L.; Tyler, B.J.; Weng, L.-T. Secondary ion mass spectrometry. *Nat. Rev. Methods Primers* **2024**, *4*, 32. [CrossRef]
52. Madroñero, A.; Aguado, J.; Blanco, J.M.; López, A. Uptake of hydrogen from some carbon fibres examined by Secondary Ion Mass Spectrometry. *Appl. Surf. Sci.* **2011**, *257*, 1881–1885. [CrossRef]
53. Andersen, D.; Chen, H.; Pal, S.; Cressa, L.; De Castro, O.; Wirtz, T.; Schmitz, G.; Eswara, S. Correlative high-resolution imaging of hydrogen in $Mg_2Ni$ hydrogen storage thin films. *Int. J. Hydrog. Energy* **2023**, *48*, 13943–13954. [CrossRef]
54. Hryniewicz, T.; Konarski, P.; Rokicki, R. Hydrogen Reduction in MEP Niobium Studied by Secondary Ion Mass Spectrometry (SIMS). *Metals* **2017**, *7*, 442. [CrossRef]
55. Lagator, M.; Berrueta Razo, I.; Royle, T.; Lockyer, N.P. Sensitivity enhancement using chemically reactive gas cluster ion beams in secondary ion mass spectrometry (SIMS). *Surf. Interface Anal.* **2022**, *54*, 349–355. [CrossRef]
56. Francois-Saint-Cyr, H.; Martin, I.; Peres, P.; Guillermier, C.; Prosa, T.; Blanc, W.; Larson, D. Secondary Ion Mass Spectrometry (SIMS) and Atom Probe Tomography (APT): Powerful Synergetic Techniques for Materials Scientists. *Microsc. Microanal.* **2020**, *26*, 524–525. [CrossRef]
57. Liu, Y.; Lorenz, M.; Ievlev, A.V.; Ovchinnikova, O.S. Secondary Ion Mass Spectrometry (SIMS) for Chemical Characterization of Metal Halide Perovskites. *Adv. Funct. Mater.* **2020**, *30*, 2002201. [CrossRef]
58. Gao, Y.-Y.; Ren, T.-X.; Williams, I.S.; Ireland, T.R.; Long, T.; Rienitz, O.; Pramann, A.; Wang, S.; Song, P.-S.; Wang, J. Molar mass measurement of a $^{28}Si$-enriched silicon crystal with high precision secondary ion mass spectrometry (SIMS). *J. Anal. At. Spectrom.* **2022**, *37*, 2546–2555. [CrossRef]
59. Munteshari, O.; Zhou, Y.; Mei, B.-A.; Pilon, L. Theoretical validation of the step potential electrochemical spectroscopy (SPECS) and multiple potential step chronoamperometry (MUSCA) methods for pseudocapacitive electrodes. *Electrochim. Acta* **2019**, *321*, 134648. [CrossRef]
60. Palagonia, M.S.; Erinmwingbovo, C.; Brogioli, D.; La Mantia, F. Comparison between cyclic voltammetry and differential charge plots from galvanostatic cycling. *J. Electroanal. Chem.* **2019**, *847*, 113170. [CrossRef]
61. Nara, H.; Yokoshima, T.; Osaka, T. Technology of electrochemical impedance spectroscopy for an energy-sustainable society. *Curr. Opin. Electrochem.* **2020**, *20*, 66–77. [CrossRef]
62. Matsubara, Y. A Small yet Complete Framework for a Potentiostat, Galvanostat, and Electrochemical Impedance Spectrometer. *J. Chem. Educ.* **2021**, *98*, 3362–3370. [CrossRef]
63. Iwamoto, R.T.; Adams, R.N.; Lott, H. Drop-scale chronopotentiometry. *Anal. Chim. Acta* **1959**, *20*, 84–88. [CrossRef]
64. Lin, Y.; Lian, C.; Berrueta, M.U.; Liu, H.; van Roij, R. Microscopic Model for Cyclic Voltammetry of Porous Electrodes. *Phys. Rev. Lett.* **2022**, *128*, 206001. [CrossRef] [PubMed]
65. Lazanas, A.C.; Prodromidis, M.I. Electrochemical Impedance Spectroscopy—A Tutorial. *ACS Meas. Sci. Au* **2023**, *3*, 162–193. [CrossRef]
66. Moradighadi, N.; Nesic, S.; Tribollet, B. Identifying the dominant electrochemical reaction in electrochemical impedance spectroscopy. *Electrochim. Acta* **2021**, *400*, 139460. [CrossRef]
67. Cruz-Manzo, S.; Greenwood, P.; Chen, R. An Impedance Model for EIS Analysis of Nickel Metal Hydride Batteries. *J. Electrochem. Soc.* **2017**, *164*, A1446. [CrossRef]
68. Lindberg, A.; Eriksson, B.; Börjesson Axén, J.; Sandra, A.P.; Lindbergh, G. Gas phase composition of a NiMH battery during a work cycle. *RSC Adv.* **2024**, *14*, 19996–20003. [CrossRef]
69. Lota, K.; Swoboda, P.; Acznik, I.; Sierczyńska, A.; Mańczak, R.; Kolanowski, Ł.; Lota, G. Electrochemical properties of modified negative electrode for Ni-MH cell. *Curr. Appl. Phys.* **2020**, *20*, 106–113. [CrossRef]
70. Yang, C.C.; Wang, C.C.; Li, M.M.; Jiang, Q. A start of the renaissance for nickel metal hydride batteries: A hydrogen storage alloy series with an ultra-long cycle life. *J. Mater. Chem. A* **2017**, *5*, 1145–1152. [CrossRef]
71. Edalati, P.; Mohammadi, A.; Li, Y.; Li, H.-W.; Floriano, R.; Fuji, M.; Edalati, K. High-entropy alloys as anode materials of nickel-metal hydride batteries. *Scr. Mater.* **2022**, *209*, 114387. [CrossRef]
72. Wu, J.; Liu, Z.; Zhang, H.; Zou, Y.; Li, B.; Xiang, C.; Sun, L.; Xu, F.; Yu, T. Hydrogen storage performance of $MgH_2$ under catalysis by highly dispersed nickel-nanoparticle–doped hollow spherical vanadium nitride. *J. Magnes. Alloys* **2024**, in press. [CrossRef]
73. Rej, S.; Mascaretti, L.; Santiago, E.Y.; Tomanec, O.; Kment, Š.; Wang, Z.; Zbořil, R.; Fornasiero, P.; Govorov, A.O.; Naldoni, A. Determining Plasmonic Hot Electrons and Photothermal Effects during $H_2$ Evolution with TiN-Pt Nanohybrids. *ACS Catal.* **2020**, *10*, 5261–5271. [CrossRef]
74. Ross, D.J.; Halls, M.D.; Nazri, A.G.; Aroca, R.F. Raman scattering of complex sodium aluminum hydride for hydrogen storage. *Chem. Phys. Lett.* **2004**, *388*, 430–435. [CrossRef]
75. Alessandri, I.; Lombardi, J.R. Enhanced Raman Scattering with Dielectrics. *Chem. Rev.* **2016**, *116*, 14921–14981. [CrossRef]

76. Eslami, S.; Palomba, S. Integrated enhanced Raman scattering: A review. *Nano Converg.* **2021**, *8*, 41. [CrossRef]
77. Min, W.; Gao, X. The Duality of Raman Scattering. *Acc. Chem. Res.* **2024**, *57*, 1869–1905. [CrossRef]
78. Liebel, M.; Pazos-Perez, N.; van Hulst, N.F.; Alvarez-Puebla, R.A. Surface-enhanced Raman scattering holography. *Nat. Nanotechnol.* **2020**, *15*, 1005–1011. [CrossRef]
79. Balcerzak, M.; Runka, T.; Sniadecki, Z. Influence of carbon catalysts on the improvement of hydrogen storage properties in a body-centered cubic solid solution alloy. *Carbon* **2021**, *182*, 422–434. [CrossRef]
80. Vellingiri, L.; Annamalai, K.; Kandasamy, R.; Kombiah, I. Characterization and hydrogen storage properties of $SnO_2$ functionalized MWCNT nanocomposites. *Int. J. Hydrog. Energy* **2018**, *43*, 10396–10409. [CrossRef]
81. Reed, D.; Book, D. Recent applications of Raman spectroscopy to the study of complex hydrides for hydrogen storage. *Curr. Opin. Solid State Mater. Sci.* **2011**, *15*, 62–72. [CrossRef]
82. Valero-Pedraza, M.J.; Gascón, V.; Carreón, M.A.; Leardini, F.; Ares, J.R.; Martín, Á.; Sánchez-Sánchez, M.; Bañares, M.A. Operando Raman-mass spectrometry investigation of hydrogen release by thermolysis of ammonia borane confined in mesoporous materials. *Microporous Mesoporous Mater.* **2016**, *226*, 454–465. [CrossRef]
83. Lipinski, G.; Jeong, K.; Moritz, K.; Petermann, M.; May, E.F.; Stanwix, P.L.; Richter, M. Application of Raman Spectroscopy for Sorption Analysis of Functionalized Porous Materials. *Adv. Sci.* **2022**, *9*, 2105477. [CrossRef] [PubMed]
84. Liu, A.; Song, Y. In Situ High-Pressure and Low-Temperature Study of Ammonia Borane by Raman Spectroscopy. *J. Phys. Chem. C* **2012**, *116*, 2123–2131. [CrossRef]
85. Bleda-Martínez, M.J.; Pérez, J.M.; Linares-Solano, A.; Morallón, E.; Cazorla-Amorós, D. Effect of surface chemistry on electrochemical storage of hydrogen in porous carbon materials. *Carbon* **2008**, *46*, 1053–1059. [CrossRef]
86. Kalashnikov, D.A.; Paterova, A.V.; Kulik, S.P.; Krivitsky, L.A. Infrared spectroscopy with visible light. *Nat. Photonics* **2016**, *10*, 98–101. [CrossRef]
87. Lim, Y.; Hong, S.J.; Cho, Y.; Bang, J.; Lee, S. Fourier Surfaces Reaching Full-Color Diffraction Limits. *Adv. Mater.* **2024**, *36*, e2404540. [CrossRef]
88. Hashimoto, K.; Nakamura, T.; Kageyama, T.; Badarla, V.R.; Shimada, H.; Horisaki, R.; Ideguchi, T. Upconversion time-stretch infrared spectroscopy. *Light Sci. Appl.* **2023**, *12*, 48. [CrossRef]
89. Lassaline, N.; Brechbühler, R.; Vonk, S.J.W.; Ridderbeek, K.; Spieser, M.; Bisig, S.; le Feber, B.; Rabouw, F.T.; Norris, D.J. Optical Fourier surfaces. *Nature* **2020**, *582*, 506–510. [CrossRef]
90. Muthu, R.N.; Rajashabala, S.; Kannan, R. Hydrogen storage performance of lithium borohydride decorated activated hexagonal boron nitride nanocomposite for fuel cell applications. *Int. J. Hydrog. Energy* **2017**, *42*, 15586–15596. [CrossRef]
91. Pei, Z.; Bai, Y.; Wang, Y.; Wu, F.; Wu, C. Insight to the Thermal Decomposition and Hydrogen Desorption Behaviors of NaNH2–NaBH4 Hydrogen Storage Composite. *ACS Appl. Mater. Interfaces* **2017**, *9*, 31977–31984. [CrossRef]
92. Kern, J.; Alonso-Mori, R.; Tran, R.; Hattne, J.; Gildea, R.J.; Echols, N.; Glöckner, C.; Hellmich, J.; Laksmono, H.; Sierra, R.G.; et al. Simultaneous Femtosecond X-ray Spectroscopy and Diffraction of Photosystem II at Room Temperature. *Science* **2013**, *340*, 491–495. [CrossRef] [PubMed]
93. McCusker, L.B. Electron diffraction and the hydrogen atom. *Science* **2017**, *355*, 136. [CrossRef] [PubMed]
94. Wang, Y.; Lan, Z.; Huang, X.; Liu, H.; Guo, J. Study on catalytic effect and mechanism of MOF (MOF = ZIF-8, ZIF-67, MOF-74) on hydrogen storage properties of magnesium. *Int. J. Hydrog. Energy* **2019**, *44*, 28863–28873. [CrossRef]
95. Ma, Z.; Zhang, Q.; Panda, S.; Zhu, W.; Sun, F.; Khan, D.; Dong, J.; Ding, W.; Zou, J. In situ catalyzed and nanoconfined magnesium hydride nanocrystals in a Ni-MOF scaffold for hydrogen storage. *Sustain. Energy Fuels* **2020**, *4*, 4694–4703. [CrossRef]
96. Zhang, L.; Nyahuma, F.M.; Zhang, H.; Cheng, C.; Zheng, J.; Wu, F.; Chen, L. Metal organic framework supported niobium pentoxide nanoparticles with exceptional catalytic effect on hydrogen storage behavior of $MgH_2$. *Green Energy Environ.* **2023**, *8*, 589–600. [CrossRef]
97. Chen, L.; Wang, B.; Zhang, W.; Zheng, S.; Chen, Z.; Zhang, M.; Dong, C.; Pan, F.; Li, S. Crystal Structure Assignment for Unknown Compounds from X-ray Diffraction Patterns with Deep Learning. *J. Am. Chem. Soc.* **2024**, *146*, 8098–8109. [CrossRef]
98. Zlotea, C.; Sow, M.A.; Ek, G.; Couzinié, J.P.; Perrière, L.; Guillot, I.; Bourgon, J.; Møller, K.T.; Jensen, T.R.; Akiba, E.; et al. Hydrogen sorption in TiZrNbHfTa high entropy alloy. *J. Alloys Compd.* **2019**, *775*, 667–674. [CrossRef]
99. Jensen, T.R.; Andreasen, A.; Vegge, T.; Andreasen, J.W.; Ståhl, K.; Pedersen, A.S.; Nielsen, M.M.; Molenbroek, A.M.; Besenbacher, F. Dehydrogenation kinetics of pure and nickel-doped magnesium hydride investigated by in situ time-resolved powder X-ray diffraction. *Int. J. Hydrog. Energy* **2006**, *31*, 2052–2062. [CrossRef]
100. Dewhurst, C.D.; Grillo, I. Neutron imaging using a conventional small-angle neutron scattering instrument. *J. Appl. Crystallogr.* **2016**, *49*, 736–742. [CrossRef]
101. Zu, T.; Tang, Y.; Huang, Z.; Qin, S.; Li, J.; He, Q.; Cao, L.; Wu, H. Treatments of Thermal Neutron Scattering Data and Their Effect on Neutronics Calculations. *Front. Energy Res.* **2021**, *9*, 779261. [CrossRef]
102. Mühlbauer, S.; Honecker, D.; Périgo, E.A.; Bergner, F.; Disch, S.; Heinemann, A.; Erokhin, S.; Berkov, D.; Leighton, C.; Eskildsen, M.R.; et al. Magnetic small-angle neutron scattering. *Rev. Mod. Phys.* **2019**, *91*, 015004. [CrossRef]
103. Nazirkar, N.P.; Shi, X.; Shi, J.; N'Gom, M.; Fohtung, E. Coherent diffractive imaging with twisted X-rays: Principles, applications, and outlook. *Appl. Phys. Rev.* **2024**, *11*, 021302. [CrossRef]
104. Cao, C.; Toney, M.F.; Sham, T.-K.; Harder, R.; Shearing, P.R.; Xiao, X.; Wang, J. Emerging X-ray imaging technologies for energy materials. *Mater. Today* **2020**, *34*, 132–147. [CrossRef]

105. Schriber, E.A.; Paley, D.W.; Bolotovsky, R.; Rosenberg, D.J.; Sierra, R.G.; Aquila, A.; Mendez, D.; Poitevin, F.; Blaschke, J.P.; Bhowmick, A.; et al. Chemical crystallography by serial femtosecond X-ray diffraction. *Nature* **2022**, *601*, 360–365. [CrossRef]
106. Yu, X.; Cheng, Y.; Li, Y.; Polo-Garzon, F.; Liu, J.; Mamontov, E.; Li, M.; Lennon, D.; Parker, S.F.; Ramirez-Cuesta, A.J.; et al. Neutron Scattering Studies of Heterogeneous Catalysis. *Chem. Rev.* **2023**, *123*, 8638–8700. [CrossRef]
107. Ponthieu, M.; Cuevas, F.; Fernández, J.F.; Laversenne, L.; Porcher, F.; Latroche, M. Structural Properties and Reversible Deuterium Loading of $MgD_2$–$TiD_2$ Nanocomposites. *J. Phys. Chem. C* **2013**, *117*, 18851–18862. [CrossRef]
108. Ramirez-Cuesta, A.J.; Jones, M.O.; David, W.I.F. Neutron scattering and hydrogen storage. *Mater. Today* **2009**, *12*, 54–61. [CrossRef]
109. Sato, T.; Orimo, S.-I. Hydrogen Vibration in Hydrogen Storage Materials Investigated by Inelastic Neutron Scattering. *Top. Catal.* **2021**, *64*, 614–621. [CrossRef]
110. Zhang, X.; Sun, Y.; Xia, G.; Yu, X. Light-weight solid-state hydrogen storage materials characterized by neutron scattering. *J. Alloys Compd.* **2022**, *899*, 163254. [CrossRef]
111. Jeffries, C.M.; Ilavsky, J.; Martel, A.; Hinrichs, S.; Meyer, A.; Pedersen, J.S.; Sokolova, A.V.; Svergun, D.I. Small-angle X-ray and neutron scattering. *Nat. Rev. Methods Primers* **2021**, *1*, 70. [CrossRef]
112. Yusuf, S.M.; Kumar, A. Neutron scattering of advanced magnetic materials. *Appl. Phys. Rev.* **2017**, *4*, 031303. [CrossRef]
113. Korin, E.; Froumin, N.; Cohen, S. Surface Analysis of Nanocomplexes by X-ray Photoelectron Spectroscopy (XPS). *ACS Biomater. Sci. Eng.* **2017**, *3*, 882–889. [CrossRef] [PubMed]
114. Greczynski, G.; Hultman, L. X-ray photoelectron spectroscopy: Towards reliable binding energy referencing. *Prog. Mater. Sci.* **2020**, *107*, 100591. [CrossRef]
115. Das, T.K.; Banerjee, S.; Sharma, P.; Sudarsan, V.; Sastry, P.U. Nitrogen doped porous carbon derived from EDTA: Effect of pores on hydrogen storage properties. *Int. J. Hydrog. Energy* **2018**, *43*, 8385–8394. [CrossRef]
116. Pei, P.; Whitwick, M.B.; Kureshi, S.; Cannon, M.; Quan, G.; Kjeang, E. Hydrogen storage mechanism in transition metal decorated graphene oxide: The symbiotic effect of oxygen groups and high layer spacing. *Int. J. Hydrog. Energy* **2020**, *45*, 6713–6726. [CrossRef]
117. Zhao, Y.; Liu, F.; Tan, J.; Li, P.; Wang, Z.; Zhu, K.; Mai, X.; Liu, H.; Wang, X.; Ma, Y.; et al. Preparation and hydrogen storage of Pd/MIL-101 nanocomposites. *J. Alloys Compd.* **2019**, *772*, 186–192. [CrossRef]
118. Smardz, L.; Nowak, M.; Jurczyk, M. XPS valence band studies of hydrogen storage nanocomposites. *Int. J. Hydrog. Energy* **2012**, *37*, 3659–3664. [CrossRef]
119. Kumar, S.; Kojima, Y.; Kain, V. XPS study on the vanadocene-magnesium system to understand the hydrogen sorption reaction mechanism under room temperature. *Int. J. Hydrog. Energy* **2019**, *44*, 2981–2987. [CrossRef]
120. Selvam, P.; Viswanathan, B.; Srinivasan, V. XPS and XAES studies on hydrogen storage magnesium-based alloys. *Int. J. Hydrog. Energy* **1989**, *14*, 899–902. [CrossRef]
121. Xing, X.; Liu, Y.; Zhang, Z.; Liu, T. Hierarchical Structure Carbon-Coated CoNi Nanocatalysts Derived from Flower-Like Bimetal MOFs: Enhancing the Hydrogen Storage Performance of $MgH_2$ under Mild Conditions. *ACS Sustain. Chem. Eng.* **2023**, *11*, 4825–4837. [CrossRef]
122. Xie, X.; Zhang, B.; Kimura, H.; Ni, C.; Yu, R.; Du, W. Morphology evolution of bimetallic Ni/Zn-MOFs and derived $Ni_3ZnC_{0.7}$/Ni/ZnO used to destabilize $MgH_2$. *Chem. Eng. J.* **2023**, *464*, 142630. [CrossRef]
123. Zhang, J.; Wang, W.; Chen, X.; Jin, J.; Yan, X.; Huang, Z. Single-Atom Ni Supported on $TiO_2$ for Catalyzing Hydrogen Storage in $MgH_2$. *J. Am. Chem. Soc.* **2024**, *146*, 10432–10442. [CrossRef] [PubMed]
124. Silva, B.H.; Almeida, J.M.; Hernandes, A.C.; Goncalves, R.V.; Zepon, G. Pulsed laser activation method for hydrogen storage alloys. *Int. J. Hydrog. Energy* **2024**, *53*, 885–890. [CrossRef]
125. Barroo, C.; Wang, Z.-J.; Schlögl, R.; Willinger, M.-G. Imaging the dynamics of catalysed surface reactions by in situ scanning electron microscopy. *Nat. Catal.* **2019**, *3*, 30–39. [CrossRef]
126. Bianco, E.; Kourkoutis, L.F. Atomic-Resolution Cryogenic Scanning Transmission Electron Microscopy for Quantum Materials. *Acc. Chem. Res.* **2021**, *54*, 3277–3287. [CrossRef]
127. Kim, P.Y.; Ribbe, A.E.; Russell, T.P.; Hoagland, D.A. Visualizing the Dynamics of Nanoparticles in Liquids by Scanning Electron Microscopy. *ACS Nano* **2016**, *10*, 6257–6264. [CrossRef]
128. Donald, A.M. The use of environmental scanning electron microscopy for imaging wet and insulating materials. *Nat. Mater.* **2003**, *2*, 511–516. [CrossRef]
129. McKernan, S. Environmental Scanning Electron Microscopy:-Advantages and Disadvantages. *Microsc. Microanal.* **1997**, *3*, 381–382. [CrossRef]
130. Niania, M.; Podor, R.; Britton, T.B.; Li, C.; Cooper, S.J.; Svetkov, N.; Skinner, S.; Kilner, J. Correction: In situ study of strontium segregation in $La_{0.6}Sr_{0.4}Co_{0.2}Fe_{0.8}O_{3-\delta}$ in ambient atmospheres using high-temperature environmental scanning electron microscopy. *J. Mater. Chem. A* **2018**, *6*, 14464. [CrossRef]
131. Zhang, L.; Zhu, J.; Wilke, K.L.; Xu, Z.; Zhao, L.; Lu, Z.; Goddard, L.L.; Wang, E.N. Enhanced Environmental Scanning Electron Microscopy Using Phase Reconstruction and Its Application in Condensation. *ACS Nano* **2019**, *13*, 1953–1960. [CrossRef]
132. Zhu, J.; Zhang, L.; Li, X.; Wilke, K.L.; Wang, E.N.; Goddard, L.L. Quasi-Newtonian Environmental Scanning Electron Microscopy (QN-ESEM) for Monitoring Material Dynamics in High-Pressure Gaseous Environments. *Adv. Sci.* **2020**, *7*, 2001268. [CrossRef] [PubMed]

133. Ren, L.; Zhu, W.; Zhang, Q.; Lu, C.; Sun, F.; Lin, X.; Zou, J. MgH$_2$ confinement in MOF-derived N-doped porous carbon nanofibers for enhanced hydrogen storage. *Chem. Eng. J.* **2022**, *434*, 134701. [CrossRef]
134. Schulz, F.; Ritala, J.; Krejci, O.; Seitsonen, A.P.; Foster, A.S.; Liljeroth, P. Elemental Identification by Combining Atomic Force Microscopy and Kelvin Probe Force Microscopy. *ACS Nano* **2018**, *12*, 5274–5283. [CrossRef] [PubMed]
135. Collins, L.; Liu, Y.; Ovchinnikova, O.S.; Proksch, R. Quantitative Electromechanical Atomic Force Microscopy. *ACS Nano* **2019**, *13*, 8055–8066. [CrossRef]
136. Oinonen, N.; Xu, C.; Alldritt, B.; Canova, F.F.; Urtev, F.; Cai, S.; Krejci, O.; Kannala, J.; Liljeroth, P.; Foster, A.S. Electrostatic Discovery Atomic Force Microscopy. *ACS Nano* **2022**, *16*, 89–97. [CrossRef]
137. Singh, A. Towards resolving proteomes in single cells. *Nat. Methods* **2021**, *18*, 856. [CrossRef]
138. Songen, H.; Bechstein, R.; Kuhnle, A. Quantitative atomic force microscopy. *J. Phys. Condens. Matter* **2017**, *29*, 274001. [CrossRef]
139. Kalisvaart, W.P.; Luber, E.J.; Poirier, C.; Harrower, C.T.; Teichert, A.; Wallacher, D.; Grimm, N.; Steitz, R.; Fritzsche, H.; Mitlin, D. Probing the Room Temperature Deuterium Absorption Kinetics in Nanoscale Magnesium Based Hydrogen Storage Multilayers Using Neutron Reflectometry, X-ray Diffraction, and Atomic Force Microscopy. *J. Phys. Chem. C* **2012**, *116*, 5868–5880. [CrossRef]
140. Ke, X.; Zhang, M.; Zhao, K.; Su, D. Moire Fringe Method via Scanning Transmission Electron Microscopy. *Small Methods* **2022**, *6*, e2101040. [CrossRef]
141. Kuei, B.; Aplan, M.P.; Litofsky, J.H.; Gomez, E.D. New opportunities in transmission electron microscopy of polymers. *Mater. Sci. Eng. R Rep.* **2020**, *139*, 100516. [CrossRef]
142. Lei, X.; Zhao, J.; Wang, J.; Su, D. Tracking lithiation with transmission electron microscopy. *Sci. China Chem.* **2023**, *67*, 291–311. [CrossRef]
143. Schwartz, O.; Axelrod, J.J.; Campbell, S.L.; Turnbaugh, C.; Glaeser, R.M.; Muller, H. Laser phase plate for transmission electron microscopy. *Nat Methods* **2019**, *16*, 1016–1020. [CrossRef] [PubMed]
144. Dick, K.A. Gas-phase materials synthesis in environmental transmission electron microscopy. *MRS Bull.* **2023**, *48*, 833–841. [CrossRef]
145. Han, Z.; Yang, F.; Li, Y. Dynamics of metal-support interface revealed by environmental transmission electron microscopy. *Matter* **2022**, *5*, 2531–2533. [CrossRef]
146. Parent, L.R.; Pham, C.H.; Patterson, J.P.; Denny, M.S.; Cohen, S.M.; Gianneschi, N.C.; Paesani, F. Pore Breathing of Metal-Organic Frameworks by Environmental Transmission Electron Microscopy. *J. Am. Chem. Soc.* **2017**, *139*, 13973–13976. [CrossRef]
147. Stach, E.A.; Zakharov, D.; Akatay, M.C.; Baumann, P.; Ribeiro, F.; Zvienevich, Y.; Li, Y.; Frenkel, A. Developments in environmental transmission electron microscopy for catalysis research. *Microsc. Microanal.* **2013**, *19*, 1174–1175. [CrossRef]
148. Tanaka, N.; Fujita, T.; Takahashi, Y.; Yamasaki, J.; Murata, K.; Arai, S. Progress in environmental high-voltage transmission electron microscopy for nanomaterials. *Philos. Trans. R. Soc. A Math. Phys. Eng. Sci.* **2020**, *378*, 20190602. [CrossRef]
149. Nakamura, E.; Sommerdijk, N.; Zheng, H. Transmission Electron Microscopy for Chemists. *Acc. Chem. Res.* **2017**, *50*, 1795–1796. [CrossRef]
150. Wu, R.; Zhang, X.; Liu, Y.; Zhang, L.; Hu, J.; Gao, M.; Pan, H. A Unique Double-Layered Carbon Nanobowl-Confined Lithium Borohydride for Highly Reversible Hydrogen Storage. *Small* **2020**, *16*, 2001963. [CrossRef]
151. Liu, X.; Zhang, C.; Li, Y.; Niemantsverdriet, J.W.; Wagner, J.B.; Hansen, T.W. Environmental Transmission Electron Microscopy (ETEM) Studies of Single Iron Nanoparticle Carburization in Synthesis Gas. *ACS Catal.* **2017**, *7*, 4867–4875. [CrossRef]
152. Zhang, D.; Jin, C.; Li, Z.Y.; Zhang, Z.; Li, J. Oxidation behavior of cobalt nanoparticles studied by in situ environmental transmission electron microscopy. *Sci. Bull.* **2017**, *62*, 775–778. [CrossRef] [PubMed]
153. Adams, J.D.; Erickson, B.W.; Grossenbacher, J.; Brugger, J.; Nievergelt, A.; Fantner, G.E. Harnessing the damping properties of materials for high-speed atomic force microscopy. *Nat. Nanotechnol.* **2016**, *11*, 147–151. [CrossRef] [PubMed]
154. Ando, T. High-speed atomic force microscopy. *Curr. Opin. Chem. Biol.* **2019**, *51*, 105–112. [CrossRef] [PubMed]
155. Brown, B.P.; Picco, L.; Miles, M.J.; Faul, C.F.J. Opportunities in High-Speed Atomic Force Microscopy. *Small* **2013**, *9*, 3201–3211. [CrossRef]
156. Fukui, T.; Uchihashi, T.; Sasaki, N.; Watanabe, H.; Takeuchi, M.; Sugiyasu, K. Direct Observation and Manipulation of Supramolecular Polymerization by High-Speed Atomic Force Microscopy. *Angew. Chem. Int. Ed.* **2018**, *57*, 15465–15470. [CrossRef]
157. Das, S.K.; Badal, F.R.; Rahman, M.A.; Islam, M.A.; Sarker, S.K.; Paul, N. Improvement of Alternative Non-Raster Scanning Methods for High Speed Atomic Force Microscopy: A Review. *IEEE Access* **2019**, *7*, 115603–115624. [CrossRef]
158. Verma, A.; Wilson, N.; Joshi, K. Solid state hydrogen storage: Decoding the path through machine learning. *Int. J. Hydrog. Energy* **2024**, *50*, 1518–1528. [CrossRef]

**Disclaimer/Publisher's Note:** The statements, opinions and data contained in all publications are solely those of the individual author(s) and contributor(s) and not of MDPI and/or the editor(s). MDPI and/or the editor(s) disclaim responsibility for any injury to people or property resulting from any ideas, methods, instructions or products referred to in the content.

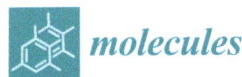 

Article

# Sintering Behavior of Molybdenite Concentrate During Oxidation Roasting Process in Air Atmosphere: Influences of Roasting Temperature and K Content

Jiangang Liu [1], Lu Wang [2,*] and Guohuan Wu [3,*]

1. College of Mechanical and Electrical Engineering, Wuyi University, Wuyishan 354300, China; liujiangang87@126.com
2. Key Laboratory for Ferrous Metallurgy and Resources Utilization of Ministry of Education, Wuhan University of Science and Technology, Wuhan 430081, China
3. School of Intelligent Manufacturing, Wenzhou Polytechnic, Wenzhou 325035, China
* Correspondence: wanglu@wust.edu.cn (L.W.); wugh@wzpt.edu.cn (G.W.)

**Abstract:** Sintering is a common phenomenon, which often takes place during the oxidation roasting process of molybdenite concentrate in multiple-hearth furnaces. The occurrence of sintering phenomena has detrimental effects on the product quality and the service life of the furnace. In this work, the influence of two key factors (roasting temperature and K content) on the sintering behavior is investigated using molybdenite concentrate as the raw material. Different technologies such as XRD, FESEM-EDS, and phase diagrams are adopted to analyze the experimental data. The results show that the higher the roasting temperature is, the greater the mass loss and the more serious the sintering degree will be. The results also show that with the increase in K content, the mass loss of the raw material is first increased and then decreased, while its sintering degree is still gradually increased. The sintering products obtained during the oxidation roasting process are often tightly combined with the bottom of the used crucible with a smooth and dense surface structure, while their internal microstructures are very complicated, which not only includes numerous $MoO_3$ species, but also unoxidized $MoS_2$, Mo sub-oxide, $SiO_2$, and a variety of molybdates. Among them, both $MoO_3$ and molybdates can be easily dissolved into the ammonia solution, leading to a residue mainly composed of $SiO_2$ and $CaMoO_4$. This study also finds that the sintering phenomenon is caused by the increase in local temperature and the formation of various low-melting-point eutectics. It is suggested that decreasing the roasting temperature and K content, especially the K content, are effective methods for reducing the sintering degree of molybdenite concentrate during the oxidation roasting process.

**Keywords:** molybdenite concentrate; oxidation roasting; sintering behavior; temperature; K content

## 1. Introduction

The oxidation roasting of molybdenite concentrate in multiple-hearth furnaces is an important process for preparing molybdenum calcine and the subsequent molybdenum products [1–7]. Data in the literature show that this process is composed of two main steps: the oxidation of $MoS_2$ to $MoO_2$ (Reaction (1)) and the further oxidation of $MoO_2$ to $MoO_3$ (Reaction (2)) [8–11]. However, the sintering phenomenon always occurs during the process, which makes the prepared molybdenum calcine become dense and hard. The occurrence of the sintering phenomenon will also cause some other adverse effects, such as the incomplete oxidation of molybdenite concentrate and the increase in residual sulfur content. In addition, the target teeth and target arm of the multiple-hearth furnace may be damaged if the sintering phenomenon is serious enough, which will even lead to the occurrence of a "dead furnace". In order to enhance the product quality of molybdenum

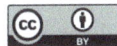

calcine and improve the service life of multiple-hearth furnaces, a systematic analysis of the sintering mechanism, therefore, is important.

$$MoS_2 + 3O_2 = MoO_2 + 2SO_2 \tag{1}$$

$$MoO_2 + 0.5O_2 = MoO_3 \tag{2}$$

Numerous papers about the sintering behaviors of molybdenite concentrate have been reported [12,13], and they found that the main influencing factors include roasting temperature, impurity type and content, sample thickness, stirring speed, reaction time, oxidation atmosphere and pressure, etc. [14–17]. For example, our previous work [18] demonstrated that sintering phenomena will not occur when adopting air as the oxidation atmosphere at 600 °C, whereas when oxygen is adopted, the sintering phenomenon will occur. The influence of different factors (roasting temperature, impurity type, and content) on the sintering degree of pure $MoS_2$ were also investigated [19], and the results showed that impurities such as elements Al and Si had no obvious effect on the sintering behavior; as for the impurities such as elements Ca, Fe, Pb, Mg, Cu, and K, however, the effects were serious. Similar results were also reported by Bu et al. [20], in which molybdenite concentrate was used as the raw material.

Even though many valuable conclusions about the sintering behavior have been drawn in recent decades, some issues still exist. For example, research concerning the influence of different factors on the regular phase transition of the sintering product is lacking; as to the morphology evolution behavior, related research is also scarce. In order to make up for these gaps, the current work was initiated. On one hand, K impurities were reported to have serious influences on the sintering behavior [19]; on the other hand, it was considered as a harmful element on the product performance of Mo-based alloys [21,22]. Therefore, K impurities were selected as the main study object in this work. In addition, the influence of roasting temperature on the sintering behavior of molybdenite concentrate during the oxidation roasting process was also investigated.

## 2. Results

*2.1. Mass Loss and Sintering Degree*

The mass loss of the mixed sample and the mass of the sintering product were calculated by the following equations:

$$m_{\text{mass loss}} = m_{\text{total}} - m_{\text{residual sample}} \tag{3}$$

$$m_{\text{sintering product}} = m_{\text{residual sample}} - m_{\text{surface loose}} \tag{4}$$

where $m_{\text{mass loss}}$ is the mass loss of the mixed sample, g; $m_{\text{residual sample}}$ and $m_{\text{surface loose}}$ are the masses of the residual sample and the surface loss sample after the roasting reaction, respectively, g; $m_{\text{total}}$ is the initial mass of the used mixed sample; $m_{\text{sintering product}}$ is the mass of the sintering product that adhered tightly to the bottom of crucible.

The sintering degree of the used mixed sample was defined as the ratio of the sintering product mass to the residual sample mass, see Equation (5):

$$\beta = \frac{m_{\text{sintering product}}}{m_{\text{residual sample}}} \tag{5}$$

2.1.1. Influence of Roasting Temperature

Figure 1 shows the influence of roasting temperature on the mass loss and sintering degree of the used mixed sample. When the roasting temperature is 550 °C, the mass loss and sintering product mass are both small, which may be due to the low roasting temperature and reaction rate. When the roasting temperature increased from 550 °C to

700 °C, the values of mass loss and sintering product mass are both gradually increased. At 700 °C, the sintering product mass reaches its peak value (0.6803 g). When the roasting temperature increased to 750 °C, the mass loss is still increased, while the sintering product mass begins to decrease, which may be due to the strong sublimation effect of $MoO_3$ at higher-temperature atmospheres [23–25]. As for the sintering degree, the results show that its value is gradually increased until reaching 1 at 700 °C; that is to say, when the roasting temperature is higher than 700 °C, the residual samples are all sintering products and they are all firmly glued to bottom of the crucible.

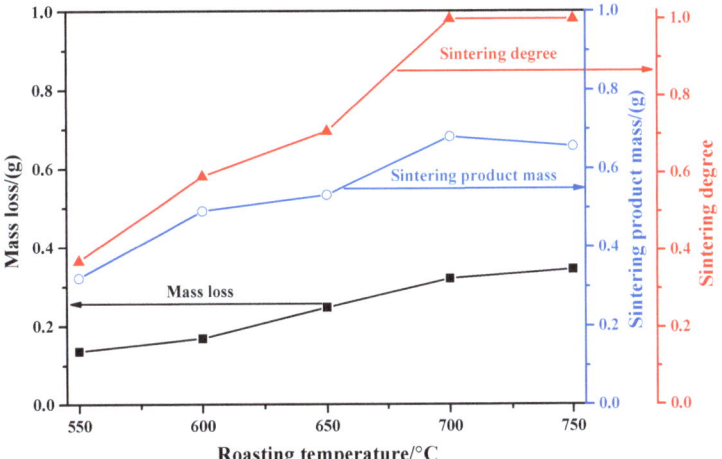

**Figure 1.** Influence of roasting temperature on the mass loss and sintering degree of the used mixed sample (K content: 2%).

2.1.2. Influence of K Content

Figure 2 shows the influence of K content on the mass loss and sintering degree of the used mixed sample. From this figure, it can be found that K content has significant influences on the mass loss: when the K content is below 1%, the mass loss is gradually increased; however, due to the small amount of $K_2CO_3$, the release rate of gaseous products is relatively slow, and thus the increase rate of mass loss is relatively slow. When the K content is in the range of 1% to 3.5%, the results show that the mass loss is increased with a relatively fast increase rate, which may be due to the higher release rate of gaseous products, especially for $SO_2$ and $CO_2$. Moreover, the maximum mass loss of 0.4532 g will be reached at a K content of 3.5%. Strangely, when the K content is further increased (above 3.5%), the mass loss begins to decrease. For this phenomenon, we have conducted several trials with the same experimental samples and procedures in order to verify the result, and the obtained mass losses are all similar to those that displayed in Figure 2, which indicates that the displayed results have a good reproducibility. Herein, the reason for the decrease in the mass loss at a higher K content may mainly result from the strong sintering behavior and the incomplete oxidation of molybdenite concentrate. Figure 2 also shows that the sintering product's mass and sintering degree are both increased with the increasing K content: when the K content is 3.5%, the sintering product mass is 0.5468 g and the sintering degree reaches 1, which indicates that under these conditions the residual samples are all becoming sintering products. Further increasing the K content, the sintering product mass is still increased, and the sintering degree always remains constant at 1. Herein, the ever-increasing sintering product mass is another important reason for the ever-decreasing mass loss under the conditions of a K content above 3.5%.

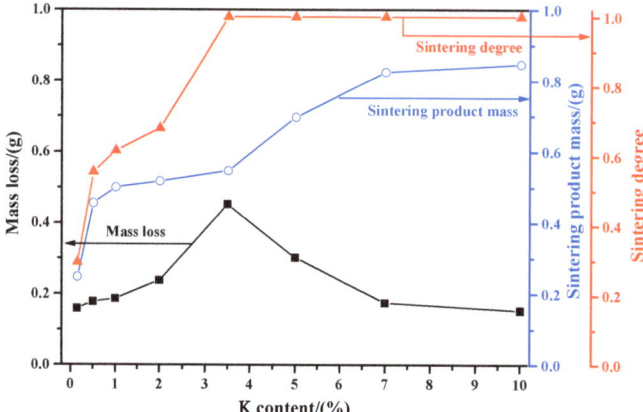

**Figure 2.** Influence of K content on the mass loss and sintering degree of the used mixed sample (roasting temperature: 650 °C).

*2.2. Phase Composition of Sintering Product*

The phase composition of the surface loss sample after the roasting reaction is first checked, and the result shows that it is mainly composed of $MoO_3$; in addition, its morphological structure is observed, and the results demonstrate that it will transform from an irregular granular structure to a platelet-shaped structure as the roasting temperature increases. The results agree well with our previous work [18]. However, since the main task of this work is to investigate the influence of roasting temperature and K content on the sintering behavior of molybdenite concentrate during the oxidation roasting process, the systematic analysis of the two factors on the phase composition of the sintering product is therefore the focus.

2.2.1. Influence of Roasting Temperature

Figure 3 shows the influence of roasting temperature on the phase composition of the sintering product. As observed in Figure 3a, the raw material before the roasting reaction is only $MoS_2$, and the other impurity components are not detected due to their low amount. When the roasting temperature is 550 °C, the result shows that the sintering product is mainly composed of $MoO_3$; in addition, small amounts of $MoS_2$, $MoO_2$, $Mo_4O_{11}$, $K_{0.3}MoO_3$, $K_2MoO_4O_{13}$, and $SiO_2$ also exist (see Figure 3b). Increasing the roasting temperature to 600 °C, the result is similar to that obtained at 550 °C; however, the intensity of the diffraction peak of $MoS_2$ is greatly weakened (see Figure 3c), indicating most of the $MoS_2$ is oxidized. No diffraction peak of $MoS_2$ is detected when the roasting temperature increases to 650 °C. This suggests that all the $MoS_2$ has been completely oxidized or there is little left; even so, the sintering product is still not only composed of $MoO_3$, but also some molybdenum sub-oxides and molybdates (see Figure 3d). When the roasting temperature is 700 °C, the sintering product not only includes all the phases that existed at low temperatures, but some new phases such as $K_4SiO_4$ and $CaSiO_3$ are also observed (see Figure 3e). The appearance of the new phases may be due to the complicated chemical reactions that only occur at high temperatures. Figure 3e also shows that the intensity of the diffraction peak of $SiO_2$ is much stronger than that observed at low temperatures, meaning its relative amount is increased. Further increasing the roasting temperature to 750 °C, it can be seen that the intensity of the diffraction peak of $MoO_3$ is weakened, while that of $K_2MoO_4O_{13}$ is enhanced (see Figure 3f). This result indicates that the amount of $MoO_3$ is decreased and that of $K_2Mo_4O_{13}$ is increased. The reasons for this phenomenon may be due to the strong sublimation effect of $MoO_3$ and the favorable formation conditions for $K_2Mo_4O_{13}$.

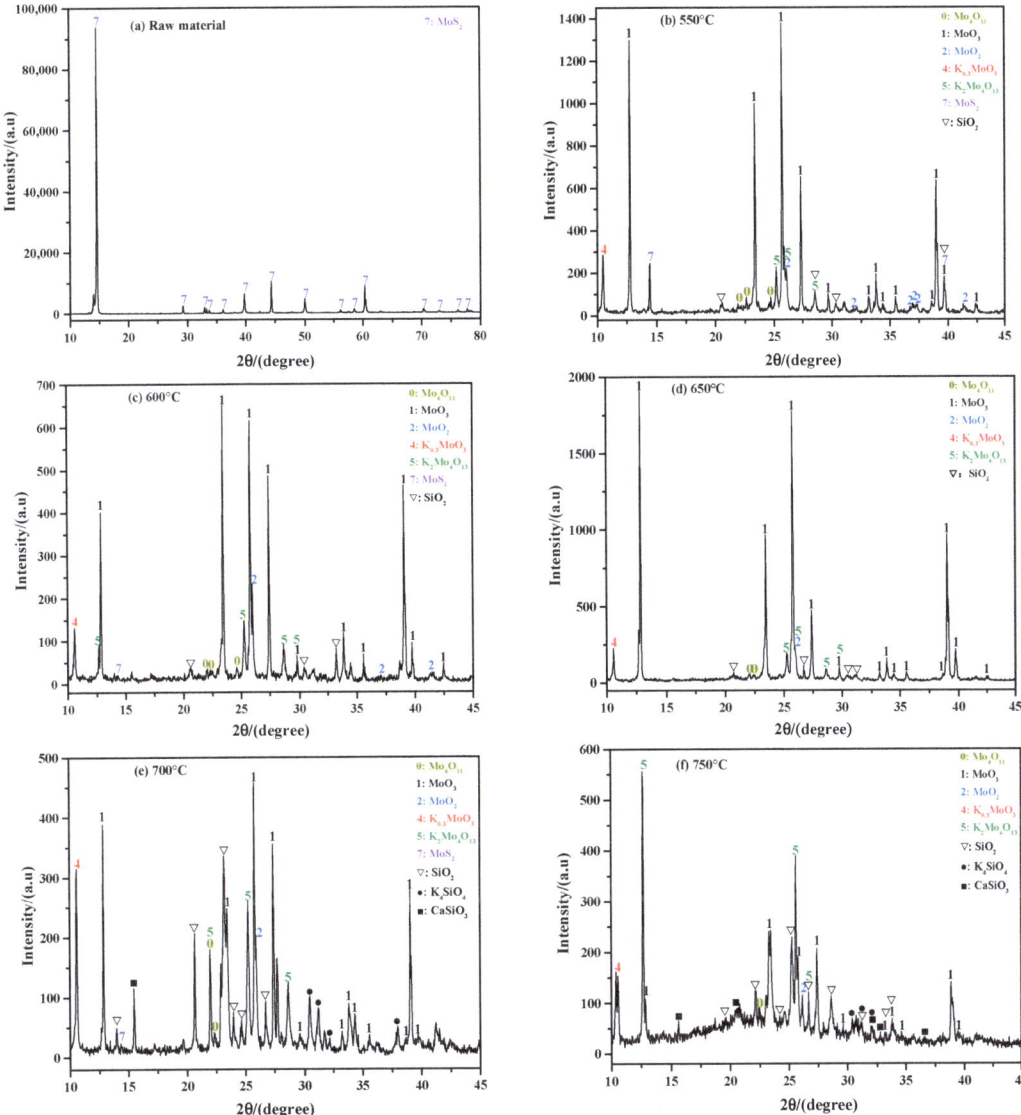

**Figure 3.** XRD patterns of sintering product obtained at different roasting temperatures: (**a**) raw material; (**b**) 550 °C; (**c**) 600 °C; (**d**) 650 °C; (**e**) 700 °C; (**f**) 750 °C. K content: 2%.

2.2.2. Influence of K Content

Figure 4 shows the influence of the K content on the phase composition of the sintering product. When the raw material is used ($\varepsilon_K$ = 0.14%), the results show that the sintering product is mainly $MoO_3$ (see Figure 4a); however, a small amount of other phases such as $MoO_2$ and $K_{0.3}MoO_3$ also exist. The results for the case with $\varepsilon_K$ = 0.5% and 1% are nearly the same as the raw material (see Figure 4b). When the K content increases to 2% ($\varepsilon_K$ = 2%), the result begins to differ, in which the sintering product not only includes all the phases that are observed at low K contents, but some new phases such as $K_2Mo_4O_{13}$ and $SiO_2$ are also detected, as shown in Figure 3d. Further increasing the K content to 3.5% ($\varepsilon_K$ = 3.5%), the phase compositions become more complicated: on one hand, the amount of $K_2Mo_4O_{13}$

is significantly increased; on the other hand, some new molybdates such as $K_2Mo_3O_{10}$ and $K_2Mo_7O_{22}$ appear (see Figure 4c). When the K content is 5% ($\varepsilon_K$ = 5%), the result is similar to that obtained at $\varepsilon_K$ = 3.5%; however, it can also be found that the relative intensity of the $MoO_3$ diffraction peak is significantly decreased, while that of $K_2Mo_4O_{13}$ is increased (see Figure 4d); this indicates that the relative amount of $MoO_3$ in the sintering product is decreased, while that of $K_2Mo_4O_{13}$ increased. The above phenomena become more obvious at a higher K content, where $MoO_3$ could even disappears at $\varepsilon_K$ = 10% (see Figure 4e,f). In addition to molybdates, a large amount of $SiO_2$ and $CaMoO_4$ are also observed at the higher K content conditions, which indicates that the impurities have been enriched at this moment.

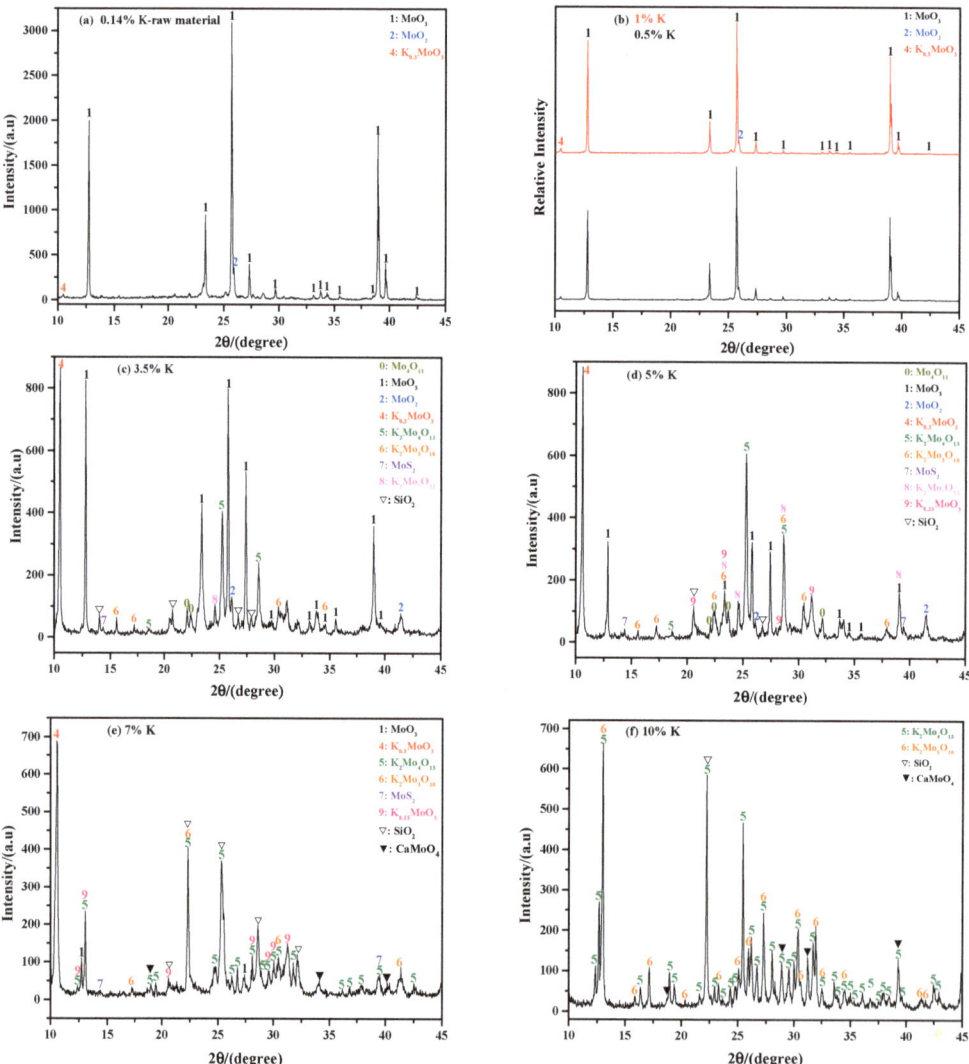

**Figure 4.** XRD patterns of sintering product obtained at different K contents: (**a**) $\varepsilon_K$ = 0.14%, raw material; (**b**) $\varepsilon_K$ = 0.5% and 1%; (**c**) $\varepsilon_K$ = 3.5%; (**d**) $\varepsilon_K$ = 5%; (**e**) $\varepsilon_K$ = 7%; (**f**) $\varepsilon_K$ = 10%. Roasting temperature: 650 °C.

## 2.3. Morphological Structure of Sintering Product

### 2.3.1. Influence of Roasting Temperature

Figure 5 shows the influence of roasting temperature on the morphological structure of the sintering product. From this figure, it can be observed that roasting temperature has no obvious influence on the microstructure, and all of products exhibit a smooth and dense surface structure. The XRD results in Figure 3 show that the main phase composition of the sintering product is $MoO_3$, so it can be deduced that the smooth surface particles are $MoO_3$. Figure 5f is the macroscopic image of the residual sample after the roasting reaction, from which it can be observed that when the roasting temperature is low (550 °C and 600 °C), the residual sample exhibits a golden-yellow color and its surface is relatively loose. When the roasting temperature increases to 650 °C and 700 °C, the results show that the residual sample becomes a light grey color, and a smooth and dense surface structure formed by liquid solidification is clearly observed; in this case, the residual sample is hard to remove from the bottom of the crucible. When the roasting temperature increases to 750 °C, the results show that the mass of the residual sample is very small due to the strong sublimation effect of $MoO_3$, and no obvious smooth structure is observed, while the residual sample is still tightly bound to the bottom of the crucible.

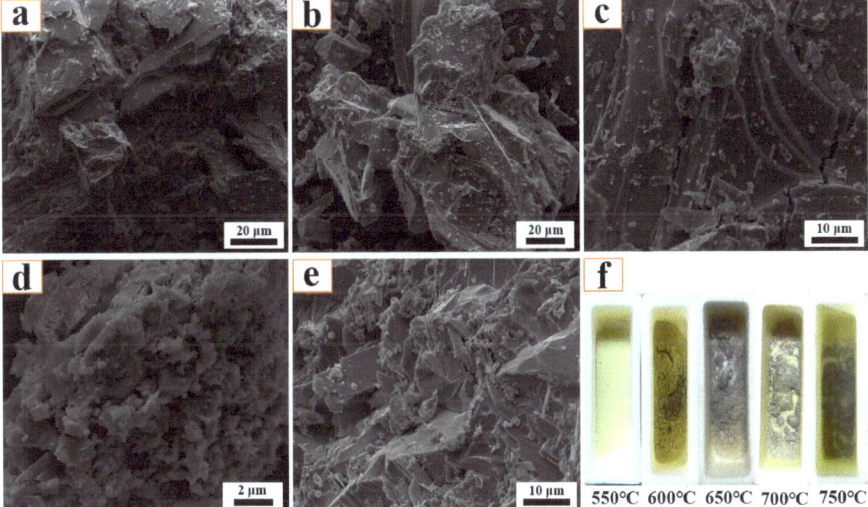

**Figure 5.** Morphological structure of sintering product obtained at different roasting temperatures: (**a**) 550 °C; (**b**) 600 °C; (**c**) 650 °C; (**d**) 700 °C; (**e**) 750 °C; (**f**) Macroscopic image of the residual sample. K content: 2%.

### 2.3.2. Influence of K Content

Figure 6 shows the influence of K content on the morphological structure of the sintering product. Unlike the influence of roasting temperature, Figure 6 demonstrates that the K content has a certain influence on the microscopic structure. When the K content is relatively low (0.14–2%), the results show that the sintering product mainly exhibits a platelet-shaped structure with a large dimension. Combining the XRD results and other references [18], the platelet-shaped product can be deduced to be $MoO_3$. Increasing the K content to a relatively high value (5–10%), the sintering product becomes coarse and the amount of platelet-shaped particles is relatively small, which indicates that the amount of $MoO_3$ is decreased. The above results agree well with the XRD results shown in Figure 4.

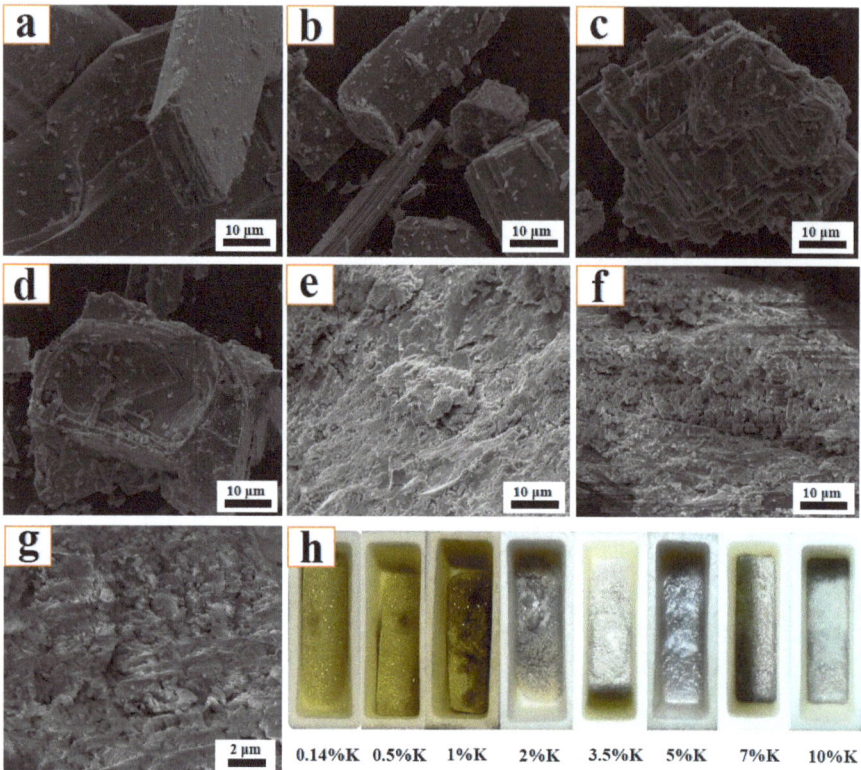

**Figure 6.** Morphological structure of sintering product obtained at different K contents: (**a**) $\varepsilon_K$ = 0.14%, raw material; (**b**) $\varepsilon_K$ = 0.5%; (**c**) $\varepsilon_K$ = 1%; (**d**) $\varepsilon_K$ = 2%; (**e**) $\varepsilon_K$ = 5%; (**f**) $\varepsilon_K$ = 7%; (**g**) $\varepsilon_K$ = 10%; (**h**) Macroscopic image of the residual sample. Roasting temperature: 650 °C.

Figure 6h is a macroscopic image of the residual sample after the roasting reaction. It shows that the residual sample exhibits a golden-yellow color when the K content is below 3.5%, while the surface structure is smoother and denser when the K content is 2% and 3.5%, indicating a large amount of liquid has formed. When the K content increases to 5%, the product's surface appears grey, with the grey color becoming lighter when the K content is further increased (7–10%).

2.3.3. Cross-Section Microstructure

Both Figures 5 and 6 show the three-dimensional microstructure of the sintering product, and the results are beneficial to the qualitative analysis of the sintering degree. To gain insight into the sintering mechanism of molybdenite concentrate, the cross-section microstructure of the sintering product is also analyzed. Herein, the sintering products obtained under the following conditions are selected as the experimental samples: 650 °C and 2% K, 650 °C and 5% K, 650 °C and 7% K, 650 °C and 10% K, as well as 750 °C and 2% K. The corresponding results are displayed in Figure 7. It shows that all the samples reveal various color regions, such as black, light-grey, and light-white, which indicates that the phase composition of the sintering product is complex. From Figure 7, it can also observe that the black phase (which is identified to be $SiO_2$) is not closely connected with the other phases and many cracks/fissures (yellow square area) exist, while the light-grey phase and light-white phase are tightly bonded. The reason for the phenomenon may be due to the different wettabilities between different phases.

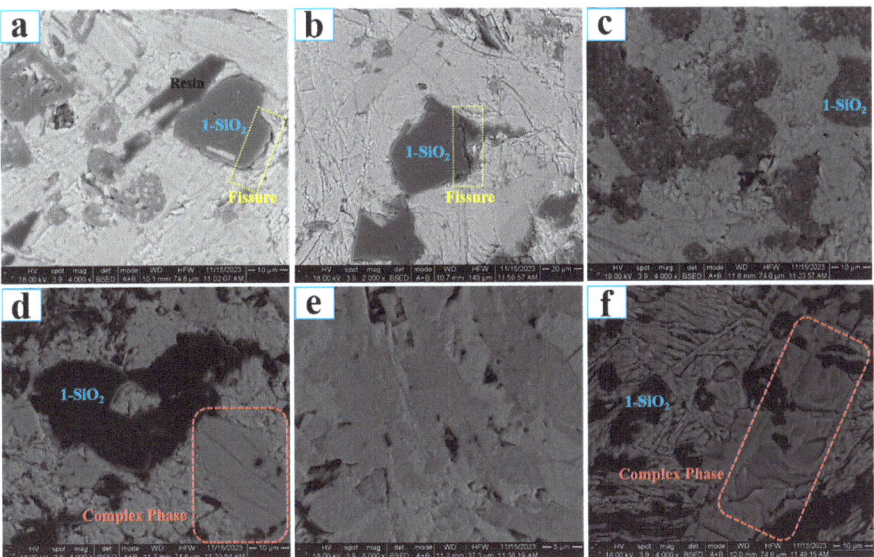

**Figure 7.** FESEM backscattering micrographs of the cross-section of the sintering product obtained under different conditions: (**a**) 650 °C, $\varepsilon_K$ = 2%; (**b**) 650 °C, $\varepsilon_K$ = 5%; (**c**) 650 °C, $\varepsilon_K$ = 7%; (**d**) 650 °C, $\varepsilon_K$ = 10%; (**e**) 650 °C, $\varepsilon_K$ = 10%; (**f**) 750 °C, $\varepsilon_K$ = 2%.

In order to identify the elemental distribution and possible phase composition of different color areas, EDS area scanning maps are used. In this section, sintering products obtained under the following conditions were selected as the experimental samples: 650 °C and 2% K, 650 °C and 10% K, as well as 750 °C and 2% K. The corresponding map scanning results are presented in Figures 8–10, respectively. In the case of 650 °C and 2% K, Figure 8 shows that the main elements are O and Si in the black area, indicating the existence of $SiO_2$. The oxidation roasting of molybdenite concentrate in air/oxygen atmosphere was investigated in our previous work [18], and the results found that $SiO_2$ also existed in the molybdenum calcine. If the molybdenum calcine contains $SiO_2$, undoubtedly, the $SiO_2$ will also remain in the sintering product. As for the light-grey and light-white areas, Figure 8 shows that the main elements are Mo and S, indicating the existence of unreacted $MoS_2$; furthermore, partial K, Ca, and Mg are also detected in the two regions. Al and Fe are uniformly distributed in the whole field of view. With the increase in the K content to 10%, the main elements in the black area are O, Si, and Al (see Figure 9). The appearance of the additional Al element may be due to the complicated chemical reaction that occurred under the higher K content condition. Some overlapping areas between elements, namely Al and Fe, are also observed (marked by red squares in Figure 7d), indicating that the two elements could combine with each other to form a eutectic. In the case of 750 °C and 2% K, the results show that the phase of the black region is $SiO_2$, and Al and Fe also have some overlapping regions (see Figure 10), which is similar to the results shown in Figure 9. However, in this case, elements Al and Si have no obvious overlapping regions. According to the above results, it can be inferred that a higher K content is the prerequisite for the mutual solution of Al and Si; the above results also suggest that the K content has a more significant influence on the sintering behavior than roasting temperature. However, the elements of Al, Fe, and Mg are not detected in the XRD patterns, which may be due to their low amounts, which can even be below the detection limits of XRD measurement.

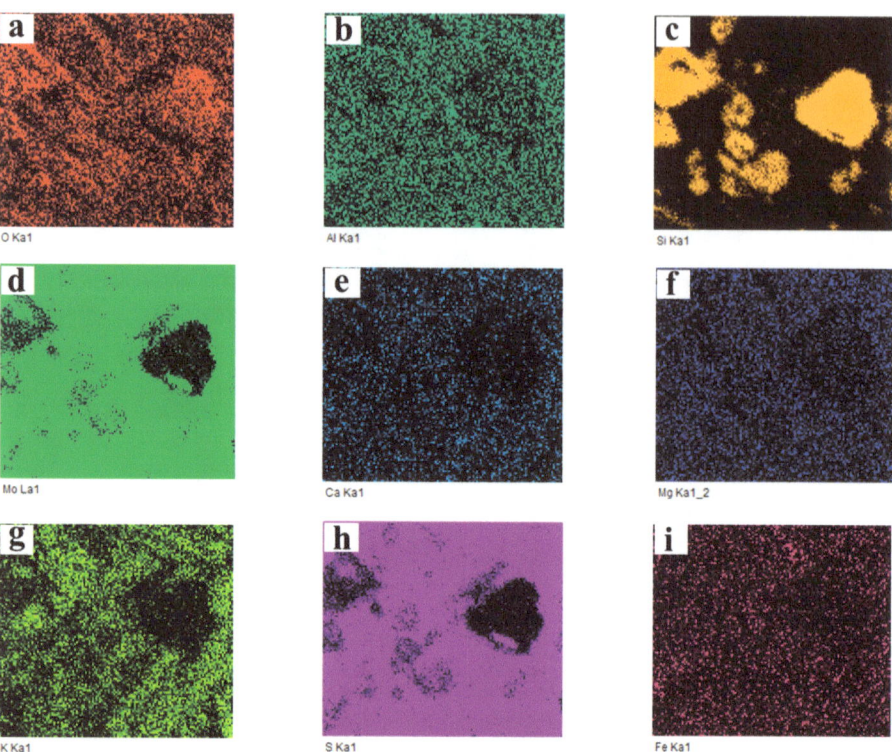

**Figure 8.** Map scanning result of the cross-section of the sintering product shown in Figure 7a: (**a**) O; (**b**) Al; (**c**) Si; (**d**) Mo; (**e**) Ca; (**f**) Mg; (**g**) K; (**h**) S; (**i**) Fe. (650 °C, $\varepsilon_K = 2\%$).

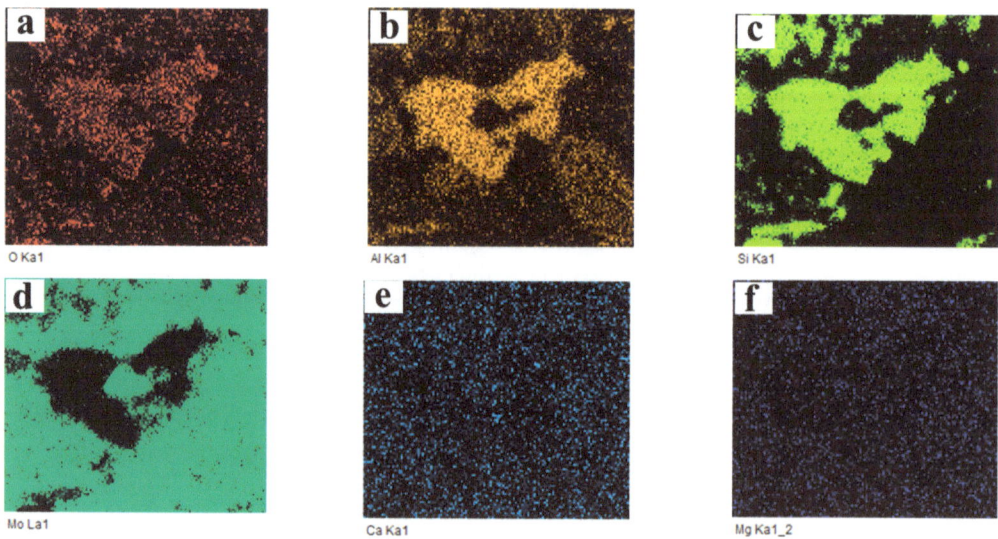

**Figure 9.** *Cont.*

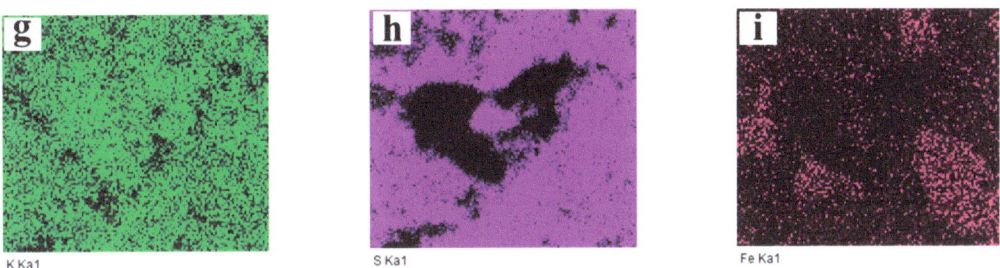

**Figure 9.** Map scanning result of the cross-section of the sintering product shown in Figure 7d: (**a**) O; (**b**) Al; (**c**) Si; (**d**) Mo; (**e**) Ca; (**f**) Mg; (**g**) K; (**h**) S; (**i**) Fe. (650 °C, $\varepsilon_K$ = 10%).

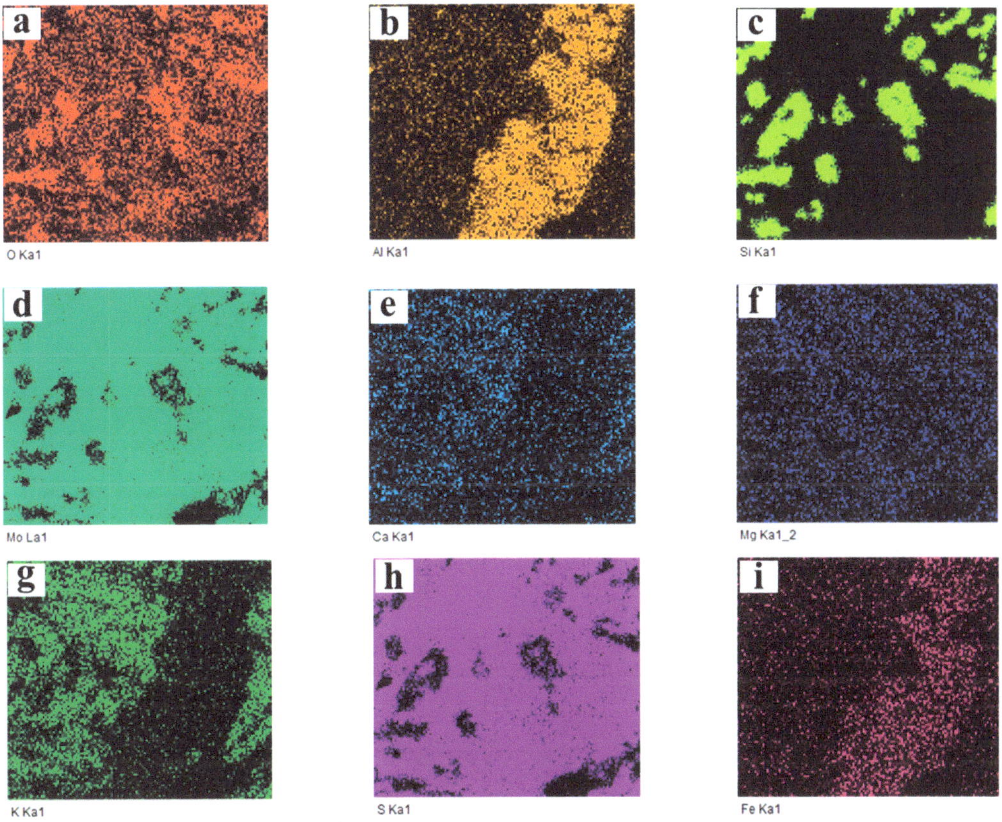

**Figure 10.** Map scanning result of the cross-section of the sintering product shown in Figure 7f: (**a**) O; (**b**) Al; (**c**) Si; (**d**) Mo; (**e**) Ca; (**f**) Mg; (**g**) K; (**h**) S; (**i**) Fe. (750 °C, $\varepsilon_K$ = 2%).

## 3. Discussion

### 3.1. Ammonia Leaching of Sintering Product

As mentioned above, the phase composition of the sintering product is very complicated, as it not only includes various molybdenum oxides, but also unreacted $MoS_2$ and other impurities. To analyze the sintering product and illustrate the sintering mechanism in detail, an ammonia leaching treatment is conducted. The treating process is described as follows: first, a certain amount of sintering product is mixed with 20 mL ammonia solution, with a stirring time of 2 h; second, the mixed solution is filtered by a vacuum filter and washed with deionized water and anhydrous ethanol several times; then, the leaching residue is dried at 110 °C in a drying oven for 8 h; finally, the masses of the used sintering product and obtained ammonia leaching residue are recorded, respectively. After that, the leaching rate (defined as the ratio of the leached mass to the initial mass of used sintering product) of the sintering product is calculated.

3.1.1. Influence of Roasting Temperature

Figure 11 shows the ammonia leaching rates of the sintering products obtained at different roasting temperatures. From this figure, it can be found that the leaching rate is gradually increased with the increase in roasting temperature at a value below 700 °C. Specifically, when the roasting temperatures are 550 °C, 600 °C, 650 °C, and 700 °C, their leaching rates are 79.57%, 88.58%, 91.59%, and 92.34%, respectively. On one hand, both $MoO_3$ and partial molybdates can be dissolved in ammonia solution; on the other hand, the amount of $MoO_3$ dominates in the sintering product according to the above XRD results, so the value of the leaching rate may be considered as the amount of exiting $MoO_3$ (in fact, it is a litter bigger). That is, the higher the roasting temperature is, the larger the amount of existing $MoO_3$ will be. However, when the roasting temperature is increased to 750 °C, the leaching rate is decreased to a value of only 66.58%. The XRD results in Figure 3f show that the intensity of the $MoO_3$ diffraction peak is extremely weak, which also indicates that the amount of $MoO_3$ in the sintering product obtained at 750 °C is relatively small. All in all, the results of the ammonia leaching rates are consistent with the XRD results shown in Figure 3.

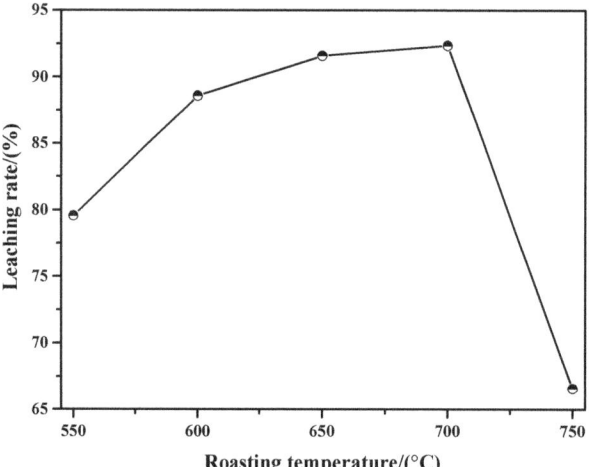

**Figure 11.** Results of the ammonia leaching rate of sintering product obtained at different roasting temperatures.

3.1.2. Influence of K Content

Figure 12 shows the results of the ammonia leaching rates of the sintering products obtained at different K contents. From this figure, it can be found that the ammonia leaching rate is gradually decreased with the increase in K content. Specifically, when the K contents are 0.14% (raw material), 0.5%, 2%, 5%, 7%, and 10%, the values are 93.96%, 93.65%, 91.59%, 91.13%, 90.33%, and 90.05%, respectively. The results also show that the amount of $MoO_3$ in the sintering product is gradually decreased with the increasing K content. The reason for this phenomenon may be due to the rapid formation of insoluble $CaMoO_4$ between

MoO$_3$ and Ca containing impurities. Similarly, the current results agree well with the XRD results shown in Figure 4.

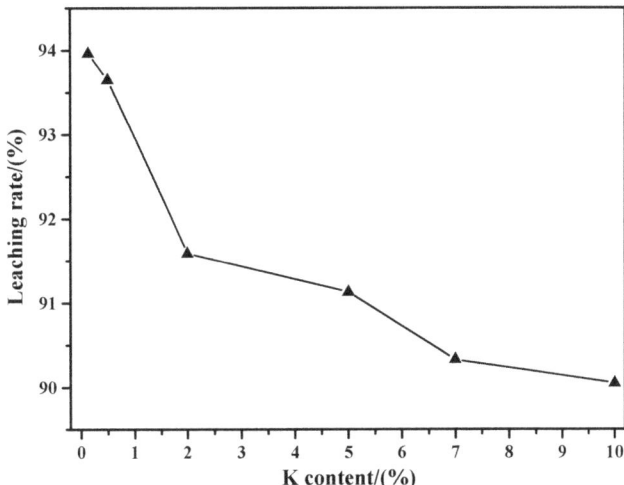

**Figure 12.** Results of the ammonia leaching rate of sintering products obtained at different K contents.

*3.2. Phase Composition of Ammonia Leaching Residue*

3.2.1. Influence of Roasting Temperature

Figure 13 shows the phase compositions of the ammonia leaching residues of sintering products obtained at different roasting temperatures. At 550 °C, the XRD results show that the intensity of the MoO$_2$ diffraction peak is the strongest, indicating that MoO$_2$ is the main component of the ammonia leaching residue; in addition, small amounts of MoS$_2$, SiO$_2$, and Mo$_4$O$_{11}$ are also included (see Figure 13a). When compared with the XRD result in Figure 3b, it is found that the components of MoO$_3$, K$_{0.3}$MoO$_3$, and K$_2$Mo$_4$O$_{13}$ are absent, which indicates that the three components are easily soluble in ammonia solution. When the roasting temperature is 600 °C, the results show that MoO$_2$ still has the largest amount, and the components of MoS$_2$, SiO$_2$, and Mo$_4$O$_{11}$ still exist (see Figure 13b). The only difference is that a lot of CaMoO$_4$ appears at this temperature. However, the phase of CaMoO$_4$ is not detected in the sintering product according to Figure 3c; the reason for this phenomenon may be due to its extremely low amount in the sintering product. The above results also indicate that the ammonia leaching treatment could not only estimate the content of phase that could be dissolved in ammonia solution, but could also enrich and identify potential phases with present in relatively low amounts. When the roasting temperature is 700 °C, the phase composition of the ammonia leaching residue is the same as that obtained at 600 °C, while the main components are transformed into SiO$_2$ and CaMoO$_4$ instead, which can be clearly deduced from their strong diffraction peak intensities (see Figure 13c). Further increasing the roasting temperature to 750 °C, both SiO$_2$ and CaMoO$_4$ are still the main components, while the amount of CaMoO$_4$ dominates (see Figure 13d). In combination with Figure 3e,f, it can be observed that the phases of K$_4$SiO$_4$ and CaSiO$_3$ disappear, suggesting that both of them have a strong solubility in ammonia solution.

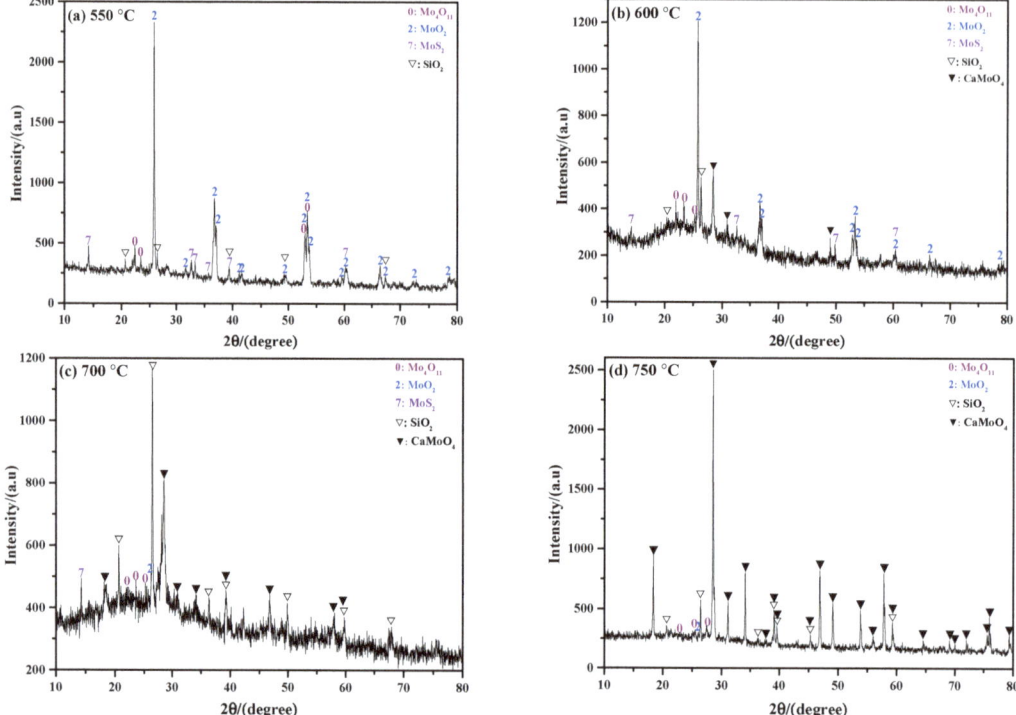

**Figure 13.** Phase composition of the ammonia leaching residue of sintering products obtained at different roasting temperatures: (**a**) 550 °C; (**b**) 600 °C; (**c**) 700 °C; (**d**) 750 °C. K content: 2%.

3.2.2. Influence of K Content

To analyze the influence of K content on the phase composition of ammonia leaching residue, the sintering products obtained at the K contents of 2%, 3.5%, 7%, and 10% were selected as reference materials, and the corresponding XRD results are presented in Figure 14. From the figure, it can be seen that the main phase compositions are $SiO_2$, $CaMoO_4$, $Mo_4O_{11}$, and $MoO_2$; among them, the amount of $SiO_2$ dominates in the ammonia leaching residue. In fact, partial $MoS_2$ may also be present, although it is not detected due to its relatively small amount. Combining Figures 13 and 14, it can be concluded that roasting temperature has a more significant influence than K content on the phase composition of the ammonia leaching residue: when the roasting temperatures are in the range of 550–600 °C, 650–700 °C, and above 750 °C, the dominant phases in the ammonia leaching residue are $MoO_2$, $SiO_2$, and $CaMoO_4$, respectively.

*3.3. Sintering Mechanism Analysis*

During the oxidation roasting process of molybdenite concentrate, the higher the roasting temperature is, the faster the formation rate of $MoO_3$ will be; thus, there will also be a higher content of $MoO_3$ in sintering product. In addition, due to the strong exothermic effect of the oxidation roasting process of molybdenite concentrate, at a higher roasting temperature, more heat will be released, which may lead to a rapid increase in the local reaction temperature. Once the temperature is higher than the melting point of $MoO_3$ (795 °C) [26–28], the generated $MoO_3$ will be melted. The liquid $MoO_3$ can adsorb the incompletely oxidized $MoS_2$ and other solid impurity particles around it, resulting in the occurrence of the sintering phenomenon. During the sintering process, the incompletely oxidized $MoS_2$ can react with $MoO_3$ to form $MoO_2$ (see Equation (6)) [29–31]. This is an important reason for the existence of MoO$_2$ in the sintering product. Therefore, in order to reduce the occurrence of the sintering phenomenon, the roasting temperature should not be too high. However, if the roasting temperature is too low, the oxidation rate of molybdenite concentrate will be greatly decreased and then a longer time is required for the completion of the oxidation reaction; In addition, a low roasting temperature can easily lead to the incomplete oxidation of MoS$_2$, which will not only reduce the production efficiency, but also increase the amount of residual sulfur in molybdenum calcine. Therefore, the roasting temperature should also not be too low [32]. According to the results of the current work and the practices in industrial production, this work believes that 650 °C is a good choice.

$$MoS_2 + 6MoO_3 = 7MoO_2 + 2SO_2 \qquad (6)$$

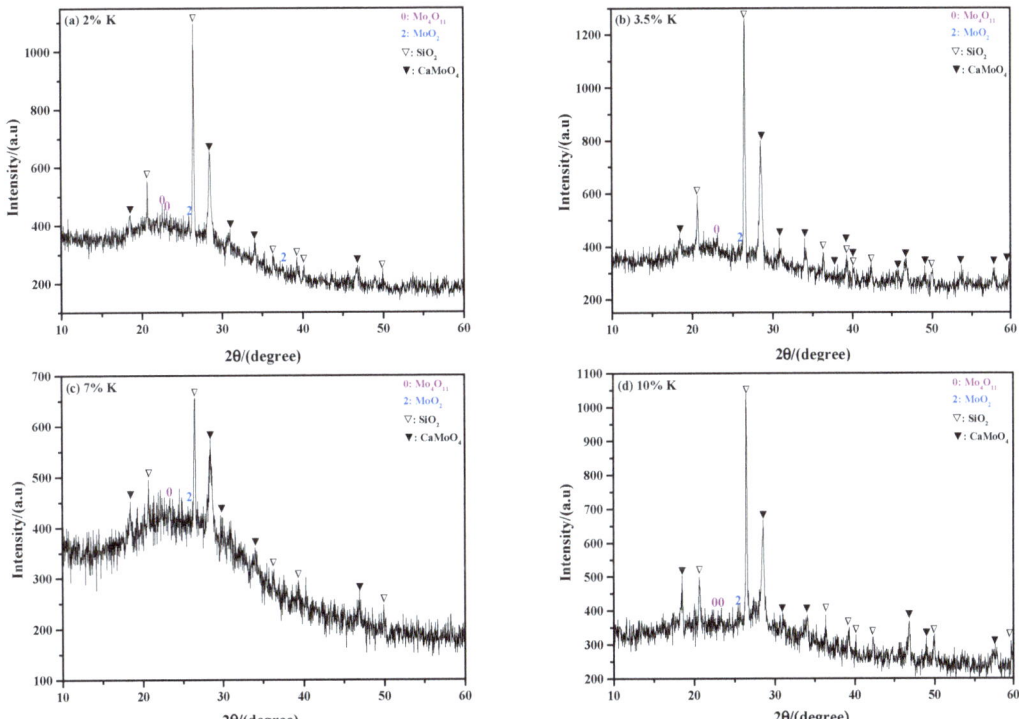

**Figure 14.** Phase composition of the ammonia leaching residues of sintering products obtained at different K contents: (**a**) 2% K; (**b**) 3.5% K; (**c**) 7% K; (**d**) 10% K. Roasting temperature: 650 °C.

K$_2$CO$_3$ is easily decomposed into potassium oxide in a high-temperature environment; in this situation, the reactive activity of the newly formed potassium oxide is relatively high, which will make it easy to react with MoO$_3$ to form K$_2$MoO$_4$ during the oxidation roasting process of molybdenite concentrate. The generated K$_2$MoO$_4$ may further react with MoO$_3$ again to form various eutectics, as can be supported by the binary phase diagram between K$_2$MoO$_4$ and MoO$_3$ see Figure 15 [19,20,33], which shows that the eutectics such as K$_2$Mo$_4$O$_{13}$ (3MoO$_3$·K$_2$MoO$_4$), K$_2$Mo$_3$O$_{10}$ (2MoO$_3$·K$_2$MoO$_4$), and K$_2$Mo$_2$O$_7$ (MoO$_3$·K$_2$MoO$_4$) can be formed with the increase in K$_2$MoO$_4$). Figure 15 also shows that when the contents of K$_2$MoO$_4$ are 21%, 28%, 48%, and 62%, the melting points of the eutectics are 558 °C, 542 °C, 490 °C, and 480 °C, respectively. These temperatures are not only lower than the melting point of MoO$_3$, but also lower than the used experimental temperatures. In other words, K$_2$MoO$_4$ can form a variety of low-melting-point eutectics with MoO$_3$, and their melting points are gradually decreased with the increase in K$_2$MoO$_4$. Once the above low-melting-point eutectics are formed, they will be rapidly melted within the temperature range of this work. Obviously, their melting speeds are faster than that of MoO$_3$. After melting, the liquid low-melting-point eutectics are more likely to entrain the solid particles (MoO$_2$, SiO$_2$, and MoS$_2$, etc.) around them to form complex molten salt mixtures, in which some reactions may occur to produce various silicates (such as K$_4$SiO$_4$ and CaSiO$_3$) and molybdates (such as CaMoO$_4$). Therefore, with the increase in K content, the sintering phenomenon will become more and more serious.

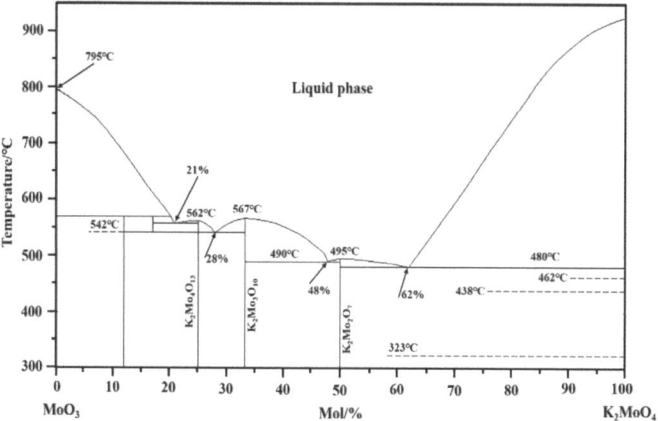

**Figure 15.** Phase diagram for the K$_2$MoO$_4$–MoO$_3$ binary system [19,20,33].

In our previous work [19], the influence of K content on the sintering behavior of pure MoS$_2$ during the oxidation roasting process was investigated, and the results showed that the sintering degree was 0.6 under the conditions of 650 °C and 2% K. In the current work, the sintering degree is 0.68 under the same temperature and K content conditions, which is higher than the value reported in our previous work. Moreover, the sample mass used in the previous work is 5 g, while that used in the current work is 1 g; that is to say, the sample thickness used in our previous work was thicker than that used in the current work under the same crucible conditions. When the used sample (molybdenite concentrate) has the same thickness as our previous work, Bu's work [20] found that the sintering degree was up to 0.8 under the same temperature and K content conditions. The results of the current and previous work once again conclude that sample thickness and impurity elements have important influences on the occurrence of sintering phenomena. In addition, the interactions between different impurities (such as Ca, Fe, Pb, Al, etc.) will also occur, and thus a eutectic composed of three or four elements or even more may be formed. This speculation can be confirmed by the images of the cross-section microstructures of the sintering products shown in Figures 7–10. The melting point of the multicomponent eutectic may be much lower than that of the binary system. In this case, they are easier to melt, leading to the occurrence of sintering phenomena, which is another reason why the sintering degree is higher when molybdenite concentrate is used as the raw material.

Due to the fact that both SiO$_2$ and MoO$_3$ are acidic oxides, no reactions between them will occur during the sintering process. In addition, due to the insolubility of SiO$_2$ in ammonia solution, the excess Si can exist in the form of SiO$_2$ in both the sintering product and the ammonia leaching residue. Ca impurities in the molybdenite concentrate generally exist in the form of alkaline oxide or sulfide, and its sulfide will be oxidized into an oxide during the process, so Ca impurities can combine with MoO$_3$ to form CaMoO$_4$, which can remain in the ammonia leaching residue due to its insolubility in ammonia solution. The XRD results in Figure 13d show that the relative amount of CaMoO$_4$ is higher under the high-temperature conditions, so it can be speculated that increasing the roasting temperature is conducive to the formation of CaMoO$_4$. Even if Ca impurities have a certain influence on the sintering behavior of molybdenite concentrate, as reported by [19,20], when compared with K impurities, the degree of influence of Ca is negligible. In fact, it is difficult for us to completely abolish the occurrence of sintering phenomena during the industrial production process; however, decreasing the degree of sintering is still possible. Herein, the work believes that decreasing the roasting temperature and the content of elemental impurities, especially for K, are effective choices.

## 4. Materials and Experimental Procedure

### 4.1. Materials

Molybdenite concentrate from Jinduicheng Molybdenum Industry Co., Ltd., Xi'an, China, was used as the raw material. The main elemental components of molybdenite are Mo and S with respective contents of 54.89% and 33.27%. In addition, other impurities components such as Pb (0.08%), Si (1.83%), Cu (0.07%), Ca (0.28%), Fe (1.12%), Al (0.19%), K (0.14%), Ti (0.04%), C (0.17%), and P (0.01%) are also included. The XRD results show that the raw material is mainly composed of MoS$_2$, and the FESEM imaging shows that it has a layered structure with a wide size distribution ranging from several microns to 100 μm [18].

To investigate the influence of K content on the sintering behavior, a small amount of extra K was added into the raw material in the form of K$_2$CO$_3$. According to the content of K, the mass of the added K$_2$CO$_3$ was calculated using the following Equation (7):

$$m_{K_2CO_3} = \frac{M_{K_2CO_3}}{2M_K} \cdot m_{total} \cdot \varepsilon_K \quad (7)$$

where $m_{K_2CO_3}$ is the mass of added K$_2$CO$_3$, g; $M_{K_2CO_3}$ is the relative molecular mass of K$_2$CO$_3$, g/mol; $M_K$ is the relative atomic mass of element K, g/mol; $m_{total}$ is the total mass of molybdenite concentrate and added K$_2$CO$_3$ (herein, its value is fixed to be 1 g); and $\varepsilon_K$ is the total content of element K, %.

Since the initial K content (0.14%) in molybdenite concentrate is lower than the XRD detection limit, to explore the evolution behavior of K-containing compounds during the roasting process, the K content must be enlarged. Moreover, a higher K content could lead to a larger mass of the sintering product; in this case, weighing errors can be greatly reduced and the sintering degree can be easily evaluated. Therefore, the K content was selected from 1 to 10% in this work. Based on the different K contents, the masses of molybdenite concentrate and added K$_2$CO$_3$ can be calculated, and the corresponding results are listed in Table 1.

**Table 1.** The masses of used molybdenite concentrate and added K$_2$CO$_3$.

| Total K Content, $\varepsilon_K$/% | 0.14 | 0.5 | 1 | 2 | 3.5 | 5 | 7 | 10 |
|---|---|---|---|---|---|---|---|---|
| Mass of molybdenite concentrate/g | 1 | 0.9936 | 0.9847 | 0.9670 | 0.9405 | 0.9138 | 0.8783 | 0.8251 |
| Mass of added K$_2$CO$_3$/g | 0 | 0.0064 | 0.0153 | 0.0330 | 0.0595 | 0.0862 | 0.1217 | 0.1749 |

Note: 0.14% is the initial K content in the raw material.

### 4.2. Experimental Procedure

In order to simulate the oxidation roasting process of molybdenite concentrate in multiple-hearth furnace, muffle furnace was selected as the experimental equipment in the work. In each of the experimental run, the mass of molybdenite concentrate and required K$_2$CO$_3$ were first weighed according to Table 1, and then the mixture of them were put into an agate mortar and grinded for 30 min; after that, the mixed sample was loaded into an alumina crucible with the dimension of 50 mm × 20 mm × 20 mm, and then the sample-containing crucible was put into the center of muffle furnace, the temperature of which is aforehand raised to the desired value. When the sample was oxidized completely (herein, the roasting time was enough, about 3 h), taking out the reaction product and cooling it to room temperature. The masses of the residual sample and the surface loose sample were weighed, respectively. To explore the influence of roasting temperature on the sintering behavior, the mixed sample with the K content of 2% was used as the reference material, and the roasting temperatures were set as 550 °C, 600 °C, 650 °C, 700 °C, and 750 °C.

*4.3. Characterization Methods*

The phase composition of the sintering product was analyzed by X-ray diffraction analyzer (XRD; XPert PRO MPD PANalytical; Netherlands; sweep speed: 10°/min; operation voltage: 30 kV; operation current: 30 mA). The morphological structure of the sintering product was observed by field emission scanning electron microscope (FESEM; Thermo Fisher, Waltham, MA, USA; FEI Corporation, Hillsboro, OR, USA; operation voltage: 18 kV).

## 5. Conclusions

In this work, the influence of roasting temperature and K content on the sintering behavior of molybdenite concentrate during the oxidation roasting process in an air atmosphere was investigated. The following conclusions are drawn:

(1) When the roasting temperature is in the range of 550 °C to 700 °C, the mass loss of the molybdenite concentrate, the mass of the sintering product, and the sintering degree are all increased with the increase in roasting temperature. Meanwhile, when the roasting temperature is above 750 °C, the mass of the sintering product is decreased due to the intense sublimation effect of $MoO_3$.

(2) With the increase in K content, the mass loss of molybdenite concentrate is increased first and then gradually decreased. The maximum mass loss is reached at a K content of 3.5% with a sintering degree close to 1. This work also found that the sintering product mass is continuously increased with the increase in K content.

(3) The phase composition of sintering product has a certain relationship with the roasting temperature and K content. In general, the sintering product not only contains a large amount of $MoO_3$, but also contains numerous unoxidized $MoS_2$, molybdenum suboxide, $SiO_2$, and various molybdates; among these, most of the $MoO_3$ and molybdates can be removed after ammonia leaching treatment.

(4) The occurrence of the sintering phenomenon is due to the increase in local reaction temperature and the formation of various low-melting-point eutectics. This work also finds that decreasing the roasting temperature and K content, especially the K content, are effective strategies to reduce the sintering degree of molybdenite concentrate during the oxidation roasting process.

**Author Contributions:** J.L.: writing—review and editing, funding acquisition; L.W.: conceptualization, methodology, investigation, writing—original draft, funding acquisition, project administration; G.W.: validation, data curation. All authors have read and agreed to the published version of the manuscript.

**Funding:** The authors gratefully acknowledge the financial support for this work from the Fujian Natural Science Foundation (2024J01911) and the National Natural Science Foundation of China (52104310).

**Institutional Review Board Statement:** Not applicable.

**Informed Consent Statement:** Not applicable.

**Data Availability Statement:** The raw data can be provided as requested upon reasonable request.

**Conflicts of Interest:** The authors declare no conflicts of interest.

## References

1. Fu, X.K.; Sun, B.; Yang, M.; Yan, J.; Han, X.B.; Zhai, Y.H.; Wang, W.A.; Li, X.M. Thickening mechanism of furnace bed bottom material of multi-hearth furnace oxidation roasting for molybdenum concentrate metallurgy. *China Nonferr. Metall.* **2023**, *52*, 73–80.
2. Liu, H.Z.; Wang, H.F.; Zhang, B.; Wang, W.; Cao, Y.H.; Liu, L.; Wang, H.L. Distribution characteristic of Re during molybdenum concentrate roasting in multiple heart furnace. *Nonferr. Met. (Extr. Metall.)* **2020**, *6*, 48–52.
3. Li, H.X.; Wang, L.; Xue, Z.L. A novel way for preparing hexagonal-shaped $Mo_2N$ by $NH_3$ reduction of Fe-doped $h-MoO_3$. *Metall. Mater. Trans. B* **2024**, *55*, 2378–2387. [CrossRef]
4. Yang, H.; Ding, Z.; Li, Y.T.; Li, S.Y.; Wu, P.K.; Hou, Q.H.; Zheng, Y.; Gao, B.; Huo, K.F.; Du, W.J. Recent advances in kinetic and thermodynamic regulation of magnesium hydride for hydrogen storage. *Rare Met.* **2023**, *42*, 2906–2927. [CrossRef]
5. Rakass, S.; Oudghiri Hassani, H.; Abboudi, M.; Kooli, F.; Mohmoud, A.; Aljuhani, A.; Al Wadaani, F. Molybdenum trioxide: Efficient nanosorbent for removal of methylene blue dye from aqueous solutions. *Molecules* **2018**, *23*, 2295. [CrossRef]
6. Liu, X.; Wang, L.; Xue, Z.L. Parameter optimization of ultrafine molybdenum powder during hydrogen reduction of $MoO_2$ based on central composite design method. *Int. J. Refract. Met. Hard Mater.* **2024**, *124*, 106845. [CrossRef]
7. Ding, Z.; Li, Y.; Yang, H.; Lu, Y.; Tan, J.; Li, J.; Li, Q.; Chen, Y.; Shaw, L.L.; Pan, F. Tailoring $MgH_2$ for hydrogen storage through nanoengineering and catalysis. *J. Magnes. Alloys* **2022**, *10*, 2946–2967. [CrossRef]
8. Wang, L.Y.; Zhang, J.F.; Cai, J.J.; Sun, H.C.; Liu, Y. Study on mechanism of molybdenum concentrate roasting. *China Molybdenum Ind.* **2011**, *35*, 17–19. [CrossRef]
9. Utigard, T. Oxidation mechanism of molybdenite concentrate. *Metall. Mater. Trans. B* **2009**, *40*, 490–496. [CrossRef]
10. Wang, Q.; Liu, C.H.; Zhang, L.B.; Gao, J.Y.; Wang, F.; Dai, Y. Preparation and mechanism of molybdenum trioxide by microwave oxidation roasting of molybdenite. *Chin. J. Nonferr. Met.* **2023**, *33*, 2015–2030.
11. Gan, M.; Fan, X.H.; Zhang, L.; Jiang, T.; Qiu, G.Z.; Wang, Y.; Deng, Q.; Chen, X.L. Reaction behavior of low grade molybdenum concentrates in oxidation roasting process. *Chin. J. Nonferr. Met.* **2014**, *24*, 3115–3122.
12. Sun, H.; Li, G.H.; Bu, Q.Z.; Fu, Z.Q.; Liu, H.B.; Zhang, X.; Luo, J.; Rao, M.J.; Jiang, T. Features and mechanisms of self-sintering of molybdenite during oxidative roasting. *Trans. Nonferr. Met. Soc. China* **2022**, *32*, 307–318. [CrossRef]
13. Li, X.M.; Zhai, Y.H.; Zou, C.; Wang, W.A.; Lin, B. Effect of impurity compounds on sintering behavior of molybdenum concentrate during roasting process. *Chin. J. Nonferr. Met.* **2024**, *34*, 549–560.
14. Ammann, P.R.; Loose, T.A. The oxidation kinetics of molybdenite at 525° to 635 °C. *Metall. Trans.* **1971**, *2*, 889–893. [CrossRef]
15. Marin, T.; Utigard, T.; Hernandez, C. Roasting kinetics of molybdenite concentrates. *Can. Metall. Q.* **2009**, *48*, 73–80. [CrossRef]
16. Fu, Y.F.; Xiao, Q.G.; Gao, Y.Y.; Ning, P.G.; Xu, H.B.; Zhang, Y. Pressure aqueous oxidation of molybdenite concentrate with oxygen. *Hydrometallurgy* **2017**, *174*, 131–139. [CrossRef]
17. Blanco, E.; Sohn, H.Y.; Han, G.; Hakobyan, K.Y. The kinetics of oxidation of molybdenite concentrate by water vapor. *Metall. Mater. Trans. B* **2007**, *38*, 689–693. [CrossRef]
18. Wang, L.; Zhang, G.H.; Dang, J.; Chou, K.C. Oxidation roasting of molybdenite concentrate. *Trans. Nonferr. Met. Soc. China* **2015**, *25*, 4167–4174. [CrossRef]
19. Wang, L.; Zhang, G.H.; Wang, J.S.; Chou, K.C. Influences of different components on agglomeration behavior of $MoS_2$ during oxidation roasting process in Air. *Metall. Mater. Trans. B* **2016**, *47*, 2421–2432. [CrossRef]
20. Bu, C.Y.; Cao, W.C.; Wang, L.; Zhang, G.H.; Sun, G.D.; Wang, D.H.; Chang, H.Q.; Song, C.M.; Zhou, G.Z.; He, K. Study on the sintering phenomenon during the roasting processes of molybdenite by air. *China Molybdenum Ind.* **2018**, *42*, 8–11.
21. Liu, Q.H.; Tian, S.Z.; Yang, S.P.; Wang, L.D.; He, K. Potassium release mechanism of potassium-bearing minerals in ammonium molybdate production process. *Chin. J. Process Eng.* **2022**, *22*, 1271–1278.
22. Liu, Q.H.; Liu, R.L.; Yang, S.P.; He, K.; Wang, L.D. Thermodynamic behavior and analysis of typical impurity elements in the roasting process of molybdenum concentrate. *J. Chongqing Univ.* **2023**, *46*, 89–100.
23. Li, G.H.; Huang, J.H.; Sun, H.; Mang, C.Y.; Hou, Y.R.; Luo, J. Phase and structure optimizations of MoS2 concentrate pellets with $Al_2O_3$-$SiO_2$ additives during oxidative and volatilizing roasting process. *JOM* **2023**, *75*, 5167–5175. [CrossRef]
24. Sun, H.; Li, G.; Yu, J.; Luo, J.; Rao, M.; Peng, Z.; Zhang, Y.; Jiang, T. Preparation of high purity $MoO_3$ through volatilization of technical-grade Mo calcine in water vapor atmosphere. *Int. J. Refract. Met. Hard Mater.* **2018**, *77*, 1–7. [CrossRef]
25. Chychko, A.; Teng, L.; Seetharaman, S. $MoO_3$ evaporation studies from binary systems towards choice of Mo precursors in EAF. *Steel Res. Int.* **2010**, *81*, 784–791. [CrossRef]
26. Shibata, K.; Tsuchida, K.; Kato, A. Preparation of ultrafine molybdenum powder by vapour phase reaction of the $MoO_3$-$H_2$ system. *J. Less Common Met.* **1990**, *157*, L5–L10. [CrossRef]
27. Chiang, T.H.; Yeh, H.C. The synthesis of α-$MoO_3$ by ethylene glycol. *Materials* **2013**, *6*, 4609–4625. [CrossRef]
28. Silveira, J.; Moura, J.; Luz-Lima, C.; Freire, P.; Souza Filho, A. Laser-induced thermal effects in hexagonal $MoO_3$ nanorods. *Vib. Spectrosc.* **2018**, *98*, 145–151. [CrossRef]
29. Zhang, S.M.; Jiang, D.S.; Song, J.X.; Che, Y.S.; He, J.L. Investigation of the roasting behavior of mixtures of molybdenum trioxide and molybdenum concentrates. *ACS Sustain. Chem. Eng.* **2022**, *10*, 16150–16158. [CrossRef]
30. Lee, J.R.; Kim, Y.H.; Won, Y.S. Solid-state reaction between $MoS_2$ and $MoO_3$ in a fluidized bed reactor. *Korean J. Chem. Eng.* **2021**, *38*, 1791–1796. [CrossRef]

31. Wilkomirsky, I.; Sáez, E. Kinetics and mechanism of formation of $MoO_2$ by solid state reaction between $MoS_2$ and $MoO_3$. *Can. Metall. Q.* **2020**, *59*, 41–50. [CrossRef]
32. Li, X.L.; Wang, Z.; Wang, Y.F.; Zhang, B.S. Experimental study on oxidation and roasting of molybdenite. *China Resour. Compr. Util.* **2017**, *35*, 29–31, 39.
33. Caillet, P. Anhydrous sodium or potassium polymolybdates and polytungstates. *Bull. Soc. Chim. Fr.* **1967**, *12*, 4750–4755.

**Disclaimer/Publisher's Note:** The statements, opinions and data contained in all publications are solely those of the individual author(s) and contributor(s) and not of MDPI and/or the editor(s). MDPI and/or the editor(s) disclaim responsibility for any injury to people or property resulting from any ideas, methods, instructions or products referred to in the content.

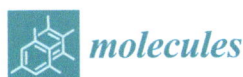

*Review*

# Research Progress in Strategies for Enhancing the Conductivity and Conductive Mechanism of LiFePO₄ Cathode Materials

Li Wang, Hongli Chen, Yuxi Zhang, Jinyu Liu * and Lin Peng

School of Chemistry and Chemical Engineering, Hebei Minzu Normal University, Chengde 067000, China
* Correspondence: liujinyu@hbun.edu.cn

**Abstract:** $LiFePO_4$ is a cathode material for lithium (Li)-ion batteries known for its excellent performance. However, compared with layered oxides and other ternary Li-ion battery materials, $LiFePO_4$ cathode material exhibits low electronic conductivity due to its structural limitations. This limitation significantly impacts the charge/discharge rates and practical applications of $LiFePO_4$. This paper reviews recent advancements in strategies aimed at enhancing the electronic conductivity of $LiFePO_4$. Efficient strategies with a sound theoretical basis, such as in-situ carbon coating, the establishment of multi-dimensional conductive networks, and ion doping, are discussed. Theoretical frameworks underlying the conductivity enhancement post-modification are summarized and analyzed. Finally, future development trends and research directions in carbon coating and doping are anticipated.

**Keywords:** lithium iron phosphate; conductivity; carbon coating; doping

Citation: Wang, L.; Chen, H.; Zhang, Y.; Liu, J.; Peng, L. Research Progress in Strategies for Enhancing the Conductivity and Conductive Mechanism of LiFePO₄ Cathode Materials. *Molecules* **2024**, *29*, 5250. https://doi.org/10.3390/molecules29225250

Academic Editor: Federico Bella

Received: 28 May 2024
Revised: 30 September 2024
Accepted: 8 October 2024
Published: 6 November 2024

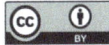

**Copyright:** © 2024 by the authors. Licensee MDPI, Basel, Switzerland. This article is an open access article distributed under the terms and conditions of the Creative Commons Attribution (CC BY) license (https://creativecommons.org/licenses/by/4.0/).

## 1. Introduction

Currently, the research and development of high-energy-density cathode materials is a crucial focus within battery material science, with a parallel emphasis on battery safety. Since its initial report in 1997, olivine-type $LiFePO_4$ has emerged as a leading contender in power battery and energy storage applications due to its exceptional thermal stability and safety [1–4]. However, inherent structural limitations impede the free diffusion of electrons and Li ions within the $LiFePO_4$ olivine framework. Notably, Li-ion movement along the c-axis is obstructed, restricting ions to a non-linear zigzag pathway along the b-axis. Because of the structural limitations, $LiFePO_4$ exhibits low electronic conductivity and Li-ion diffusion coefficients, hampering its potential for achieving high energy density and rapid charge–discharge performance [5–7]. A key strategy to enhance the electrochemical performance of $LiFePO_4$ is carbon coating, which involves enveloping $LiFePO_4$ particles with a carbon layer and interconnecting them with a conductive carbon network. This approach significantly enhances the external conductive environment of the particles, thereby enhancing the electrochemical performance of the material. Additionally, the presence of carbon materials effectively inhibits the growth of particles, creating excellent conditions for particle nanoization. Different from surface coating, ion doping involves introducing metal or non-metal ions into various positions within the $LiFePO_4$ structure to reduce band gap width, generate lattice defects, change semiconductor properties, broaden ion transport pathways, add ionic conductive materials, construct defects in carbon layers, etc. [8–14]. Thus, this review highlights recent advancements in enhancing the conductivity of $LiFePO_4$ materials, encompassing strategies such as in situ carbon coating, the establishment of multi-dimensional conductive networks, and ion doping.

## 2. The Effectiveness of Modification and Ion Doping

In the stable internal spatial structure of lithium iron phosphate, electrons and lithium ions are difficult to diffuse and shuttle freely, the movement of ions in the c-axis direction is hindered, and they can only perform a non-linear sawtooth-like shuttle motion in the b-axis direction [1]. Furthermore, relevant theoretical calculations have shown that lithium iron phosphate is a semiconductor with low electronic conductivity [12]. The above shortcomings completely limit the large-scale application of lithium iron phosphate, and are also the theoretical basis for surface modification and internal doping of lithium iron phosphate. In power batteries and energy storage devices, it is also necessary to consider the kinetic characteristics and thermodynamic stability of the particle transport process [15–17]. Through thermodynamic and kinetic simulation analysis, materials can be purposefully designed. The strategy for modifying and doping materials requires the selection of efficient and effective implementation methods and characterization methods. Compared to traditional simple physical mixed calcination carbon coating, in situ nanoparticle growth carbon coating, the construction of a multi-dimensional conductive system, and ion doping will be emphasized in this review.

*2.1. Strategy for Surface Modification*

2.1.1. In Situ Carbon Coating

Carbon coating involves applying a layer of carbon material with excellent electrical conductivity onto the surface of $LiFePO_4$ particles using various methods. This enhances the electronic conductivity between particles and stabilizes the coated cathode material during electrolyte and electrochemical reactions [18,19]. The carbon sources utilized include organic and inorganic carbon materials, carbon fibers, and carbon nanomaterials [20–24]. In addition to improving the electron conductivity, a uniform carbon layer on nanoparticles prevents uneven conduction due to material agglomeration.

The in-situ carbon coating method yields superior coating results by significantly enhancing particle-to-collector fluid contact, thus improving electron conductivity. The introduction of the carbon source before particle formation prevents particle growth during high-temperature sintering, controlling particle size and enhancing material electrochemical activity [25]. In situ carbon coating can be understood as two aspects: (1) the in-situ growth of $LiFePO_4$ particles on the surface of carbon materials (such as graphene and carbon nanotubes) [26,27]; (2) the in-situ growth of carbon-containing materials on the surface of $LiFePO_4$ [21]. Regardless of the selection of raw materials, the purpose of in situ coating is to achieve chemical bonding between carbon and $LiFePO_4$, achieving good conductivity.

Graphene is a typical graphite carbon structure material which has a regular layered carbon structure and can construct an excellent 2D conductive carbon network and elastic structure [28]. The distinctive two-dimensional configuration, irregular surface topography, impurities from different atoms, enhanced contact between the electrode and the electrolyte, augmented spacing between layers, and heightened electrical conductivity all contribute to swift surface lithium-ion absorption and extremely rapid lithium-ion diffusion along with electron transfer [29,30].

Yang [26] studied an in-situ growth method, growing $LiFePO_4$ nanoparticles on monolayer graphene with excellent dispersion (Figure 1a). Monolayer graphene provides a high-quality three-dimensional (3D) conductive network, enabling each $LiFePO_4$ particle to attach to the conductive layer (Figure 1a). This method substantially improves material electrical conductivity, leading to enhanced electrochemical properties. The initial discharge capacity reached 166.2 mAh $g^{-1}$ (98% of theoretical value).

Xu [31] studied the in-situ coating of zeolite-imidazole ZIF-8 on commercial $LiFePO_4$ material with a thickness of ~10 nm. The study analyzed coating structure and metal zinc (Zn) distribution on the $LiFePO_4$ (LFP) surface (Figure 1b). Nucleation and crystal growth of ZIF-8 nanoparticles on $LiFePO_4$ surfaces were followed by new graphite-like carbon appearance and generation post-calcination. The results indicated that the LFP/$C_{ZIF-8}$ material exhibited a heterogeneous electrical conductivity mechanism, and the graphitic carbon in the material exhibited exceptional electrical conductivity because of the ordered $sp^2$ carbon and free electrons (yellow sphere, FE I in Figure 2). An optimal carbon coating material should maximize free electrons, facilitating inter-regional electron flow to enhance electrochemical material properties.

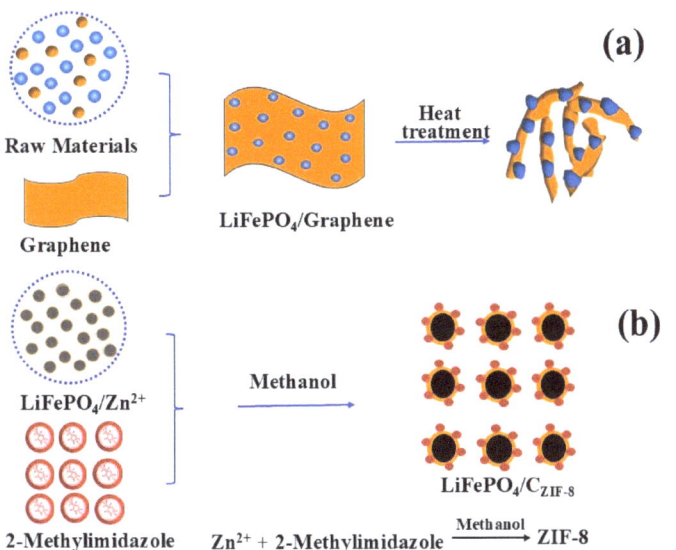

**Figure 1.** (**a**) Schematic image of LiFePO$_4$ growth on unfolded graphene [26]. Adapted from [26]. (**b**) Schematic image of C$_{ZIF-8}$ growth on the surface of LiFePO$_4$ [31]. Adapted from [31].

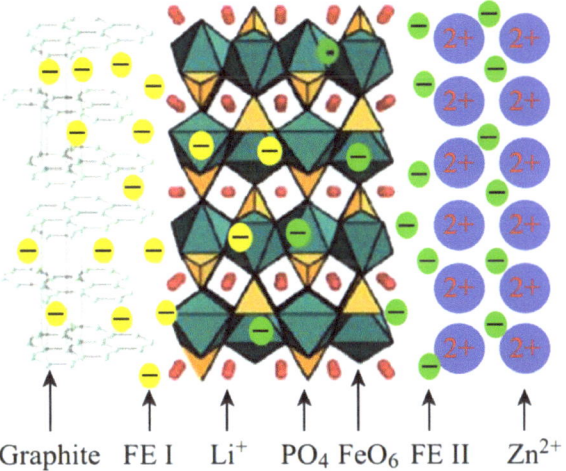

**Figure 2.** Mechanism of conductivity improvement. FE I represents free electron in graphite; FE II is free electron in metal zinc [31]. Reprinted from [31].

The carbon coating process represents material surface modification. The carbon layer serves as an interface between the cathode material and electrolyte, facilitating electron and Li-ion transfer crucial to material performance. The binding force between C and LiFePO$_4$ and the mechanism of enhanced conductivity have become a focus of attention after carbon coating.

Recent studies have elucidated how defective graphene oxide (GO) coating enhanced LiFePO$_4$ conductivity through theoretical calculations. Chen [32] investigated the electronic structure of GO parallel to the LiFePO$_4$ surface using first-principles density functional theory calculations within the DFT+U framework. The results indicated that the emergence of bands in gap states originated from graphene coating. Furthermore, GO was attached to LiFePO$_4$ (010) through C-O and Fe-O bonds, instead of the attraction of van der Waals forces. The chemical bonds (Fe-O-C) are shown in Figure 3. Thus, the LFP/GO interface facilitated the electronic conductivity of the interface.

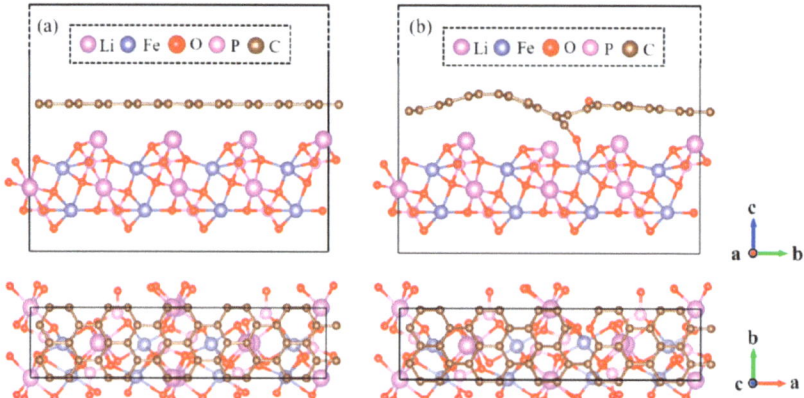

**Figure 3.** The relaxed atomic structures of (**a**) LFP/G and (**b**) LFP/GO [32]. Reprinted from [32].

The electronic energy band calculations (Figure 4) indicate increased density in valence and conduction bands owing to GO interaction with LiFePO$_4$ (010), indicating Fe-O-C bond existence. This review elucidates the principle and advantages of in situ carbon coating, enhancing the surface conductivity of LiFePO$_4$ materials, and offering theoretical support for carbon coating modification of other similar materials.

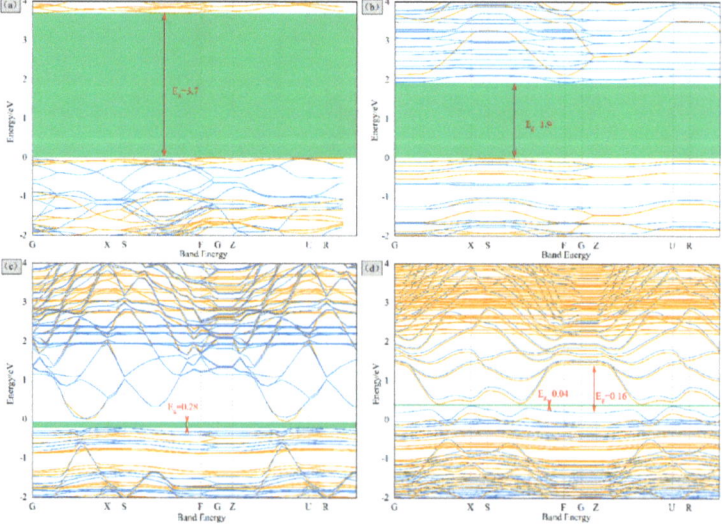

**Figure 4.** Band structure at the Fermi level for (**a**) LFP bulk, (**b**) LFP (010), (**c**) G on LFP (010), and (**d**) GO on LFP (010) [32]. Reprinted from [32].

Graphite carbon has excellent electrical conductivity, which is why researchers choose this type of material for carbon coating. In addition to graphene, other carbon materials can also be processed to achieve graphite carbon, and their conductivity can be optimized through improvements in the manufacturing process. Apart from graphene, other carbon materials can also be processed to obtain graphite carbon, and their electrical conductivity can be maximized through advancements in the manufacturing process. Raman analysis can be used to detect the degree of graphitization of the carbon layer coated on the surface of materials. The use of this technique makes the design of materials more superior [33,34].

In summary, the in-situ carbon coating strategy is an excellent method for enhancing the surface and conductivity of materials. However, before implementing carbon coating, a detailed analysis and explanation of the conductive mechanism should be conducted to enhance coating material design and structural optimization. In situ carbon coating holds promise for modifying surface conductivity in other insulators or semiconductor materials, achieving dual electronic conduction and material application effects.

2.1.2. Surface Carbon Layer Doping and LiFePO$_4$ Modification

In research on some non-in situ carbon coating processes, researchers have devoted considerable effort to doping the carbon layer with non-metal atoms. The main non-metal elements used and their primary functions in carbon layer doping are listed in Table 1 below.

Table 1. Elements used to dope the carbon layer and their primary functions.

| Materials | Doped Atoms | Functions | Discharge Capacity (High Rate) | Conductivity/ $\times 10^{-2}$ S cm$^{-1}$ | Ref. |
|---|---|---|---|---|---|
| Egg white (1 mL) | N | offer superior electronic transportation between LiFePO$_4$ active particles | 120 mAh g$^{-1}$ (LFP/C+N at 5 C) 113 mAh g$^{-1}$ (LFP/C at 5 C) | | [35,36] |
| Polyvinylidene fluoride (5% wt) | F | play a vital role in the improvement of electron transfer kinetics | 121.5 mAh g$^{-1}$ (LFP@FC-II at 10 C) approaching 120.0 mAh g$^{-1}$ (LFP at 0.1 C) | | [37] |
| Sulfur-doped graphene sheet | S | promote the transportation of electrons and Li-ions; prevent volume change during the Li$^+$ intercalation/deintercalation procedure | 130.5 mAh g$^{-1}$ (LiFePO$_4$@C/S-doped graphene at 10 C) 116.5 mAh g$^{-1}$ LiFePO$_4$@C | | [38,39] |
| Oxalic acid and benzyl disulfide | S | promote the electronic conductivity and defect level of the carbon | 137 mAh g$^{-1}$ (LiFePO$_4$/SC at 5 C) 128.5 mAh g$^{-1}$ (LiFePO$_4$/C at 5 C) | | [40] |
| Triphenylphosphine (0.2 g mL$^{-1}$ was mixed with 4 g LiFePO$_4$/C) | P | benefit the graphitization of the carbon; decrease transfer resistance | 124.0 mAh g$^{-1}$ (LFP/C-P3 at 20 C) 105.4 mAh g$^{-1}$ (LFP/C at 20 C) | | [41] |
| Melamine, boric acid | N+B | electron-type and the hole-type carriers donated by nitrogen and boron atoms generate the synergistic effect to greatly elevate the high-rate capacity | 121.6 mAh g$^{-1}$ (LFP/C-N+B at 20 C) 101.1 mAh g$^{-1}$ (LFP/C at 20 C) | 13.6 (LFP/C-N+B) 2.56 (LFP/C) | [42] |
| Methionine | S+N | good ionic and electronic conductivities | 103 mAh g$^{-1}$ (NSC@LFP at 2 C) 63 mAh g$^{-1}$ (pristine LFP at 2 C) | | [43] |

It was reported that additional electrons contributed by the N atom can provide electron carriers for the conduction band, which can contribute to the electrical conductivity of the material by introducing N into the carbon structures [35,36]. The F atom has a higher electronegativity than other anions, and F doping will accelerate the decrease in the interfacial resistance of the battery [37]. Coating lithium iron phosphate with sulfur-doped graphene nanosheets can create an electronic conductive network and can also promote the transportation of electrons and Li-ions [38–40]. Phosphorus-doped carbon layers can decrease transfer resistance and are good at the graphitization of the carbon [41]. The multi-element doping of carbon layers can achieve higher electronic conductivity and lower migration activation energy [42]. The main function of carbon coating and carbon layer doping is to enhance the electronic conductivity of the material. Investigations have demonstrated that the application of electrochemically active electron-conducting polymer coatings on LiFePO$_4$ particles could potentially replicate the roles of carbon coatings, while also being applicable under less stringent conditions and offering the extra benefit of improved ionic conductivity within the active material [44,45].

Data from Table 1 demonstrate that the electrochemical performance and electronic conductivity of lithium iron phosphate (LFP) materials are significantly enhanced after doping the carbon layer with certain non-metal elements. By doping the carbon layer with heteroatoms such as nitrogen (N), sulfur (S), and boron (B), the conductivity of the carbon layer can be increased. For example, nitrogen doping can introduce additional electrons, thereby enhancing the electronic conductivity of the carbon layer. On the other hand, non-metal elements can assist in forming a conductive network within the carbon layer: doping with heteroatoms can promote the formation of a more comprehensive conductive network, thereby increasing the electron transfer rate of the electrode material. Furthermore, doping the carbon layer can improve the ion diffusion pathways: doping with heteroatoms can alter the surface structure of the material, providing lithium ions with shorter diffusion paths and thus enhancing the migration rate of ions. For instance, co-doping the carbon layer with nitrogen and boron can greatly enhance the electrochemical performance: at a rate of 20 C, the co-doped sample can increase the discharge capacity of LFP/C from 101.1 mAh g$^{-1}$ to 121.6 mAh g$^{-1}$ [42].

2.1.3. Ion Conductive Materials

Charging and discharging reactions of a battery are the result of the combined migration of ions and electrons. Especially during high-current charging and discharging, it is necessary to consider both the transport of electrons and the migration of ions. If the combined effects of both can be taken into account comprehensively, it will greatly enhance the electrochemical performance of the material. The main ways to improve the electrical conductivity include coating and modification with conductive carbon materials on the surface and doping with ions inside the material. To increase the migration rate of lithium ions, it is common to reduce the particle size of the material and construct special structures [46,47].

The ion conductive materials can enhance the electrochemical performances of LiFePO$_4$ because of their high ionic conductivity and lithium ionic storage ability. Typically, graphene is often regarded as an excellent electronic conductor which can significantly enhance the electronic conductivity on the surface of LiFePO$_4$. Most layered structures of graphene without defects would hinder the transition of Li$^+$ [48]. The enhancement of ionic conductivity requires more attention. Incorporating GO (graphene oxide) contributes to the preservation of material stability and the augmentation of lithium ion diffusion coefficients since the lithium ions have lower insertion and extraction potentials along the [010] facet in LiFePO$_4$ [32,49]. After being coated with graphene or GO, the average Fe-O bonds on the LiFePO$_4$ (010) surface underwent significant changes, which led to the expansion of the Li$^+$ channel, facilitating the insertion and extraction of migrating Li$^+$. In addition to the lithium ions provided by LiFePO$_4$ itself, incorporating lithium-ion conductive materials into the material can provide additional support for the intercalation and deintercalation of lithium ions, which will greatly enhance the material's rate performance and cycling performance. Some ion conducting materials have a special three-dimensional structure that can facilitate rapid diffusion of Li$^+$ [50]. Chien [51] designed a LiFePO$_4$/Li$_3$V$_2$(PO$_4$)$_3$/C composite cathode material to help enhance the diffusion properties of lithium ions. Essentially, the enhancement of ionic conductivity of coated materials is contingent upon their unique post-modification structures. Materials that facilitate lithium-ion conduction possess both high ionic conductivity and lithium-ion storage capability, thereby significantly boosting the ionic conductivity of LiFePO$_4$.

## 2.2. Strategy for Building a Multi-Dimensional Conductive Network

Nanoparticles of LiFePO$_4$ are expected to be used as the cathode material of high-performance lithium-ion batteries [52]. The design and preparation of nanocomposites can effectively improve the low thermal stability and multiple surface side reactions of nanoparticles [53]. The design and the construction of conductive network structures have been the main focus of research in recent years [27,54–60]. Constructing a multi-dimensional conductive network is one of the effective means to enhance the electronic conductivity of LiFePO$_4$. The construction of conductive networks generally uses one-dimensional materials [27] and two-dimensional materials [61] to provide a conductive skeleton in combination with two-dimensional methods. LiFePO$_4$ is then used to gradually fill the surface and interior of the skeleton, achieving multi-dimensional conductive effects. A typical multi-dimensional conductive network is shown on Table 1. The main network structure could include a porous structure [54], a hierarchically porous structure [59], a highly meso-porous structure [60], a 3D conducting network [56], a distinctive loose and scaffolded structure [27], etc.

Typical conductive network images are shown in Table 2.

**Table 2.** Characteristic, function, and network structure of multi-dimensional conductive network.

| Chemical Formula | Network Structure | Characteristic/ Function | Electrical Conductivity | Discharge Capacity (High Rate) | Ref. |
|---|---|---|---|---|---|
| C@LFP/CNTs | | Porous structure/provides favorable kinetics for both electrons and Li$^+$ | $7.71 \times 10^{-2}$ S cm$^{-1}$ (Conductivity of C@LFP/CNTs) $5.91 \times 10^{-3}$ S cm$^{-1}$ (Conductivity of C@LFP) | 102 mAh g$^{-1}$ (C@LFP/CNTs at 20 C) 50 mAh g$^{-1}$ (C@LFP at 20 C) | [54] |
| LFP@C/G | | 3D "sheets-in-pellets" and "pellets-on-sheets" conducting network structure/highly conductive and plentiful mesopores promote electronic and ionic transport | 28.4 Ω ($R_{ct}$ values for LFP@C/G) 75.5 Ω ($R_{ct}$ values for LFP@C) | 81.2 mAh g$^{-1}$ (LFP@C/G at 20 C) | [56] |
| CNT/LFP | | Distinctive loose and scaffolded composite structure/enhances the overall conductivity of the composite | 32.47 Ω ($R_{ct}$ values for LFP-CNT-G) 46.23 Ω ($R_{ct}$ values for LFP) | 143 mAh g$^{-1}$ (LFP-CNT at 20 C) | [27] |
| LFP-CNT-G | | 3D conducting networks/faster electron transfer and lower resistance during the Li-ions' reversible reaction | 50.17 Ω ($R_{ct}$ values for LFP-CNT-G) 103.93 Ω ($R_{ct}$ values for LFP-CNT) | 115.8 mAh g$^{-1}$ (LFP-CNT-G at 20 C) 99.4 mAh g$^{-1}$ (LFP-CNT at 20 C) | [58] |

Table 2. Cont.

| Chemical Formula | Network Structure | Characteristic/ Function | Electrical Conductivity | Discharge Capacity (High Rate) | Ref. |
|---|---|---|---|---|---|
| LFP@C/MXene | | Hierarchically porous structure and "dot-to-surface" conductive network/fast ion and electron transfer for redox reactions | 17.26 Ω ($R_{ct}$ values for LFP@C/MX-3.0) 93.32 Ω ($R_{ct}$ values for LFP@C) | 140.3 mA h·g$^{-1}$ (LFP@C/MX-3.0 at 20 C) 86.6 mA h·g$^{-1}$ (LFP@C at 20 C) | [59] |
| LFP/R-GO | | Highly meso-porous structure/good electronic conductivity and high electrolyte permeability | 25 Ω ($R_{ct}$ values for LiFePO$_4$/R-GO) 50 Ω ($R_{ct}$ values for LiFePO$_4$) | 135 mAh g$^{-1}$ (LiFePO$_4$/R-GO at 5 C) | [60] |
| LFP/MXene/ CNT/Cellulose | | 3-dimensional MXene-Carbon nanotubes-Cellulose- LiFePO$_4$ (3D-MCC-LFP)/faster electronic/ionic transport | 26.6 Ω ($R_{ct}$ values for 3D-MCC-LFP10) 32.2 Ω ($R_{ct}$ values for Con-LFP10) | 159.5 mAh g$^{-1}$ (3D-MCC-LFP$_{120}$ at 1 mA cm$^{-2}$) | [61] |
| LFP/Ti$_3$C$_2$Tx/ CNTs | | 1D single-walled carbon nanotubes (CNTs)/bound together using 2D MXene (Ti$_3$C$_2$Tx) nanosheets/highlights the ability of multi-dimensional conductive fillers to realize simultaneously superior electrochemical and mechanical properties | 27.7 Ω ($R_{ct}$ values for LFP/CNT/Ti$_3$C$_2$Tx) 32.2 Ω ($R_{ct}$ values for LFP/Ti$_3$C$_2$Tx) | | [62] |

Data from Table 2 clearly indicate that the construction of a 3D conductive network significantly enhances the electrical conductivity and high-rate discharge capacity of lithium iron phosphate (LFP) materials. The excellent electrochemical performance is attributed to the following factors: (i) increased contact between particles, enhancing the efficiency of electron transport within the material; (ii) providing a larger surface area for electrochemical reactions; (iii) allowing more lithium ions to participate in the charging and discharging process. The following text provides a more detailed narrative.

Wu [63] designed a new LiFePO$_4$ nanoparticle, which exhibited two types of carbon complexes, including amorphous carbon coating and a graphitized conductive structure (Figure 5). Furthermore, compared with the original LFP@C and LFP/CNT coatings, the initial carbon layer evenly coated all nanoscale LiFePO$_4$ particles due to the synergistic effect of amorphous carbon. This stabilized the interface of LiFePO$_4$ nanoparticles, thereby enhancing electrical conductivity and Li diffusion.

Dong and colleagues [61] designed a 3D-MCC-LFP material with a high load rate, exceptional mechanical properties, and excellent electrical conductivity using an assembly method (Figure 6). In this structure, 2D MXene served as a key component, providing sites for LiFePO$_4$ particle loading, connecting materials, and facilitating simultaneous electron and ion transport. One-dimensional carbon nanotubes served as conductive agents, enabling full interconnectivity of the scaffold and thereby enhancing electronic conductivity. One-dimensional cellulose served as a reinforcing filler, preserving the mechanical properties and structural integrity of 3D-MCC-LFP while accommodating a large amount of LiFePO$_4$ material.

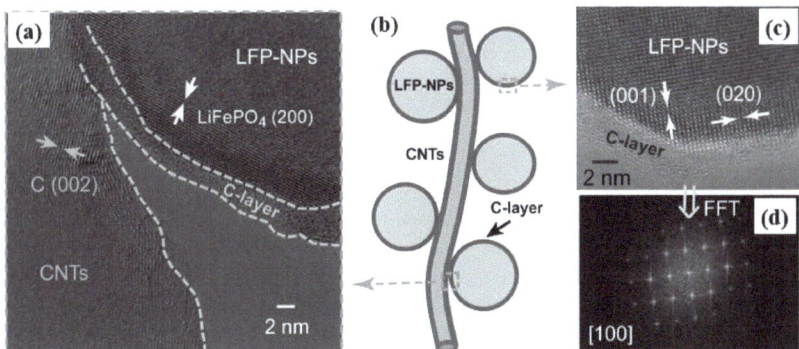

Figure 5. (a,c) HRTEM images and (b) a schematic illustration of the prepared LFP@C/CNT nanocomposite. (d) The corresponding FFT of the HRTEM in (c) [63]. Reprinted from [63].

The author employed SnO$_2$-NF as the negative electrode material to test the performance of the assembled battery, and due to its excellent conductivity and high loading capacity of LiFePO$_4$, the electrochemical properties of 3D-MCC-LFP materials surpassed those prepared using traditional methods.

Similarly, Checko [62] designed a new multi-dimensional network to enhance local electrical transport across the LiFePO$_4$ surface (Figure 7). This structure is consistent with single-walled carbon nanotubes (1D) and MXene nanosheet (2D) bound together. The CNTs facilitated local electron transport across the LiFePO$_4$ surface, while Ti$_3$C$_2$T$_x$ nanosheets provided conductive pathways through the bulk of the electrode. The electrochemical characterization supported by numerical simulation verified the charge transfer characteristics of this multi-dimensional conductive network.

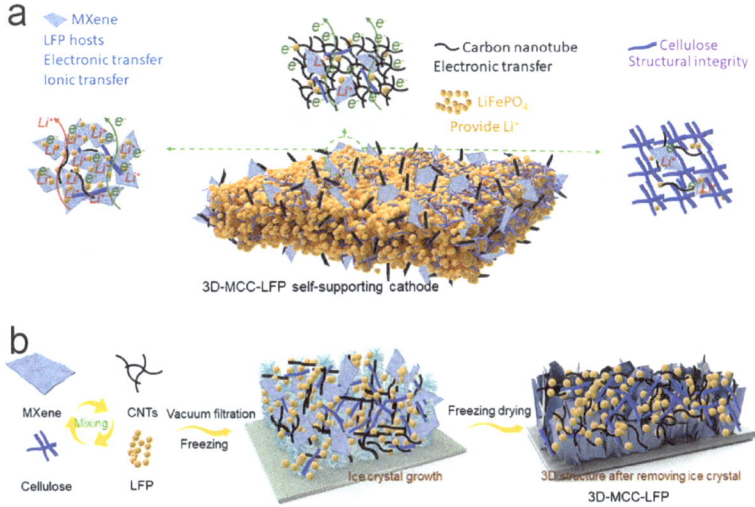

Figure 6. Schematic illustration of the structure (a) and fabrication process (b) of 3D-MCC-LFP cathode [61]. Reprinted from [61].

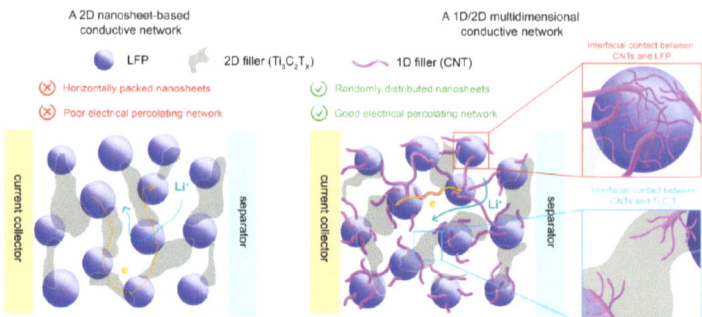

**Figure 7.** Schematic illustration depicting electrode characteristics in a 2D nanosheet-based conductive network (**left**) and a 1D/2D multi-dimensional conductive network (**right**) with inset schemes showing magnified views of the interfacial contacts between CNTs and LFP particles (**top**) and between CNTs and Ti3C2Tx (**bottom**) in the multi-dimensional conductive network [62]. Reprinted from [62].

Contrastingly, Luo [64] exploited N-doped graphene (NG)-modified LiFePO$_4$ material with a 3D conductive network structure for Li-ion batteries. In this structure, NG effectively coated and connected LiFePO$_4$ particles, and N doping reduced electrode polarization, enhancing electrochemical reaction reversibility. The special structure constructed with NG provided faster and more efficient 3D transport channels for Li$^+$ and electrons.

The construction of a multi-dimensional conductive network is an efficient approach for rapid transmission on and between particle surfaces. The dual connected channel composed of a solid phase network channel and an internal cavity channel with a conductive network structure achieves rapid electron and ion transport, and also ensures uniform contact between the electrolyte and the positive electrode, thereby forming a good interface. The porous structure can achieve effective infiltration of electrolytes, which is beneficial for improving the lithium diffusion rate and reaction kinetics. However, critical factors to consider include the mechanical stability of the structure, electronic transmission efficiency, and compatibility between the conductive network and the material interface.

In addition to intrinsic material properties, achieving excellent carbon coating is essential to fully utilize electrochemical performance. A uniform and effective carbon skeleton conductive network should form between particles, emphasizing molecular-level mixing of carbon skeleton and LiFePO$_4$. Conventional physical coating methods with simple processes and low costs may struggle to achieve accurate carbon coating requirements. Therefore, they have become a prospective technology to study new carbon coating methods with controlled nano-growth mechanisms.

### 2.3. Strategy for Ion Doping

The purpose of in situ carbon coating and the construction of a multi-dimensional conductive network on particle surfaces is to enhance electrical conductivity both within and between particles, representing a physical modification of battery materials. However, ion doping constitutes a chemical modification aimed at enhancing intrinsic electrical conductivity [65,66]. Specific doping locations include iron (Fe), phosphorus (P), and Li sites, among which Fe-site doping is the most prevalent [66–71]. Additionally, various doping elements have been studied, including manganese (Mn), nickel (Ni), niobium (Nb), magnesium (Mg), cobalt (Co), vanadium (V), and others [72–77]. However, Fe-site doping serves a dual purpose. First, it narrows the band gap between the conduction and valence bands of semiconductor material (LiFePO$_4$), thereby increasing material conductivity. Second, ion doping induces Li or Fe vacancies, forming charge compensation defects, and the conductivity of electrons is enhanced. Zhang [78] studied the electronic properties of LiFePO$_4$ doped with Mn, Co, Nb, Mo, and other elements using first-principles calculations.

The results (Figure 8) indicated reduced band gaps with the doping of these elements, facilitating electron transitions. Notably, Co and Nb doping exhibited obvious enhancement effects. Moreover, studies have shown that doped materials inhibit microcracks, prevent electrode polarization, and enhance overall material performance. Furthermore, doping with Mn, Nb, Mo, and Co also enhances the mechanical stability of LiFePO$_4$, altering parameters such as material structure, M-O (metal–oxygen) bond energy, and band gap width, thereby enhancing both electrical and mechanical properties.

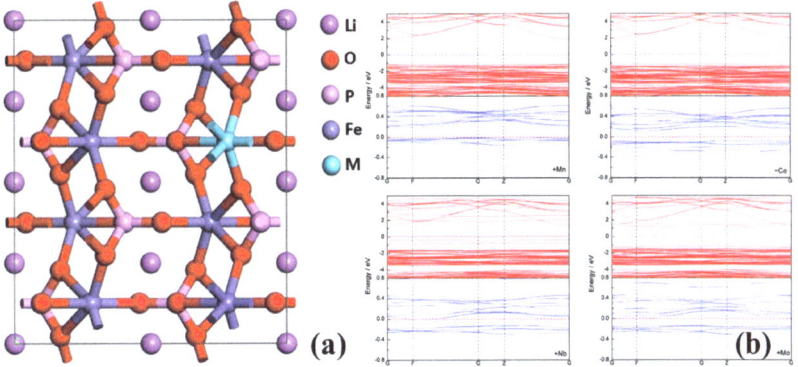

**Figure 8.** (**a**) Bulk model of M-doped LiFePO$_4$ (M = Mn, Co, Nb, Mo). (**b**) Band structures of LiFePO$_4$. The red and blue lines represent majority spin states and minority spin states, respectively (for interpretation of the references to color in this figure legend, the reader is referred to the web version of this article) [78]. Reprinted from [78].

Dou [12] examined the electronic structure of LiFe$_x$Mn$_{1-x}$PO$_4$ doped with different Mn contents using first-principles density functional methods. The study found that LiFe$_{0.75}$Mn$_{0.25}$PO$_4$ exhibited the smallest bandgap width with a Mn doping amount of $x = 0.25$. This was attributable to the Fe3d electron contributions dominating the density of states (DOS) near the Fermi plane of LiFePO$_4$, while Mn3d electrons become predominant upon Mn incorporation, increasing the DOS near the Fermi level in LiFe$_{0.75}$Mn$_{0.25}$O$_2$ and enhancing material conductivity. Conversely, introducing Mn lengthened Fe-O bonds and weakened Fe-O bond energy, widening Li-ion migration channels and facilitating ion diffusion.

Ban et al. [79] studied the co-doping of "donor-acceptor" charge compensation, combining theoretical calculations with experiments to significantly enhance material rate performance. It was observed that P and O sites co-doped with silicon (Si) and fluorine (F) altered the conduction band edge of LiFePO$_4$, enhancing material conductivity by at least two to three orders of magnitude compared with pre-doping levels. This approach facilitated the positive magnification performance of LiFePO$_4$.

In addition to theoretical studies, replacing and occupying the spatial structure of an element in LiFePO$_4$ using doping elements to create lattice defects broadens ion transport channels, enhancing material intrinsic conductivity. Marnix [80] studied the doping of hypervalent ions in LiFePO$_4$, observing that the ions that occupied Li positions maintained a positive bivalent state in Fe, thus contributing to improved material conductivity.

Recently, the doping of rare earth elements into positive electrode materials has also been widely studied [81,82]. The ionic radius of rare earth elements is larger than that of transition metal elements, resulting in an increased material cell volume and a reduced band gap after doping with rare earth elements. This increase in mobility and carrier concentration significantly enhances the electrical conductivity of the final material [83,84]. Studies have shown that doping Li ion phosphate with rare earth element ions such as erbium (Er$^{3+}$), yttrium (Y$^{3+}$), and Nd$^{3+}$ leads to Fe replacement by rare earth ions, resulting in increase in material conductivity of four orders of magnitude. This occurred because the electron-deficient rare earth element ions created holes that readily exited full electrons to the hole level, transforming the material from a N-type to a P-type semiconductor [85,86]. Qiu Peng [87] studied the effects of lanthanum (La), Nd, and Y doping on the structure and electrochemical properties of LiFePO$_4$. The results indicated increased cell parameters and volume, smaller particle size, and uniform, tightly bonded pores in the doped material. In comparison with pure Li–Fe phosphate, the electrical conductivity of the doped material increased by four orders of magnitude, owing to enhanced Li-ion diffusion facilitated by the small particle size and internal lattice defects created by the doped elements. Studies have shown that rare earth element-doped materials exhibit smaller particle sizes [88–93].

Notably, enhancing the diffusion performance of Li-ions is also an important purpose of doping, and its double effect was achieved through the co-doping method [94,95]. Wang [96] successfully synthesized Y-F co-doped LiFePO$_4$/C material using a high-temperature solid-phase method. The introduction of F enhanced the electron-cloud rearrangement of PO$_4^{3-}$, significantly enhancing conductivity. Simultaneously, Y was introduced into Li$^+$ vacancy, reducing spatial resistance to Li-ion diffusion and comprehensively enhancing material ionic conductivity. Additionally, X-ray diffraction analysis results revealed weakened Li-O bonds and widened Li-ion diffusion tunnels due to Y-F doping, leading to Li-ion diffusion rates. As a result, the material exhibited excellent electrochemical properties, that is, its specific discharge capacity reached a 179.3 mAh·g$^{-1}$ capacity at a 0.1 C current density and a 135.5 mAh·g$^{-1}$ capacity at 10 C.

The doping method theoretically optimized the structure of the crystal, and the conductivity of the material was fundamentally improved. However, the mechanism by which doping changes the electrochemical properties of materials remains unclear. The electronic conduction within the crystal of the material was very complicated, and whether the doped element fulfilled its designed role remains uncertain, with assessments largely based on macro-level performance. The particle size reduction following rare earth element doping lacks detailed analysis, indicating a partial absence of a relevant theoretical basis. Therefore, careful selection of doping elements and the acquisition of necessary theoretical support are essential prerequisites for material doping research.

## 3. New Carbon Coating Technologies and LiFePO$_4$ Batteries

Some new carbon coating technologies are rapidly developing which not only apply to lithium iron phosphate materials but also provide new ideas for surface coating modification of other materials with poor conductivity.

Flash Joule heating (FJH): Using an ex situ carbon coating method, the precursor could rapidly decompose through flash Joule heating (FJH) technology. By depositing carbon heteroatom materials within a limited space in just 10 s, a uniform amorphous carbon layer can be obtained on LFP; at the same time, different heteroatoms can be introduced into the surface carbon layer. Solvent-free, versatile cathode surface modification is the highlight of this technology [97]. Supercritical CO$_2$-enhanced surface modification: Employing supercritical CO$_2$ (SCCO$_2$) for a proficient ex situ carbon coating method on lithium iron phosphate (LFP) results in a superior carbon coating layer with a higher graphite carbon content and reduced oxygen-derived functional groups, significantly improving electron transfer efficiency [98]. Spray coating technology: Using spray coating technology to produce LiFePO$_4$-coated carbon fiber (CF) as a structural battery cathode component can yield substantial electrochemical performance for the battery. The use of spray coating technology stands out as an innovative method for manufacturing electrodes in structural batteries, highlighting its capacity to enhance the efficiency of multifunctional energy storage systems [22]. Ultrafast nonequilibrium high-temperature shock technology: This technology introduces Li-Fe anti-site defects and controllable tensile strain into the LiFePO$_4$ lattice. This design allows for research on the impact of strain fields on performance to extend from theoretical calculations to experimental perspectives [99]. Recycling and reuse technology for spent LiFePO$_4$: This is a direct regeneration of LiFePO$_4$ based on a doping strategy, a highly efficient additive for direct reactivation of waste LiFePO$_4$, prilling, and a cocoating collaborative strategy [100–102].

## 4. Conclusions

The carbon layer structure significantly affects the conductivity of LiFePO$_4$. To achieve optimal electrochemical performance, it is necessary to incorporate highly graphitized carbon (sp$^2$ hybrid state) to enhance its conductivity. However, traditional organic or inorganic carbon struggles to achieve a high degree of graphitization at sintering temperatures of 500–800 °C. Therefore, while in situ growth of LiFePO$_4$ on a single layer of graphene proves promising, the development and adoption of this technology must overcome challenges related to cost and synthesis methods. Furthermore, the quest for new carbon materials with enhanced graphitization remains imperative. Additionally, modifying crystal structures through cationic or anionic doping offers optimization potential. However, the mechanisms and effects of doping reactions on material properties require more comprehensive investigation. The analysis of substitution sites and doping quantities necessitates refined proof methods. Finally, future efforts concerning LiFePO$_4$ and other types of cathode (anode) materials with poor conductivity must be focused on achieving high energy and vibration densities alongside stable cycling, excellent rate performance, and low-temperature capabilities. This trajectory underscores the imperative for ongoing advancements in material science and electrochemistry.

**Author Contributions:** L.W.: Writing (original draft, resources, investigation); H.C.: Conceptualization; Y.Z.: Writing (review and editing); J.L.: Conceptualization, Writing (review and editing); L.P.: Writing (review and editing). All authors have read and agreed to the published version of the manuscript.

**Funding:** This work was funded by the Science and Technology Project of Hebei Education Department (grant no. QN2022203) and the S&T Program of Chengde (grant no. 202201A062).

**Institutional Review Board Statement:** Not applicable.

**Informed Consent Statement:** Not applicable.

**Data Availability Statement:** Not applicable.

**Conflicts of Interest:** The authors declare no conflict of interest.

## References

1. Padhi, A.K.; Nanjundaswamy, K.S.; Goodenough, J.B. Phospho-olivines as positive-electrode materials for rechargeable lithium batteries. *J. Electrochem. Soc.* **1997**, *144*, 1188–1194. [CrossRef]
2. Guyomard, D.; Tarascon, J.M. Rocking-chair or Lithium-ion rechargeable Lithium batteries. *Adv. Mater.* **1994**, *6*, 408–412. [CrossRef]
3. Zhang, S.S.; Allen, J.L.; Xu, K.; Jow, T.R. Optimization of reaction condition for solid-state synthesis of LiFePO$_4$-C composite cathodes. *J. Power Sources* **2005**, *147*, 234–240. [CrossRef]
4. Cheng, F.Q.; Wan, W.; TAN, Z.; Huang, Y.Y.; Zhou, H.H.; Chen, J.T.; Zhang, X.X. High power performance of nano-LiFePO$_4$/C cathode material synthesized via lauric acid-assisted solid-state reaction. *Electrochim. Acta* **2011**, *56*, 2999–3005. [CrossRef]
5. Liu, W.; Gao, P.; Mi, Y.Y.; Chen, J.T.; Zhou, H.H.; Zhang, X.X. Fabrication of high tap density LiFe$_{0.6}$Mn$_{0.4}$PO$_4$/C microspheres by a double carbon coating-spray drying method for high rate lithium ion batteries. *J. Mater. Chem. A* **2013**, *1*, 2411–2417. [CrossRef]
6. Li, Y.; Wang, L.; Zhang, K.Y.; Yao, Y.C.; Kong, L.X. Optimized synthesis of LiFePO$_4$ cathode material and its reaction mechanism during solvothermal. *Adv. Powder Technol.* **2021**, *32*, 2097–2105. [CrossRef]
7. Xie, Y.; Yu, H.T.; Yi, T.F.; Zhu, Y.R. Understanding the thermal and mechanical stabilities of olivine type LiMPO$_4$ (M = Fe, Mn) as cathode materials for rechargeable lithium batteries from first principles. *ACS Appl. Mater. Interfaces* **2011**, *6*, 4033–4042. [CrossRef]
8. Ramasubramanian, B.; Sundarrajan, S.; Chellappan, V.; Reddy, M.V.; Ramakrishna, S.; Zaghib, K. Recent development in carbon-LiFePO$_4$ cathodes for lithium-ion batteries: A mini review. *Batteries* **2022**, *8*, 133. [CrossRef]
9. Chen, S.P.; Lv, D.; Chen, J.; Zhang, Y.H.; Shi, F.N. Review on defects and modification methods of LiFePO$_4$ cathode material for lithium-ion batteries. *Energy Fuels* **2022**, *36*, 1232–1251. [CrossRef]
10. Wang, J.J.; Sun, X.L. Understanding and recent development of carbon coating on LiFePO$_4$ cathode materials for lithium-ion batteries. *Energy Environ. Sci.* **2012**, *5*, 5163–5185. [CrossRef]

11. Chung, S.Y.; Blocking, J.T.; Chiang, Y.M. Electronically conductive phospho-olivines as lithium storage electrodes. *Nat. Mater.* **2002**, *1*, 123–128. [CrossRef] [PubMed]
12. Dou, J.Q.; Kang, X.Y.; Tuerdi, W.; Hua, N.; Han, Y. The first principles and experimental study on Mn doped LiFePO$_4$. *Acta Phys. Sin.* **2012**, *61*, 341–348.
13. Ruan, Y.Y.; Tang, Z.Y.; Guo, H.Z. Effects on the structure and electrochemical performance of LiFePO$_4$ by Mn$^{2+}$ doping. *J. Funct. Mater.* **2008**, *39*, 747–750.
14. Li, Y.; Wang, L.; Liang, F.; Yao, Y.C.; Zhang, K.Y. Enhancing high rate performance and cyclability of LiFePO$_4$ cathode materials for lithium ion batteries by boron doping. *J. Alloys Compd.* **2021**, *880*, 160560. [CrossRef]
15. Xiao, P.H.; Henkelman, G. Kinetic monte carlo study of Li intercalation in LiFePO$_4$. *ACS Nano* **2018**, *12*, 844–851. [CrossRef]
16. Yang, H.; Ding, Z.; Li, Y.T.; Li, S.Y.; Wu, P.K.; Hou, Q.H.; Zheng, Y.; Gao, B.; Huo, K.F.; Du, W.J.; et al. Recent advances in kinetic and thermodynamic regulation of magnesium hydride for hydrogen storage. *Rare Met.* **2023**, *42*, 2906–2927. [CrossRef]
17. Ding, Z.; Li, Y.T.; Yang, H.; Lu, Y.F.; Tan, J.; Li, J.B.; Li, Q.; Chen, Y.A.; Shaw, L.L.; Pan, F.S. Tailoring MgH$_2$ for hydrogen storage through nanoengineering and catalysis. *J. Magnes. Alloys* **2022**, *10*, 2946–2967. [CrossRef]
18. Saikia, D.; Deka, J.R.; Chou, C.J.; Lin, C.H.; Yang, Y.C.; Kao, H.M. Encapsulation of LiFePO$_4$ Nanoparticles into 3D interpenetrating ordered mesoporous carbon as a high-performance cathode for lithium-ion batteries exceeding theoretical capacity. *ACS Appl. Energy Mater.* **2019**, *2*, 1121–1133. [CrossRef]
19. Zhang, Z.; Wang, M.M.; Xu, J.F.; Shi, F.C.; Li, M.; Gao, Y.M. Modification of lithium iron phosphate by carbon coating. *Int. J. Electrochem. Sci.* **2019**, *14*, 10622–10632. [CrossRef]
20. Varzi, A.; Bresser, D.; Zamory, J.V.; Müller, F.; Passerini, S. ZnFe$_2$O$_4$-C/LiFePO$_4$-CNT: A novel high-power lithium-ion battery with excellent cycling performance. *Adv. Energy Mater.* **2014**, *4*, 1400054. [CrossRef]
21. Yao, Y.C.; Qu, P.W.; Gan, X.K.; Huang, X.P.; Zhao, Q.F.; Liang, F. Preparation of porous-structured LiFePO$_4$/C composite by vacuum sintering for lithium-ion battery. *Ceram. Int.* **2016**, *42*, 18303–18311. [CrossRef]
22. Yücel, Y.D.; Zenkert, D.; Lindström, R.W.; Lindbergh, G. LiFePO$_4$-coated carbon fibers as positive electrodes in structural batteries: Insights from spray coating technique. *Electrochem. Commun.* **2024**, *160*, 107670. [CrossRef]
23. Qin, J.D.; Zhang, Y.B.; Lowe, S.E.; Jiang, L.X.; Ling, H.Y.; Shi, G.; Liu, P.R.; Zhang, S.Q.; Zhong, Y.L.; Zhao, H.J. Room temperature production of graphene oxide with thermally labile oxygen functional groups for improved lithium ion battery fabrication and performance. *J. Mater. Chem. A* **2019**, *7*, 9646–9655. [CrossRef]
24. Wang, J.J.; Sun, X.L. Olivine LiFePO$_4$: The remaining challenges for future energy storage. *Energy Environ. Sci.* **2015**, *8*, 1110–1138. [CrossRef]
25. Wen, L.Z.; Guan, Z.W.; Wang, L.; Hu, S.T.; Lv, D.H.; Liu, X.M.; Duan, T.T.; Liang, G.C. Effect of carbon-coating on internal resistance and performance of lithium iron phosphate batteries. *J. Electrochem. Soc.* **2022**, *169*, 050536. [CrossRef]
26. Yang, J.L.; Wang, J.J.; Tang, Y.J.; Wang, D.N.; Li, X.F.; Hu, Y.H.; Li, R.Y.; Liang, G.X.; Sham, T.K.; Sun, X.L. LiFePO$_4$-graphene as a superior cathode material for rechargeable lithium batteries: Impact of stacked graphene and unfolded graphene. *Energy Environ. Sci.* **2013**, *6*, 1521–1528. [CrossRef]
27. Ren, X.G.; Li, Y.J.; He, Z.J.; Xi, X.M.; Shen, X.J. In-situ growth of LiFePO$_4$ with interconnected pores supported on carbon nanotubes via tavorite-olivine phase transition. *Ceram. Int.* **2023**, *49*, 40131–40139. [CrossRef]
28. Stankovich, S.; Dikin, D.A.; Piner, R.D.; Kohlhaas, K.A.; Kleinhammes, A.; Jia, Y.; Wu, Y.; Nguyen, S.T.; Ruoff, R.S. Synthesis of graphene-based nanosheets via chemical reduction of exfoliated graphite oxide. *Carbon* **2007**, *45*, 1558–1565. [CrossRef]
29. Dong, Y.F.; Wu, Z.S.; Ren, W.C.; Cheng, H.M.; Bao, X.H. Graphene: A promising 2D material for electrochemical energy storage. *Sci. Bull.* **2017**, *62*, 724–740. [CrossRef]
30. Geng, J.; Zhang, S.C.; Hu, X.X.; Ling, W.Q.; Peng, X.X.; Zhong, S.L.; Liang, F.G.; Zou, Z.G. A review of graphene-decorated LiFePO$_4$ cathode materials for lithium-ion batteries. *Ionics* **2022**, *28*, 4899–4922. [CrossRef]
31. Xu, X.L.; Qi, C.Y.; Hao, Z.D.; Wang, H.; Jiu, J.T.; Liu, J.B.; Yan, H.; Suganuma, K. The surface coating of commercial LiFePO$_4$ by utilizing ZIF-8 for high electrochemical performance lithium-ion batteries. *Nano-Micro Lett.* **2018**, *10*, 1. [CrossRef] [PubMed]
32. Chen, Z.X.; Wang, F.Z.; Li, T.B.; Wang, S.C.; Yao, C.; Wu, H. First-principles study of LiFePO$_4$ modified by graphene and defective graphene oxide. *J. Mol. Graph. Modell.* **2024**, *129*, 108731. [CrossRef]
33. Wu, S.Y.; Luo, E.M.; Ouyang, J.; Lu, Q.; Zhang, X.X.; Wei, D.; Han, W.K.; Xu, X.; Wei, L. Tuning the graphitization of the carbon coating layer on LiFePO$_4$ enables superior properties. *Int. J. Electrochem. Sci.* **2024**, *19*, 100450. [CrossRef]
34. Choi, J.; Zabihi, O.; Ahmadi, M.; Naebe, M. Advancing structural batteries: Cost-efficient high performance carbon fiber-coated LiFePO$_4$ cathodes. *RSC Adv.* **2023**, *13*, 30633–30642. [CrossRef]
35. Ou, J.K.; Yang, L.; Jin, F.; Wu, S.G.; Wang, J.Y. High performance of LiFePO$_4$ with nitrogen-doped carbon layers for lithium-ion batteries. *Adv. Powder Technol.* **2020**, *31*, 1220–1228. [CrossRef]
36. Wang, Y.Y.; Wang, X.L.; Jiang, A.; Liu, G.X.; Yu, W.S.; Dong, X.T.; Wang, J.X. A versatile nitrogen-doped carbon coating strategy to improve the electrochemical performance of LiFePO$_4$ cathodes for lithium-ion batteries. *J. Alloys Compd.* **2019**, *810*, 151889. [CrossRef]
37. Wang, X.F.; Feng, Z.J.; Hou, X.L.; Liu, L.L.; He, M.; He, X.S.; Huang, J.T.; Wen, Z.H. Fluorine doped carbon coating of LiFePO$_4$ as a cathode material for lithium-ion batteries. *Chem. Eng. J.* **2020**, *379*, 122371. [CrossRef]
38. Sun, M.J.; Han, X.L.; Chen, S.G. NaTi(PO$_4$)$_3$@C nanoparticles embedded in 2D sulfur-doped graphene sheets as high-performance anode materials for sodium energy storage. *Electrochim. Acta* **2018**, *289*, 131–138. [CrossRef]

39. Wang, W.; Tang, M.Q.; Yan, Z.W. Superior Li-storage property of an advanced LiFePO$_4$@C/S-doped graphene for lithium-ion batteries. *Ceram. Int.* **2020**, *46*, 22999–23005. [CrossRef]
40. Xun, D.; Wang, P.F.; Shen, B.W. Synthesis and characterization of sulfur-doped carbon decorated LiFePO$_4$ nanocomposite as high performance cathode material for lithium-ion batteries. *Ceram. Int.* **2016**, *42*, 5331–5338.
41. Zhang, J.L.; Wang, J.; Liu, Y.Y.; Nie, N.; Gu, J.J.; Yu, F.; Li, W. High-performance lithium iron phosphate with phosphorus-doped carbon layers for lithium-ion batteries. *J. Mater. Chem. A* **2015**, *3*, 2043–2049.
42. Zhang, J.L.; Nie, N.; Liu, Y.Y.; Wang, J.; Yu, F.; Gu, J.J.; Li, W. Boron and nitrogen co-doped carbon layers of LiFePO$_4$ improve the high-rate electrochemical performance for lithium-ion batteries. *ACS Appl. Mater. Interfaces* **2015**, *7*, 20134–20143. [CrossRef] [PubMed]
43. Nitheesha, S.J.; Feng, J.; Jae, Y.S.; Murugan, N.; Taehyung, K.; Byeong, J.J.; Soon, P.J.; Chang, W.L. Heteroatoms-doped carbon effect on LiFePO$_4$ cathode for Li-ion batteries. *J. Energy Storage* **2023**, *72*, 108710.
44. Chepurnaya, I.; Smirnova, E.; Karushev, M. Electrochemically active polymer components in next-generation LiFePO$_4$ cathodes: Can small things make a big difference? *Batteries* **2022**, *8*, 185. [CrossRef]
45. Rohland, P.; Schröter, E.; Nolte, O.; Newkome, G.R.; Hager, M.D.; Schubert, U.S. Redox-active polymers: The magic key towards energy storage—A polymer design guideline progress in polymer science. *Prog. Polym. Sci.* **2022**, *125*, 101474. [CrossRef]
46. Yang, Z.G.; Dai, Y.; Wang, S.P.; Yu, J.X. How to make lithium iron phosphate better: A review exploring classical modification approaches in-depth and proposing future optimizing methods. *J. Mater. Chem. A* **2016**, *47*, 18193–18656. [CrossRef]
47. Stenina, I.A.; Minakova, P.V.; Kulova, T.L.; Desyatov, A.V.; Yaroslavtsev, A.B. LiFePO$_4$/carbon nanomaterial composites for cathodes of high-power lithium-ion batteries. *Inorg. Mater.* **2021**, *57*, 620–628. [CrossRef]
48. Li, L.; Wu, L.; Wu, F.; Song, S.P.; Zhang, X.Q.; Fu, C.; Yuan, D.D.; Xiang, Y. Review-Recent research progress in surface modification of LiFePO$_4$ cathode materials. *J. Electrochem. Soc.* **2017**, *164*, A2138–A2150. [CrossRef]
49. Hana, N.H.; Munasir. Study of performance graphene oxide modification of LiFePO$_4$/C material for the cathode of Li-ion batteries. *J. Phys. Conf. Ser.* **2023**, *2623*, 012014. [CrossRef]
50. Zhong, S.K.; Wu, L.; Liu, J.Q. Sol-gel synthesis and electrochemical properties of LiFePO$_4$/Li$_3$V$_2$(PO$_4$)$_3$/C composite cathode material for lithium ion batteries. *Electrochim. Acta* **2012**, *74*, 8–15. [CrossRef]
51. Chien, W.C.; Jhang, J.S.; Wu, S.H.; Wu, Z.H.; Yang, C.C. Preparation of LiFePO$_4$/Li$_3$V$_2$(PO$_4$)$_3$/C composite cathode materials and their electrochemical performance analysis. *J. Alloys Compd.* **2020**, *847*, 156447. [CrossRef]
52. Bruce, P.G.; Scrosati, B.; Tarascon, J.M. Nanomaterials for rechargeable lithium batteries. *Angew. Chem. Int. Ed.* **2008**, *47*, 2930–2946. [CrossRef] [PubMed]
53. Liu, J.Y.; Li, X.X.; Huang, J.R.; Li, J.J.; Zhou, P.; Liu, J.H.; Huang, H.J. Three-dimensional graphene-based nanocomposites for high energy density Li-ion batteries. *J. Mater. Chem. A* **2017**, *13*, 5977–5994. [CrossRef]
54. Wang, B.; Liu, T.F.; Liu, A.M.; Liu, J.G.; Wang, L.; Gao, T.T.; Wang, D.L.; Zhao, X.S. A hierarchical porous C@LiFePO$_4$/carbon nanotubes microsphere composite for high-rate lithium-ion batteries: Combined experimental and theoretical study. *Adv. Energy Mater.* **2016**, *6*, 1600426. [CrossRef]
55. Ren, X.G.; Li, Y.G.; He, Z.J.; Xi, X.M.; Shen, X.J. In-situ growth of LiFePO$_4$ on graphene through controlling phase transition for high-performance Li-ion battery. *J. Energy Storage* **2023**, *74*, 109305. [CrossRef]
56. Wang, X.F.; Feng, Z.J.; Huang, J.T.; Deng, W.; Li, X.B.; Zhang, H.S.; Wen, Z.H. Graphene-decorated carbon-coated LiFePO$_4$ nanospheres as a high-performance cathode material for lithium-ion batteries. *Carbon* **2017**, *127*, 149–157. [CrossRef]
57. Wang, F.; Wang, F.F.; Hong, R.Y.; Lv, X.S.; Zheng, Y. High-purity few-layer graphene from plasma pyrolysis of methane as conductive additive for LiFePO$_4$ lithium ion battery. *J. Mater. Res. Technol.* **2020**, *5*, 10004–10015. [CrossRef]
58. Lei, X.L.; Chen, Y.M.; Wang, W.G.; Ye, Y.P.; Zheng, C.C.; Deng, P.; Shi, Z.C.; Zhang, H.Y. A three-dimensional LiFePO$_4$/carbon nanotubes/graphene composite as a cathode material for lithium-ion batteries with superior high-rate performance. *J. Alloys Compd.* **2015**, *626*, 280–286. [CrossRef]
59. Zhang, H.W.; Li, J.Y.; Luo, L.Q.; Zhao, J.; He, J.Y.; Zhao, X.X.; Liu, H.; Qin, Y.B.; Wang, F.Y.; Song, J.J. Hierarchically porous MXene decorated carbon coated LiFePO$_4$ as cathode material for high-performance lithium-ion batteries. *J. Alloys Compd.* **2021**, *876*, 160210. [CrossRef]
60. Mun, J.Y.; Ha, H.W.; Choi, W.C. Nano LiFePO$_4$ in reduced graphene oxide framework for efficient high-rate lithium storage. *J. Power Sources* **2014**, *251*, 386–392. [CrossRef]
61. Dong, G.H.; Mao, Y.Q.; Li, Y.Q.; Huang, P.; Fu, S.Y. M Xene-carbon nanotubes-cellulose-LiFePO$_4$ based self-supporting cathode with ultrahigh-area-capacity for lithium-ion batteries. *Electrochim. Acta* **2022**, *420*, 140464. [CrossRef]
62. Checko, S.; Ju, Z.Y.; Zhang, B.W.; Zheng, T.R.; Takeuchi, E.S.; Marschilok, A.C.; Takeuchi, K.J.; Yu, G.H. Fast-charging, binder-free lithium battery cathodes enabled via multidimensional conductive networks. *Nano Lett.* **2024**, *24*, 1695–1702. [CrossRef]
63. Wu, X.L.; Guo, Y.G.; Su, J.; Xiong, J.W.; Zhang, Y.L.; Wan, L.J. Carbon-nanotube-decorated nano-LiFePO$_4$@C cathode material with superior high-rate and low-temperature performances for lithium-ion batteries. *Adv. Energy Mater.* **2013**, *3*, 1155–1160. [CrossRef]
64. Luo, G.Y.; Gu, Y.J.; Liu, Y.; Chen, Z.L.; Huo, Y.L.; Wu, F.Z.; Mai, Y.; Dai, X.Y.; Deng, Y. Electrochemical performance of in situ LiFePO$_4$ modified by N-doped graphene for Li-ion batteries. *Ceram. Int.* **2021**, *47*, 11332–11339. [CrossRef]
65. Ren, Z.G.; Qu, M.Z.; Yu, Z.L. Synthesis and electrochemical properties of LiFeP$_{0.5}$B$_{0.05}$O$_{4-\delta}$/C cathode materials. *J. Inorg. Mater.* **2010**, *25*, 230–234. [CrossRef]

66. Islam, M.S.; Driscoll, D.J.; Fisher, C.A.J.; Slater, P.R. Atomic-scale investigation of defects, dopants, and lithium transport in the LiFePO$_4$ olivine-type battery material. *Chem. Mater.* **2005**, *17*, 5085–5092. [CrossRef]
67. Trinh, D.V.; Nguyen, M.T.T.; Dang, H.T.M.; Dang, D.T.; Le, H.T.T.; Le, H.T.N.; Tran, H.V.; Huynh, C.D. Hydrothermally synthesized nanostructured LiMn$_x$Fe$_{1-x}$PO$_4$ (x=0-0.3) cathode materials with enhanced properties for lithium-ion batteries. *Nat. Portf.* **2021**, *11*, 12280. [CrossRef]
68. Nie, X.; Xiong, J. Electrochemical properties of Mn-doped nanosphere LiFePO$_4$. *JOM* **2021**, *73*, 2525–2530. [CrossRef]
69. Sin, B.C.; Lee, S.U.; Jin, B.S.; Kim, H.S.; Kim, J.S.; Lee, S.I.; Noh, J.; Lee, Y. Experimental and theoretical investigation of fluorine substituted LiFe$_{0.4}$Mn$_{0.6}$PO$_4$ as cathode material for lithium rechargeable batteries. *Solid State Ion.* **2014**, *260*, 2–7. [CrossRef]
70. Pan, X.X.; Zhuang, S.X.; Sun, Y.Q.; Sun, G.X.; Ren, Y.; Jiang, S.U. Research progress of modified-LiFePO$_4$ as cathode materials for lithium-ion batteries. *Inorg. Chem. Ind.* **2023**, *55*, 18–26.
71. Zhang, H.H.; Zou, Z.G.; Zhang, S.C.; Liu, J.; Zhong, S.L. A review of the doping modification of LiFePO$_4$ as a cathode material for lithium-ion batteries. *Int. J. Electrochem. Sci.* **2020**, *15*, 12041–12067. [CrossRef]
72. Wu, T.; Liu, J.; Sun, L.; Cong, L.; Xie, H.; Ghany, A.A.; Mauger, A.; Julien, C.M. V-insertion in Li(Fe, Mn)FePO$_4$. *J. Power Sources* **2018**, *383*, 133–143. [CrossRef]
73. Strobridge, F.C.; Liu, H.; Leskes, M.; Borkiewicz, O.J.; Wiaderek, K.M.; Chupas, P.J.; Chapman, K.W.; Grey, C.P. Unraveling the complex delithiation mechanisms of olivine-type cathode materials, LiFe$_x$Co$_{1-x}$PO$_4$. *Chem. Mater.* **2016**, *28*, 3676–3690. [CrossRef]
74. Qing, R.; Yang, M.C.; Meng, Y.S.; Sigmund, W. Synthesis of LiNi$_x$Fe$_{1-x}$PO$_4$ solid solution as cathode materials for lithium ion batteries. *Electrochim. Acta* **2013**, *108*, 827–832. [CrossRef]
75. Wang, Y.M.; Wang, Y.J.; Liu, X.Y.; Zhu, B.; Wang, F. Solvothermal synthesis of LiFe$_{1/3}$Mn$_{1/3}$Co$_{1/3}$PO$_4$ solid solution as lithium storage cathode materials. *RSC Adv.* **2017**, *7*, 14354–14359. [CrossRef]
76. Amin, R.; Lin, C.T.; Maier, J. Aluminium-doped LiFePO$_4$ single crystals. Part II. Ionic conductivity, diffusivity and defect model. *Phys. Chem. Chem. Phys.* **2008**, *10*, 3524–3529. [CrossRef]
77. Meethong, N.; Kao, Y.H.; Speakman, S.A.; Chiang, Y.M. Aliovalent substitutions in olivine lithium iron phosphate and impact on structure and properties. *Adv. Funct. Mater.* **2009**, *19*, 1060–1070. [CrossRef]
78. Zhang, D.X.; Wang, J.; Dong, K.Z.; Hao, A. First principles investigation on the elastic and electronic properties of Mn, Co, Nb, Mo doped LiFePO$_4$. *Comput. Mater. Sci.* **2018**, *155*, 410–415. [CrossRef]
79. Ban, C.M.; Yin, W.J.; Tang, H.W.; Wei, S.H.; Yan, Y.F.; Dillon, A.C. A novel codoping approach for enhancing the performance of LiFePO$_4$ cathodes. *Adv. Energy Mater.* **2012**, *2*, 1028–1032. [CrossRef]
80. Wagemaker, M.; Ellis, B.L.; Hecht, D.L.; Mulder, F.M.; Naza, L.F. Proof of supervalent doping in olivine LiFePO$_4$. *Chem. Mater.* **2008**, *20*, 6313–6315. [CrossRef]
81. Altin, S.; Coban, M.; Altundag, S.; Altin, E. Production of Eu-doped LiFePO$_4$ by glass-ceramic technique and investigation of their thermal, structural, electrochemical performances. *J. Mater. Sci. Mater. Electron.* **2022**, *33*, 13720–13730. [CrossRef]
82. Zhang, Q.Y.; Zhou, J.; Zeng, G.C.; Ren, S. Effect of lanthanum and yttrium doped LiFePO$_4$ cathodes on electrochemical performance of lithium-ion battery. *J. Mater. Sci.* **2023**, *58*, 8463–8477. [CrossRef]
83. Hu, J.Z.; Zhao, X.B.; Yu, H.M.; Zhou, X.; Cao, G.S.; Tu, J.P. The conductivity and electrochemical perform- ance of lanthanon doped lithium iron phosphate cathode material. *J. Funct. Mater.* **2007**, *38*, 1394–1397.
84. Liu, Z.L.; Zhang, Z.Z.; Zhu, Y.M.; Gao, P. Progress in rare earth materials applied in cathode materials of Li-ion battery. *Battery Bimon.* **2019**, *49*, 520–523.
85. Chen, H.; Xiang, K.X.; Gong, W.Q.; Liu, J.H. Effect of rare earth ions doping on the structure and performance of LiFePO$_4$. *Rare Met. Mater. Eng.* **2011**, *40*, 1937–1940.
86. Bai, Y.M.; Qiu, P.; Han, S.C. Synthesis and properties of Y-doped LiFePO$_4$ as cathode material for lithium-ion batteries. *Rare Met. Mater. Eng.* **2011**, *40*, 917–920.
87. Qiu, P.; Han, S.C.; Bai, Y.M. Structure and electrochemical properties of LiFePO$_4$/C doped with La$^{3+}$, Nd$^{3+}$, Y$^{3+}$. *Chin. J. Power Sources* **2011**, *35*, 780–783.
88. Jiang, A.; Wang, X.L.; Gao, M.S.; Wang, J.X.; Liu, G.X.; Yu, W.S.; Zhang, H.B.; Dong, X.T. Enhancement of electrochemical properties of niobium-doped LiFePO$_4$/C synthesized by sol-gel method. *J. Chin. Chem. Soc.* **2018**, *65*, 977–981. [CrossRef]
89. Zhao, X.; Tang, X.Z.; Zhang, L.; Zhao, M.S.; Zhai, J. Effects of neodymium aliovalent substitution on the structure and electro-chemical performance of LiFePO$_4$. *Electrochim. Acta* **2010**, *55*, 5899–5904. [CrossRef]
90. Zhang, Q.M.; Qiao, Y.Q.; Zhao, M.S.; Wang, L.M. Structure and electrochemical properties of Sm-doped lithiumiron phosphate cathode materials. *Chin. J. Inorg. Chem.* **2012**, *28*, 67–73. [CrossRef]
91. Wang, C.X.; Xiang, K.X.; Gong, W.Q.; Chen, H.; Zeng, J.; Ji, X.X. Synthesis and performance of cathode materials Li$_{0.97}$Re$_{0.01}$FePO$_4$ for lithium-ion batteries. *J. Hunan Univ. Technol.* **2010**, *24*, 5–8.
92. Zhang, Q.M.; Qiao, Y.Q.; Zhao, M.S.; Wang, L.M. Structure and electrochemical properties of Yb-doped lithium iron phosphate cathode materials. *J. Chin. Soc. Rare Earths* **2012**, *30*, 78–85.
93. Liang, M.M.; Xiao, L.L.; Wang, J. Preparation and electrochemical performance test of rare earth gadolinium and yttrium doped LiFePO$_4$ cathode materials. *Appl. Chem. Ind.* **2017**, *46*, 829–834.
94. Zhang, B.F.; Xu, Y.L.; Wang, J.; Lin, J.; Wang, C.; Chen, Y.J. Lanthanum and cerium Co-doped LiFePO$_4$: Morphology, electrochemical performance and kinetic study from −30–+50 °C. *Electrochim. Acta* **2019**, *322*, 134686. [CrossRef]

95. Cui, Z.H.; Guo, X.; Ren, J.Q.; Xue, H.T.; Tang, F.L.; La, P.Q.; Li, H.; Li, J.C.; Lu, X.F. Enhanced electrochemical performance and storage mechanism of LiFePO$_4$ doped by Co, Mn and S elements for lithium-ion batteries. *Electrochim. Acta* **2021**, *388*, 138592. [CrossRef]
96. Wang, H.Q.; Lai, A.J.; Huang, D.Q.; Chu, Y.Q.; Hu, S.J.; Pan, Q.C.; Liu, Z.H.; Zheng, F.H.; Huang, Y.G.; Li, Q.Y. Y-F co-doping behavior of LiFePO$_4$/C nanocomposites for high-rate lithium-ion batteries. *New J. Chem.* **2021**, *45*, 5695–5703. [CrossRef]
97. Chen, J.H.; Onah, O.; Cheng, Y.; Silva, K.; Choi, C.; Chen, W.Y.; Xu, S.C.; Eddy, L.; Han, Y.; Yakobson, B.; et al. Fast-charging lithium iron phosphate cathodes by flash carbon coating. *ChemRxiv* **2024**. [CrossRef]
98. Chuang, H.C.; Teng, J.W.; Kuan, W.F. Supercritical CO$_2$-enhanced surface modification on LiFePO$_4$ cathodes through ex-situ carbon coating for lithium-ion batteries. *Colloids Surf. A* **2024**, *684*, 133110. [CrossRef]
99. Luo, J.W.; Zhang, J.C.; Guo, Z.X.; Liu, Z.D.; Wang, C.Y.; Jiang, H.R.; Zhang, J.F.; Fan, L.L.; Zhu, H.; Xu, Y.H.; et al. Coupling antisite defect and lattice tensile stimulates facile isotropic Li-ion diffusion. *Adv. Mater.* **2024**, *36*, 2405956. [CrossRef]
100. Wang, J.W.; Ji, S.J.; Han, Q.G.; Wang, F.Q.; Sha, W.X.; Cheng, D.P.; Zhang, W.X.; Tang, S.; Cao, Y.C.; Cheng, S.J. High performance of regenerated LiFePO$_4$ from spent cathodes via an in situ coating and heteroatom-doping strategy using amino acids. *J. Mater. Chem. A* **2024**, *12*, 15311–15320. [CrossRef]
101. Gou, Y.J.; Zhang, J.Y.; Liu, X.; Zhou, Z.H.; Zhang, M.D.; Song, L.; Jin, Y.C. A highly efficient additive for direct reactivation of waste LiFePO$_4$ with practical electrochemical performance. *Energy Fuels* **2024**, *38*, 6518–6527. [CrossRef]
102. Li, X.G.; Wang, M.Y.; Zhou, Q.B.; Ge, M.; Zhang, M.D.; Liu, W.F.; Shi, Z.P.; Yue, H.Y.; Zhang, H.S.; Yin, Y.H.; et al. The prilling and cocoating collaborative strategy to construct high performance of regeneration LiFePO$_4$ materials. *ACS Mater. Lett.* **2024**, *6*, 640–647. [CrossRef]

**Disclaimer/Publisher's Note:** The statements, opinions and data contained in all publications are solely those of the individual author(s) and contributor(s) and not of MDPI and/or the editor(s). MDPI and/or the editor(s) disclaim responsibility for any injury to people or property resulting from any ideas, methods, instructions or products referred to in the content.

MDPI AG
Grosspeteranlage 5
4052 Basel
Switzerland
Tel.: +41 61 683 77 34

*Molecules* Editorial Office
E-mail: molecules@mdpi.com
www.mdpi.com/journal/molecules

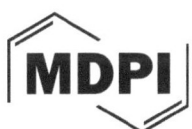

Disclaimer/Publisher's Note: The title and front matter of this reprint are at the discretion of the Guest Editors. The publisher is not responsible for their content or any associated concerns. The statements, opinions and data contained in all individual articles are solely those of the individual Editors and contributors and not of MDPI. MDPI disclaims responsibility for any injury to people or property resulting from any ideas, methods, instructions or products referred to in the content.

www.ingramcontent.com/pod-product-compliance
Lightning Source LLC
LaVergne TN
LVHW072345090526
838202LV00019B/2485